Malpractice

Malpractice

A Guide
for
Mental Health
Professionals

RONALD JAY COHEN

THE FREE PRESS
A Division of Macmillan Publishing Co., Inc.
NEW YORK

Collier Macmillan Publishers
LONDON

The Free Press
A Division of Macmillan Publishing Co., Inc.
866 Third Avenue, New York, N.Y. 10022

Collier Macmillan Canada, Ltd.

Library of Congress Catalog Card Number: 78-72147

Printed in the United States of America

printing number

1 2 3 4 5 6 7 8 9 10

Library of Congress Cataloging in Publication Data

Cohen, Ronald Jay.
    Malpractice: a guide for mental health professionals.

    Includes bibliographical references and indexes.
    1. Mental health personnel--Malpractice--United
States. 2. Psychiatry ethics. I. Title.
[DNLM: 1. Malpractice. 2. Psychiatry. WM33.1
C678m]
KF2910.P753C63   346'.73'033   78-72147
ISBN 0-02-905790-6

Excerpt, pp. 19–20, from J. Hart, R. Corriere, and J. Binder's *Going Sane* (New York: Delta, 1975), pp. 398–399, © 1975 by J. Hart, R. Corriere, and J. Binder, is reprinted by permission.

Excerpts, pp. 76 and 77, from R.J. Cohen and F.J. Smith's "Socially Reinforced Obsessing: Etiology of a Disorder in a Christian Scientist" (*Journal of Consulting and Clinical Psychology*, 1976, 44, 142–144), pp. 142 and 144 respectively, copyright 1976 by the American Psychological Association, are reprinted by permission.

Excerpt, pp. 78–79, from R.J. Cohen's "Socially Reinforced Obsessing: A Reply," (*Journal of Consulting and Clinical Psychology*, 1977, 45, 1166–1171), pp. 1169–1170, copyright 1977 by the American Psychological Association, is reprinted by permission.

Excerpts (including many paraphrased and quoted court cases) reprinted throughout from *Resident and Staff Physician* and fully cited in the References, are reprinted by permission of *Resident and Staff Physician*, © year of publication.

Excerpt, pp. 152–153, from *The Life and Work of Sigmund Freud*, Volume 3, by Ernest Jones, M.D. (New York: Basic Books, Inc., 1957), pp. 163–165. © 1957 by Ernest Jones, Basic Books, Inc., Publishers, New York; and Katherine Jones and Hogarth Press, Ltd., London.

To my parents, Edith and Harold Cohen

Contents

Preface

"I am currently heading a list of defendants in a suit in which I am personally being sued for $2 million. . . . My insurance coverage is for only $250,000. . . ." The financially crippling and otherwise potentially catastrophic effects of a malpractice suit are aptly reflected in these words of a New York psychiatrist (quoted in "What to Expect," 1974, p. 65). Cited in the same journal were the words of another doctor who focused on the feelings of apprehension attendant to each of the inevitable delays in malpractice proceedings:

> You're living under a cloud. . . . You worry about what your patients are thinking—and you get all ready to go to court and then it's postponed. One time I asked my lawyer, how long is this going to take? Oh about four months more, he said, then it'll come up. Well—it turned out to be four years. And even when you win you lose. You lose because you lose time from your practice and let's fact it—notoriety—even when it's false—never helped any doctor keep his patients. (p. 68)

In recent years, the specter of malpractice litigation has loomed as an increasing occupational hazard in the health professions. Although mental health professionals have remained relatively unscathed by this rush to the courtroom, there is evidence that they too might more frequently be named as defendants in legal actions. What accounts for this relatively recent spate of litigation? Does the rise in malpractice suits in fact reflect a rise in malpractice? What is the relationship between standards of professional ethics and the legal concept of professional liability? How can mental health professionals best protect themselves against litigation? If litigation is initiated, how can it best be dealt with?

My purpose in writing this book was to provide mental health professionals with a brief introduction to the area of malpractice. After an historical survey, general aspects of such litigation and the ethical and legal issues likely to be raised are discussed in Parts I and II. Numerous vignettes of actual malpractice proceedings against health professionals and institutions are presented in Part III. An overview of some of the legal principles involved in these cases and some guidelines for avoiding legal jeopardy appear in Part IV.

Psychiatrists, social workers, psychiatric nurses, occupational therapists, counselors, and other professionals doing applied work in the mental health field should find this book useful. It should prove particularly valuable to psychologists who work in hospitals, schools, private practice, and other applied settings, since there has been an unfortunate dearth of writing on legal and ethical matters in the clinical, counseling, educational, and industrial psychology literature. But this book, written by a psychologist, is designed only to acquaint mental health professionals with the law; it is *not* intended to be a substitute for personal legal counsel.

The general complexity of the law, the impreciseness of the legal principles in negligence law, and the vagueness of the rulings and statutes affecting mental health professionals made the review of the malpractice literature an almost prohibitive task. Still, I thoroughly enjoyed collecting and reading the material contained herein. Readers who find themselves similarly absorbed in the real-life drama of any of the cases presented are urged to visit their local law library and read the cases in the original. It is my hope that some of the information and advice contained herein will be helpful in preventing readers' names from ever appearing in volumes in law libraries or in some future edition of this book.

Acknowledgments

I have often heard fellow psychologists say, "You need a very high tolerance for ambiguity to go into clinical psychology." But then, these psychologists have never studied the law.

Helping to increase my tolerance (when they could not reduce the ambiguity of the law) were a number of people whose gracious assistance I would like to acknowledge. Lawrence A. Brenner, Esq., spent many hours doing legal research and explaining legal principles in terms understandable to a layman. It is for this reason that my first acknowledgment of help is to him. Fran H. Stern, O.T.R., helped in every which way in the preparation of the early drafts of this manuscript, and I gratefully acknowledge her assistance. I would also like to thank Carol R. Klein, B.F.A., for skillfully assisting in the preparation of the final manuscript; my family for their boundless support and encouragement—with special thanks to Barbara for her assistance in proofreading; Sidney Rosen, M.D. and Jeffrey S. Nevid, Ph.D. for their help in providing me with "hard to get" articles and books; and Paul O'Brien, Esq., Albert Podell, Esq., and William E. Mariano, Esq., for proofreading portions of the manuscript and for helpful editorial suggestions. Finally, I must thank my editor at The Free Press, Ron Chambers, for sharing my belief and confidence in this book and for helping me translate inspiration and aspiration into reality.

Note on Retrieving Legal Information

As most mental health professionals are unfamiliar with the way legal proceedings are filed and referenced in law libraries, a few words on that subject seem appropriate here. Generally speaking, case decisions are published according to the jurisdiction in which they are heard. Information concerning most proceedings are matters of public record, though in rare instances and in special cases (e.g., adoption proceedings) the court records may be sealed. Opinions (in those cases in which an opinion has been rendered) are generally available in local law libraries. Appellate-court opinions can usually be found in any law library nationwide.

Opinions and decisions pertinent to a specific case can be located in books called "reporters." Complete references to published legal proceedings typically include the name of the case or proceeding (e.g., "*Jones v. Smith*" or "*In the Matter of Goldberg*") as well as the volume, page, and title of the reporter in which the case will be found. The citation will also include the year in which the case was decided and the state in which the case was heard, though this information is not necessary for locating the reference. Consider the following citation:

Roy v. Hartogs, 381 N.Y.S.2d 350 (New York, 1975)

This citation refers to the widely publicized malpractice action that Julie Roy brought against her psychiatrist Renatus Hartogs. More information on the case could be found by consulting Volume 381 of the New York Supplement, Second Series.[1] The "350" refers to the page on which the case will be found. Now consider the following:

In the Matter of Clement, 340 N.E.2d 217 (Illinois, 1976)

The citation above refers to a hearing that was held in order to determine whether or not a Mr. Clement had been denied due process when he was civilly committed to a mental institution. Readers interested

---

[1]After varying numbers of years, different reporters will often begin a new series of volume numbers.

in learning more about Clement's civil commitment proceeding could consult Volume 340 of the Northeast (N.E.) Reporter, Second Series, page 217.

When a case appears in more than one reporter, all of the citations are usually provided. For example, a case that involved the negligent administration of electroshock therapy appeared in Volume 259 of North Carolina Reports, Volume 131 of the Southeast Reporter, Second Series, and Volume 99 of American Law Reports. The specific citation for this case as it will appear in Part III of this book[2] is as follows:

STONE V. PROCTOR
259 N.C. 633; 131 S.E.2d 297; 99 A.L.R.2d 593 (North Carolina, 1963)

Mental health professionals interested in pursuing legal references are strongly advised to enlist the aid of a librarian since there exist numerous questions (e.g., Was this decision overturned by a higher court?) and special considerations that must be kept in mind when doing serious legal research.

---

[2]Multiple citations are separated by a semicolon in this book.

BACKGROUND

In 1354, the "enormous and horrible hurt" on the right side of Thomas de Shene's jaw did not respond to physician John le Spicer's treatment. As related by H. T. Riley (cited in Sandor, 1957, p. 459), sworn testimony on the matter of "whether or not such injury was curable at the time when John le Spicer of Cornhulle took the same Thomas under his care to heal the wound" was given to the mayor, alderman, and sheriff by the masters of the Surgeons Guild. The expert surgeons testified that "if John le Spicer . . . had been expert in his craft or art, or had called in counsel and assistance . . . he might have cured the injury." The surgeons concluded that "through want of skill on the part of the said John le Spicer, the injury, under his care, had become apparently incurable."

The foregoing fourteenth-century vignette incorporates many of the elements of a modern-day malpractice proceeding. Applying current legal procedure and standards to the case, le Spicer would be held culpable for malpractice if de Shene could prove by the preponderance of the evidence that

1. le Spicer had entered into a doctor–patient relationship with him and therefore owed him a special duty of care;
2. le Spicer was negligent in the performance of his duty; and
3. damage was suffered as a result of that negligence.

The tone and content of the expert testimony adduced on de Shene's behalf makes it a reasonable inference that le Spicer would have lost the suit and de Shene would have been compensated for damages incurred as a result of his doctor's negligent treatment.

Hundreds of years later the drama of one individual's "enormous and horrible hurt" suffered at the hands of a healer is still being played out, with only the names of the litigants, witnesses, illnesses, and treatments being changed. In recent years, the number of claims filed against health professionals has risen dramatically. In Chapter 1 some of the possible reasons for this dramatic rise in malpractice litigation will be explored and the important question of whether there is more malpractice or simply more malpractice suits will be addressed. Chapter 2 is designed to provide mental health professionals with a working acquaintance with the rudiments of the legal system and the place of malpractice within that system.

1

The Malpractice Crisis

There once was a day when mental health professionals seemed to enjoy a kind of immunity from malpractice litigation. It was a day when patients respected doctors and authority in general, when psychotherapy was primarily a "talking therapy," when emotional distress was not a compensable injury, and when psychotherapy patients wanted as few people as possible to know that they were in treatment. That day is gone. We are no longer immune.

We live in increasingly litigious times. The recent rise in the number of lawsuits brought against mental health professionals is symptomatic of a general increase in litigation brought against all health professionals. Watergate, Koreagate, and numerous other revelations of scandalous activities in high places in government, business, labor unions, and elsewhere have served to make people more suspicious of authority in general (Cohen, Note 1). The net result of this growing distrust has been a greater disposition to litigation as a means of remedying perceived wrongs. Society's emphasis on human rights, patient rights, and consumer rights and the premium placed on assertiveness in general have prompted people to ask more questions than ever before about the goods and services they purchase. No one denies that there are great benefits to be achieved from such heightened consumer awareness. The problem is that the expectations aroused about the goods and especially the services one purchases are often unreasonably high, and the unfortunate result is a lawsuit. The poor economy has contributed to the problem of increasing litigation by making the idea of "easy money" through litigation all the more appealing to people. The wide publicity given to malpractice suits settled with large sums of money serves to further entice would-be litigants to contact attorneys. And "The doctor and his insurance company can afford it" is an all too familiar bromide. Furthermore, the cost of initiating a lawsuit is frequently less than the cost of a lottery ticket, since many lawyers will accept such cases on a contingency basis.

Professionals in the health care field have emerged as particularly vulnerable to litigation. Problems that would have prompted only frank doctor–patient discussions in the past now appear to be grounds for a lawsuit. In 1969, the St. Paul Fire and Marine Insurance Company had one claim pending for every twenty-three of its insured physicians; by 1974, the ratio had changed to one claim for every ten physicians (St. Paul Fire and Marine Insurance Company, Note 2). In 1970, the number of suits brought against physicians in New York State was 564; only four years later the number of suits had more than doubled (*Newsweek*, June 9, 1975, p. 59). During the fourteen-month period between January, 1974, to March, 1975, 1,010 of the 7,100 physicians in Cook County, Illinois, were sued for malpractice, and settlements in 1974 averaged about $8,000 higher than they did in 1970 (Kotulak, 1975).

Speaking at a 1976 session of the American Academy of Pediatrics, physician Robert L. Brent discussed the problem of litigation arising from the birth of congenitally malformed infants. As quoted in a *Pediatric News* article entitled "Few Suits Arising from Congenital Defects Have Factual Basis" (1976), Brent advised his audience to provide accurate information to parents as a means of preventing such cases from coming to the attention of an attorney:

> Once they get into the hands of an attorney . . . they abandon all normal priorities and their usual moral and ethical standards. The parents get so angry that lying and distortion are both acceptable and common. (p. 7)

The sheer volume of medical malpractice litigation is taken notice of with some perplexity by King (1977) in his book on medical malpractice:

> Perhaps no other area of the law, certainly no other field of personal injury law, has undergone such far-reaching change in the last several years as has the law of medical malpractice. The number and size of claims have mushroomed dramatically. There have been similar increases in liability insurance premiums and in the concomitant charges for medical services. The last twenty years have witnessed an accelerating onrush of case law that has produced an almost unmanageable dynamic in the law of medical malpractice. More recently, one finds at both the national and state levels an unprecedented degree of legislative involvement in malpractice law. This legislation is important not only for the law it contains but also to the extent that it may signal the beginnings of legislative primacy in many facets of this traditionally judicially-dominated setting.
>
> This substantial body of malpractice law evokes an ambivalent reaction from the commentator whose job it is to render it all comprehensible. On the one hand, the sheer mass and inconstancy of the law of malpractice seem to defy rational systematizing. Yet, at the same time

this mounting body of law, representing as it does the product of so much legal energy, begs ordering. (p. vii)

Included in the astronomical number of suits against health professionals are claims for the widest possible array of injuries. What is worse, there appears to be no limit to the liability doctors can incur. The range of legitimate legal actions against doctors has run the gamut from wrongful birth[1] to wrongful death[2]—and beyond. For example, in one Illinois malpractice case, the question before the court was whether or not a child could sue for alleged pre-conception injuries:

> Mother and child were originally co-plaintiffs. Then a hearing was held in circuit court, where the defendants moved to dismiss the complaint because the child was not a person or even conceived "at the time of the alleged infliction of the injury."
>
> Subsequently the mother dropped out as a plaintiff, and a court paper summed up the situation: "There is but one issue: Does a child, not conceived at the time negligent acts were committed against its mother, have a cause of action against the tort-feasors for its injuries resulting from their conduct?"
>
> That question was ultimately carried to the Illinois Supreme Court. After prolonged consideration, the seven-man court issued a close, split decision. Four voted the plaintiff had a "valid cause of action"—that is, the child had the right to sue. (Horsley, 1978a, p. 89)

Doctors have been sued not only for reassuring patients (see case 6.41 in Chapter 6) but for telling them they are going to die. In a case cited by Ledakowich (1976d) for example, legal action was taken against a doctor who told his patient that, in his professional opinion, the patient had between a year and eighteen months to live. When the patient lived longer than eighteen months the lawsuit was brought. The defendant doctor was not found to be negligent for merely expressing an opinion. If a skillful attorney arguing a similar case should convince the court that the physician's opinion represented a guarantee of sorts, we would hope that the relief granted would not be specific performance (i.e., the physician would have to see to it that the patient died within the agreed-upon time period). In actuality, of course, the relief granted would probably take the form of a monetary settlement to compensate the plaintiff for financial losses suffered as a result of early retirement. Still, the case is a fascinating example of the extent to which patients would extend their doctors' liability if they could.

Health professionals other than physicians have also become more

---

[1]See Eisberg, 1978.
[2]See page 211 in Chapter 7.

sensitized than ever before to the possibility of litigation. In his book *Pharmacy and the Law* DeMarco (1975) observed that pharmacy was a highly regulated profession, that the "risk of liability is directly proportionate to the number of standards that must be met," and that in pharmacy "the risk is high" (p. 196). Myers and Fink (1977) noted that some drug companies have begun to offer free legal advice as an inducement to pharmacists to handle their products.

Virtually no one associated with health care can boast immunity from claims of malpractice, as the following note from *MLC Commentary* ("MLC News Brief," 1975) attests:

> Not only health-care providers but clergymen are being sued for alleged malpractice. John Cardinal Cody, Catholic Bishop of Chicago, has been named as sole defendant in a medical injury suit arising from the development of retrolental fibroplasia in twin girls who received excess oxygen at birth. The suit, which seeks $2,000,000 for each plaintiff, was filed in Cook County, Illinois, nearly eighteen years after the occurrence. Michael Schaffner, Esq., attorney for the plaintiffs, stated that the children's parent was prompted to sue upon learning the outcome of a similar highly-publicized case in New York City (*Kalmowitz* v. *Brookdale Hospital*). In that case, the plaintiff settled for $165,000 moments prior to a jury verdict which would have awarded her $900,000. (p. 1)

The problem of increasing numbers of suits against health professionals has been analyzed by Crum and Forster Insurance Companies in one of their ads:

> In 1975, there were twice as many medical malpractice suits as there were in 1970. Why has this happened?
> For one thing, the new operations and miracle drugs that save lives also bring new risks. And no matter how careful a doctor or hospital may be, more and more unsatisfied patients are seeking compensation for their misfortunes. So they sue. And sympathetic juries are making bigger awards. In the last 10 years, the average award has jumped over 6 times.

Fully cognizant of the fact that sympathetic juries are making bigger and bigger awards, insurance companies seem to have resorted to a kind of "plea bargaining" with judges. As reflected in the following quotation from a chief of anesthesiology in a New York hospital, an insurance company representative was willing to pay out a small award in return for the judge's future favor:

> I was sued for $50,000 on charges of negligence in doing a spinal anesthesia that resulted in paresthesia and foot drop, which cleared up in six months. By the time the case came to trial, the signs and symptoms had cleared completely. My attorney moved for dismissal. The judge called the two attorneys for consultation and asked whether the company

would be willing to give $1,000 to the plaintiff. My attorney said he would like to please the judge in his request so that the insurance company might get a break in the future—on bigger cases. He asked my permission to agree on the settlement on the grounds that it was being made "without prejudice" to me . . . in other words, that it would not count against my record. (cited in "What to Expect," 1974, p. 66)

In addition to such extraordinary tactics, insurance companies have reacted to the malpractice crisis with more mundane strategies, such as raising premium rates. In fact, one of the most immediate consequences of the increase in malpractice litigation has been the dramatic increases doctors have had to pay for malpractice insurance. In an insurance industry white paper entitled "The Problems of Insuring Medical Malpractice," it was observed that

the recent explosion in malpractice claims and costs was totally unpredictable at the time that the (present) rates were being calculated. Past patterns of claims experience were inadequate to predict future expectations in this volatile area. New techniques for predicting the effect of changes in legal interpretations, medical science, and the social climate will have to be developed since these factors have a substantial impact on this line of insurance. (All-Industry Medical Malpractice Insurance Committee, cited in "Insurance Industry," 1976)

Professional liability insurance premiums have skyrocketed, and there is no end in sight. The vice-president of one Chicago-based brokerage firm has estimated on the basis of current trends that premiums will continue to rise between 15 and 25 percent annually, and that in the ten-year period 1976–1986, $1.5 billion will have been paid out in medical injury claims. The rising cost of medical malpractice insurance has prompted unprecedented behavior on the part of physicians. To cope with extraordinary increases in insurance premiums, doctors have gone out on strike, moved to another state, and retired in record numbers. Eleven hospitals and clinics associated with Harvard University set up their own insurance company on an island in the Bahamas in an attempt to save money on premiums. State legislatures have been prompted to reexamine and update their laws pertaining to malpractice:

The problems of malpractice law were accentuated 2 years ago when malpractice claims suddenly began to increase at a startling rate, triggering even more dramatic increases in medical liability insurance premiums. The crisis prompted legislative responses in all 50 states. "Omnibus" bills, dealing with many aspects of malpractice, were enacted in several states. (DeLeon and Borreliz, 1978, p. 475)

According to a report in *MLC Commentary* ("Going Bare," 1976) many doctors have reacted to the unwieldy insurance increases by "going bare"—a term that in this context refers to practicing medicine without medical liability insurance protection. It was reported, for example, that up to 2,000 Florida physicians remained unaccounted for with regard to medical liability insurance and that 200 of Nevada's estimated 750 physicians were believed to be going bare. Tests of the constitutionality of various states' mandatory malpractice insurance laws have begun to emerge in the courts. (See, for example, *Pennsylvania Medicine*, 1977, *80*, No. 1, p. 9.) However, doctors who believe that they are protecting themselves against a malpractice suit by not carrying insurance are mistaken. As reported in *Medical Economics*, ("Medicolegal Ruling," 1978), a recent decision by the California Supreme Court would appear to *encourage* suits against uninsured professionals by providing that they can be brought into a suit even if they were not originally named as a defendant:

> Doctors who have gone bare and those only peripherally involved in a malpractice suit face new risks as a result of a decision by the California Supreme Court. Legal experts who've studied the case say it may well encourage M.D.s in a multiple-defendant suit to try to place most of the blame on one of their co-defendants. The ruling held that parties not even named by a plaintiff—perhaps because they're uninsured—can be brought into a suit by one of the defendants. (p. 254)

MENTAL HEALTH PROFESSIONALS AND MALPRACTICE

Mental health professionals have remained relatively unscathed by claims of malpractice. Suits brought against psychologists, psychiatrists, and others have been relatively few in number, and relatively low dollar amounts have been paid in damages. It has been observed that the average American psychiatrist is sued once for every 50 to 100 years of practice, whereas the average neurosurgeon can expect to be sued once for every two years of practice. "A lawsuit against a psychiatrist by a patient is a rare event compared with the number of lawsuits brought against most other physicians" (Trent and Muhl, 1975, p. 1312). What kinds of things have psychiatrists been sued for? Table 1 presents a breakdown of twenty-eight closed (settled) claims out of a total of 109 claims filed against psychiatrists in the period 1972 to 1975.

A sampling of the claims filed against psychologists during the two-year period 1973 to 1975 appears in Table 2. At the American Psychological Association Convention in 1976, Jack Wiggins (Note 3) pointed out that for the period 1973 to 1975 the annual claims rate was less than 2 per 1,000 psychologists covered by the APA's policy and that many of the suits brought were "nuisance suits" (i.e., suits probably initiated as a

TABLE 1.
Breakdown of 28 Closed Claims Against Psychiatrists (1972–1975)

CLAIM	FREQUENCY
Improper commitment	9
Pressing for fee collection	5
Drug reaction	3
Suicide of hospitalized patient	3
Improper treatment	2
Injury incurred during EST treatment	2
Unauthorized release of confidential information	2
Improper administrative handling of insurance form	1
Sexual improprieties	1

result of a fee dispute rather than malpractice). The total dollar value of the thirty-seven claims filed against psychologists during this period was $19 million; this sum included claims for damages as low as $54 and as high as $5 million. A summary of the injuries claimed is presented in Table 2.

In quoting the figures cited in Table 2, Wiggins noted that the four breach of confidentiality claims appeared to have been the result of fee disputes and the four sexual misconduct claims appeared to have been undertaken out of spite.

In April 1976 the American Psychological Association (APA) began offering professional liability insurance to its members through a policy written by the American Home Insurance Company. At present there are about 11,000 psychologists insured with the APA-sponsored policy (or approximately 90 percent of all insured psychologists). In the period from April, 1976, to August, 1978, a total of thirty-eight claims naming psychologists as a defendant or co-defendant were filed. Many of the claims cited multiple complaints against the psychologist. A total of fifty-two complaints were contained in the thirty-eight claims, and a breakdown of those complaints appears in Table 3.

TABLE 2.
Breakdown of 37 Claims* Against Psychologists (1973–1975)

CLAIM	FREQUENCY
Libel or slander	8
Office liability	8
Breach of confidential relationship	4
Sexual misconduct	4
Improper diagnosis	3
Improper treatment	3
Breach of contract	2
Conspiracy	2
Miscellaneous (unique and appeared to be filed for nuisance value)	3

*Information unavailable as to whether or not cases are closed.

TABLE 3.
Breakdown of 52 Complaints (Alleged in 38 Claims) Filed Against Psychologists (April 1976–August 1978)

COMPLAINT	FREQUENCY
Fee dispute	11
Sexual impropriety	8
Improper treatment	7
Assault	4
Employment-related	3
Hospitalization-related	3
Breach of ethical obligation	2
Treatment with medication	2
Abuse of Privileged Communication	1
Abuse of trust	1
Breach of contract	1
Diagnosis without parental consent	1
Improper contact	1
Improper diagnosis	1
Invasion of privacy	1
Irrational (brought by paranoid patient)	1
Libel	1
Sexual discrimination	1
Violation of right to take an exam	1
Wrongful death	1

It can be seen from Table 3 that the most frequent complaint against a psychologist involved fee disputes. Included in this category were allegations of harassment by collection agencies retained by psychologists. Sexual improprieties constituted the second largest source of complaints; included here were not only complaints of improper heterosexual advances but improper homosexual advances by both male and female therapists. "Hospitalization-related" complaints is a category that needs further explanation. One of these three cases involved an involuntary hospitalization and another involved a patient who was hospitalized and then assaulted while in the hospital. The third case involved a psychologist allegedly advising the patient to stop taking a certain medication. When the patient discontinued the medication it resulted in hospitalization and loss of employment. The suit claiming "sexual discrimination" was brought against a psychologist who allegedly was biased in some practice. The "violation of right to take an examination" claim was brought against a psychologist who was a member of a state psychology board that had denied the plaintiff admission to a psychology licensing examination. The "irrational" claim was filed by a patient who was diagnosed as paranoid schizophrenic and who, during the course of therapy, had threatened the psychologist with a gun. Details on this complaint as well as the fifty-one others are scant and difficult to obtain from any source. Perhaps this is because none of the cases had come to trial as of September 1978, and any detailed pretrial disclosure of the allegations and evidence might, in some way, jeopardize the parties' rights to a fair trial.

The data presented in Tables 1 through 3 are no cause for alarm to mental health professionals. One is tempted to conclude from such data that they are relatively safe from the "rush to the courtroom" that has afflicted colleagues in other health specialties. However, according to many experts the relatively low frequency of malpractice litigation against mental health professionals may be providing such professionals with a false sense of security. The professional liability statistics do not adequately reflect the low incidence but high risk nature of a malpractice suit. This means that although the incidence of malpractice litigation may be statistically small, the potential consequences of a suit may be catastrophic. Further, the unalarming statistics may be obscuring a constellation of social forces and changing public attitudes that may engender a crisis situation for the profession. This latter point will be elaborated upon elsewhere in this chapter.

Discussion pertinent to an impending malpractice crisis in the mental health profession first began to appear in the professional literature in the early 1960s—years before the actual outbreak of a malpractice crisis in the medical profession. William Bellamy (1962) was one of the first psychiatrists to study appellate-level litigation against psychiatrists and to observe that "the courts are expecting a higher duty of care from the psychiatrist as the specialty gains status in the eyes of medicine and law; awards are beginning to appear against psychiatrists, and in increasing amounts" (p. 778). Commenting on Bellamy's paper, G. Wilse Robinson (1962), a psychiatrist who candidly admitted that he might qualify for the "unenviable position of being the most sued psychiatrist in the United States," aptly noted:

> Dr. Bellamy has pointed out that these suits may be increasing in number and certainly judgments against the defendant psychiatrists are increasing. It behooves every psychiatrist to take a good hard look at his own *modus operandi* and the techniques of his associates and juniors and to bring them into conformity with modern legal practices. Things that were acceptable 20, or even 5 years ago, are no longer so in today's courts. Every established psychiatrist who has never retained an attorney to advise him as needed has a fool for an advocate.
>
> We are no longer immune. We are considered in the eyes of the layman to be business men and, as such, we are responsible to the law. (p. 780)

In 1968, numerous and ever-increasing queries from psychiatrists prompted one instructor of clinical psychopharmacology to publish a paper on legal aspects of prescribing psychiatric medication. Some of the questions dealt with by that article were:

Is it legally dangerous to prescribe more than the manufacturer's suggested maximum dose? What legal risk is involved in starting a middle-aged woman on imipramine when she refuses a preliminary physical examination? Does a psychotherapist have to take a blood pressure reading before giving his anxious patient 400 mg. of meprobamate every four hours?...

Must physical examinations be done on these hitherto untouched psychotherapy patients? What would this do to the transference? Is it necessary to send psychotherapy patients to an internist every time some meprobamate or chlordiazepoxide is given? If not, what are the legal dangers? (Appleton, 1968, p. 877)

As early as 1965, psychologists were being formally urged to become better acquainted with the problems attendant to malpractice litigation and to "prepare themselves as a profession for legal tests" (Krauskopf and Krauskopf, 1965, p. 227). By 1975, the message to psychologists was clear:

As mental health professionals other than M.D.'s begin to make diagnoses, sign papers of commitment and independently treat those considered to be mentally ill, stricter accountability and standards of practice will be imposed on all mental health professionals. Malpractice insurance will markedly increase for everyone, and nondoctoral practitioners probably will be unable to practice independently. Such changes seem inevitable. Psychologists, social workers and educators will be required to assume much greater legal and ethical responsibility. This will mean being responsible for the practices of nondoctoral mental health practitioners, much more paper work (extensive record keeping) and a much greater awareness of legal decisions, legislative statutes and professional standards. (Atthowe, 1975, p. 35)

In December of 1975, an article published in the *American Journal of Psychiatry* by a psychiatrist and an administrator of the American Psychiatric Association Professional Liability program cautioned that "it is an educated guess that claims against psychiatrists will increase in number and that the amount of judgments and/or settlements will be higher" (Trent and Muhl, 1975, p. 1313). These authors cited "chaotic changes in the malpractice insurance market" that had come about through general inflationary trends, higher settlements and court awards, and stock market losses on insurance company investments whose earnings were to partially support claim payments:

Within the past several months, shocking and unmanageable changes have occurred in the general malpractice insurance market. After 25 years of coverage, the American Mutual Insurance Company withdrew its coverage of physicians in northern California, and Employers Insurance of Wausau withdrew its coverage of physicians in New York State.

New York's new company, Argonaut, insured physicians for an additional premium of 93 percent and then withdrew its coverage. The Professional Insurance Company of New York became insolvent, leaving many insured physicians in that state without protection under their policies. The St. Paul Insurance Company has refused to renew coverage for the State of Maryland, and the Liberty Mutual Insurance Company, after many years of coverage, has refused to continue offering insurance through the American College of Physicians. Increases of 200 percent and more in malpractice insurance premiums are not unusual throughout the United States. (pp. 1312–1313)

The spring 1976 issue of *Psychotherapy Economics* (a newsletter for independent practitioners of psychotherapy, now called *Psychotherapy Finances*) featured an article entitled "Malpractice Insurance: Are Your Rates about to Take Off?" The article stated, in part:

A few weeks ago, radio news commentator Paul Harvey told his nationwide audience that psychotherapists had lost their malpractice liability coverage because of a rising number of claims of sexual misconduct. If you heard the story you can ignore it—it simply wasn't true. But you can't ignore the fact that malpractice actions against psychotherapists will be increasing and the cost of malpractice insurance will increase with them. Some recent straws in the wind:
The new malpractice policy for American Psychological Association members has a higher premium for less coverage—and next year's rates may go higher. Claims and awards are rising. Sexual abuses are the hot area now but in the liability field success in one area leads lawyers to press in others. The spillover from physicians' malpractice can't be ignored—increases in psychiatrists' premiums should make you realize how serious the threat is. . . .
The whole area of sexual abuse is bound to get more headlines in the future. . . . (p. 1)

In 1978, two articles in the journal of the National Association of Social Workers (*Social Work*) reflected the growing concern of members of that discipline with regard to the specter of a malpractice crisis. In "Social Work and Malpractice: A Converging Course," Green and Cox (1978) argued that, although "there is no reported case law on this subject. . .certain shifts now occurring in public policy will produce situations in which the logical extension of malpractice actions to certain types of social work practice will be inevitable" (p. 100). In "Malpractice: An Ogre on the Horizon," Bernstein (1978) warned that "every social worker must have a basic knowledge of the elements of negligence and malpractice" (p. 106) and that social workers' "exposure to lawsuits by dissatisfied clients—either for acts of commission or omission—has increased" (p. 111).

One past president of the American Academy of Psychiatry and the

Law, Robert Sadoff, has remarked that "changes in law that regulate psychiatric practice have led to new areas of liability for practicing psychiatrists ... some of which are covered by malpractice insurance and others that are not" (1978, p. 31). He went on to outline some of these newer areas of professional liability:

- inappropriate involuntary hospitalization
- inappropriate retention of a patient in a hospital against his will
- inappropriate intrusion of therapy upon a patient who assumes the "right to refuse treatment"
- failure to warn in a case involving a patient who has committed violent acts against a third party
- failure to retain in a hospital a patient who later commits a violent act upon a third person
- inadequate provision of information to a patient receiving treatment—without proper informed consent

Changing laws are only one aspect of an evolving state of affairs that is sure to have a great impact on the daily practice of all mental health professionals. In addition to the previously mentioned factors of declining respect for authority in general, the popular emphasis on consumerism and assertiveness, and the consequences of a slow economy, other factors likely to make the specter of malpractice litigation more of a concern to mental health professionals than in the past include the changing public attitude toward health professionals, the new candor with which mental health problems are discussed, the changing nature of that which is done in the name of psychotherapy, the consequences of lax laws regarding the licensing of therapists, changing judicial interpretations regarding what constitutes a compensable injury and negligence, and the attractiveness of professional liability work for attorneys.

Changing Public Attitudes

When F. Michael Smith sat down to write a congratulatory letter to a close family friend who had just completed medical school, his intention was to express pride and offer encouragement. In composing the letter to his junior colleague, the full impact of the great problems confronting his contemporaries in the medical profession was felt by Dr. Smith. Noting how the "requirements of our new social order" have changed in the thirty years since he entered medicine, Smith (1975) listed activities that were once avoided by physicians (e.g., abortions) and occurrences that tended to be generally forgiven (i.e., not litigated) by the public at large (e.g., slight and ordinary negligence). He went on to comment that "citi-

zens and lawyers, who, only 30 years ago regarded with respect their local
hospitals, doctors, dentists and nurses, are suddenly getting the urge to
consider them only as bonded mechanics contractually guaranteeing
health in the Hammurabic tradition" (p. 295).

Not only are physicians expected to be the guarantors of good results,
but they are expected, as a group, to adhere to high ideals and not be
tempted by things that other mortals are tempted by. It is little wonder,
then, that "the actions of a handful of physicians have tainted the reputation of every physician in this country" (*Illinois Medical Journal*, 1977,
p. 134). Reports of medical misdeeds abound in the media, and the net
result is a publicly scarred medical profession:

> Almost daily, statements derogatory to the medical profession are made
> in the news media. Reports range from descriptions of gross insensitivity
> toward patients, to blatant fraud on the part of medical professionals. Of
> course, some of the reports are justified and can be substantiated, but
> others are untrue and the result of superficial and/or incomplete investi-
> gation. In these instances, the innocent and dedicated medical profes-
> sional is branded as the callous and unscrupulous lawbreaker. The once
> lofty prestige of the medical profession has slipped. (Sampson, 1977,
> p. 9)[3]

If the "once lofty prestige" of the medical profession has slipped,
what can be said of the "never lofty prestige" of work in the mental health
profession? Addressing himself to the current status of the relationship
between clinicians and the public, Atthowe (1975, p. 36) reflected, "The
days of the autocratic, all-wise therapist and the humble all-accepting
patient are numbered." But the public image of the mental health professional has never been enviable. The idea that work in this profession is
largely a matter of common sense has paradoxically co-existed with the
idea that such professionals are capable of mind-reading and other amazing feats—notions I have referred to elsewhere as the "Common Sense
Delusion" and the "Great Expectations Delusion" (Cohen, Note 1).

In a *University of Pittsburgh Law Review* article, Cassidy (1974)
postulated that the relative paucity of litigation against mental health
professionals was related in part to transferential issues, to the shame
attendant to such litigation, and to the interpersonal skills of the
therapist:

> It is not difficult to see why a person undergoing analysis would often be
> reluctant to sue his doctor. He has had frequent contact with the psychi-
> atrist and perhaps regards him as a friend. When you add the additional

---

[3]See also Schwartz (1978).

factor of the transference phenomenon, the state of affairs becomes quite clear. The patient may be positive that he has been mistreated or that the doctor has taken advantage of him. But still, the patient would no sooner think of suing the psychiatrist than most people would think of suing their parents. It seems that in many cases the only way a malpractice action could be brought is by a spouse or relative of the patient or else by the patient at the insistence of a relative.

Another reason that many patients would not be inclined to bring an action against their therapist is shame. To prove their case they would have to reveal their condition, the course the therapy involved, and the conduct of the therapist. There are few people who would like to reveal their psychiatric history and interpersonal relationships in a court of law.

Another factor is the psychiatrist himself. He is an expert in handling people and their emotions. If a patient should disclose dissatisfaction with the course of therapy or the results obtained, a psychiatrist is far more likely to dissuade their anger or satisfy their doubts than a surgeon would be. The psychiatrist is the "talking doctor"; perhaps by "talking" they are able to cure some of their own problems, such as dissatisfied patients. (pp. 130–131)

It would seem, though, that a strong argument could be made that such variables as the interpersonal skills of the therapist and trans-ference-related phenomena have *not* been primarily responsible for preventing litigation in the past—because these two variables have presumably remained constant as the frequency of lawsuits has steadily risen. It is true, however, that the number of persons seeking psychotherapy-related services (as well as the number of persons offering such services) has risen dramatically in recent years. Gross (1978) reported that in 1955 only 233,000 persons were being treated in psychiatric outpatient clinics. That number has swelled to a total of approximately 4 million persons being treated in outpatient clinics and federally supported community mental health centers. Additionally, it has been estimated that approximately 7 million persons in the private sector obtain psychotherapy-related services from mental health professionals and non-professionals.

Increasing public acceptance of psychotherapy as a viable avenue of personal problem solving seems to have greatly minimized the shame, embarrassment, and stigma that was once attached to psychotherapeutic treatment. In contemporary America it is not unusual to hear conversational accounts of psychotherapy sessions in business offices, restaurants, cocktail parties, and related social settings. It would seem reasonable to infer that as Americans become more willing to seek treatment and to admit that they are in therapy (even to the point of casually discussing aspects of their treatment), they will also become more willing to sue mental health professionals. Perhaps as more persons than ever before are willing to "bare their souls" to psychotherapists, they will be willing to bare them before judges and juries as well.

The Changing Nature of "Psychotherapy"

> Progress in the field of psychotherapy is hindered by a factor that is endemic in our society: an item is considered newsworthy, and accolades are accorded when claims run counter to the dictates of common sense. Thus everything from megavitamins to anal lavages and primal screams gains staunch adherents who, in their frenetic search for a panacea, often breed confusion worse confounded. (Lazarus, 1976, p. 9)

What does "psychotherapy" mean? In the heyday of psychoanalysis, the meaning of the term was quite clear (even if the theory and techniques were rather mysterious to the public). Today, exactly what is meant by "psychotherapy" can only be gleaned from knowledge of the context in which the term is being discussed. Joining psychoanalysis in the psychotherapy market place have been hundreds of varied approaches to treatment, including behavior therapy, cognitive therapy, cognitive behavior therapy, client-centered therapy, direct decision therapy, existential therapy, multimodal therapy, rational-emotive therapy, emotive-reconstructive therapy, art therapy, music therapy, and dance therapy, to name but a few. The efficacy of some of these approaches, such as behavior therapy, has been rigorously tested, while no scientifically acceptable experimentation on most others (e.g., primal therapy, jogging therapy) has been done. Of course, the efficacy of even the best-researched and experimentally proven interventions is ultimately a matter of the competence and expertise of the therapist. Unfortunately, the current state of affairs is such that any number of activities are being carried out in the name of psychotherapy by "therapists" with a motley array of professional and nonprofessional backgrounds (cf. Cohen, Note 1).

Putting aside questions of therapeutic efficacy and focusing on the nature of "psychotherapy," it seems a fair observation that the onetime "talking treatment" has become more of a veritable "trial by fire," with more active roles being taken by both patients and therapists. As practiced by many contemporary therapists, activities undertaken in the name of psychotherapy have included, for example, therapist–patient, patient–patient, and patient–surrogate touching; therapist–patient and patient–patient confrontation; in vivo and imaginal exposure to phobic objects, electric shocks and other aversive stimulation administered at the sight, smell, taste, sound, or touch of one thing or another; and a truly imaginative assortment of methods that encourage or precipitate screaming, pounding, violent emoting, and so forth. It seems reasonable to predict that as treatment moves from the traditional, verbal, insight-oriented approaches toward the more intense, physical and even violently cathartic methods psychotherapists are currently experimenting with, the greater will be the risk of malpractice litigation.

Almost from the time that Freud first introduced the "talking cure," there have been people who have attempted to improve on his techniques by adding nonverbal elements. Perhaps one of the earliest attempts to transform Freud's psychoanalytic doctrines into a theory with tangible, physical correlates was made by a disciple of Freud, Wilhelm Reich. Reich's theory of orgone energy[4] has been viewed by some authorities as the "fond creation of a good mind over-wrought with the need to physicalize Freud's abstract concept of libido" (Mann, 1973, p. 26). Today, Reichian psychiatrists as well as other "orgonomists" with widely varying professional backgrounds in terms of training and credentials are among those psychotherapists who employ touch and massage as an integral part of their treatment.

Of course, the Reichians are only one of many groups who touch and massage their patients as a routine part of therapeutic treatment. Practitioners of "bioenergetic therapy" as taught by Lowen (1958) also employ touch and massage as an integral part of their treatment, as do the Rolfing therapists, who require that the patient to be "Rolfed" be dressed in underwear or be nude. In his book describing group encounter techniques, Schutz (1967) described many exercises that require therapist–patient and patient–patient contact. The encounter group assumption that touching facilitates liking and/or disclosure has received at least partial support from some experimental research (Jourard, 1971; Boderman, Freed, and Kinnucan, 1972; Cooper and Bowles, 1973; Dies and Greenberg, 1976), though these preliminary reports should be interpreted with caution (cf. Kilmann and Sotile, 1976). Taken to its ultimate point, the encouragement of touching leads to the advocacy of sexual intimacy between patient and therapist. (See, for example, McCartney, 1966, and Shepard, 1971.) Such practices are not generally endorsed by mental health professionals, and the fact that such approaches have found outspoken advocates is a matter of concern and embarrassment to many.

Even when there is no touching, many of the methods of the newer psychotherapies demand more physical and mental exertion on the part of patients than has traditionally been the case. For example, behavioral treatment of an obsessive-compulsive patient with a phobia of dirt might employ a therapy regimen of systematic desensitization combined with encouragement (if not force) to engage in the feared act or to physically contact the feared object. In the treatment of one hospitalized compulsive handwasher, the taps in the room were shut off and the patient was required to touch various "contaminating" objects in daily sessions (Meyer, 1966). Implosive therapy (Stampfl and Levis, 1967) is a treatment

---

[4]A note on the rationale of Reich's theory of orgone energy (and the fallacy thereof) appears in Cohen (1977a). A more complete treatment appears in Mann (1973).

designed to raise the patient's anxiety level (through imaginal exposure to feared stimuli) to a point of which the patient spontaneously "implodes":

> Implosive therapy is based on the premise that extinction of anxiety can be most effectively achieved by repeated elicitation of intense emotional responses without the occurrence of physically injurious consequences. Mainly for reasons of ease, the emotional responses are activated symbolically. The therapist vividly describes the most revolting and terrifying experiences conceivable, and clients are urged to imagine themselves actively engaged in these shocking activities. A compulsive handwasher who is obsessed about dirt, for example, is asked to visualize himself reaching into a wastebasket and then withdrawing his hand, which is depicted as dripping with a sickening mixture of mucus, saliva, vomit, and feces. If the dirt phobia is believed to arise from anxiety over anal functions, the client is further instructed to imagine himself residing in a septic tank where he eats his meals, entertains his friends, and mushes around in this soggy abode. (Bandura, 1969, p. 402)

The nude marathon (Bindrim, 1968) is a form of group therapy designed to help facilitate self-disclosure and acceptance of one's physical attributes. This form of treatment has been succinctly described by Mintz (1971):

> The marathon begins with a get-acquainted period in which the participants remain clothed and are given a chance to express their anxieties about nudity. Members then retire to separate dressing rooms and remove their clothing. After this there is a period of nude encounter and experience which includes bodily contact, humming, music, and the use of stroboscopic light. This period lasts for about eight hours, after which a four-hour period of silence is enjoined, during which the participants sleep, rest, or meditate. Wine may be served ceremonially at the beginning of the silence.
>
> After the rest period, the group enters the swimming pool and participates in physical procedures designed to encourage regression through massage, holding and rocking one another in the water, and occasionally by feeding a participant with a baby bottle. (p. 255)

Using props as diverse as cribs, teddy bears, and dildos, primal therapists (Janov, 1970) encourage patients to achieve what appears to be a conscious coma, called a "primal." Countless professionals have noted that no scientifically acceptable evidence for the efficacy of this technique has ever been published. Hart, Corriere, and Binder (1975) are among those who have expressed concern over primal therapy and other procedures that are passed off to the public as therapeutic:

> Because of the persuasively simple case studies offered in *The Primal Scream*, patients enter Primal Therapy expecting to intensely regress

and utter the primal scream. Actually, most people end up imitating the examples they read about. Instead of feeling their own feelings and moving from simple expressions of disordered feelings to deeper and more complex expressions, they leap into primals.

Because a patient is said to be more "real" and closer to "cure" the more he experiences his childhood pains, patients actually learn, in Primal Therapy, a new secondary defense system where they *try* to be in pain and *try* to be out of control. "Being totally out of control permits connection because self-control *always* means suppression of self (italics ours)." This claim is nonsense, destructive nonsense. Patients who believe it will never be able to counteract old regressive impulses because that activity requires positive control. Nor will they be able to form new adult expressions which allow them a free flow of feeling. Instead they will learn a new set of regressive defenses—giving in to childish defenses and going away from the expression of present feelings.

The theory and techniques of Primal Therapy are simplistic in the extreme. A capitalized Pain is the source of every disorder and a capitalized Scream is its cure. The technique of Primal Therapy is never completely described in *The Primal Scream*, but vague intimations are given that something special will be done to patients. In fact, Primal Therapy does not use any special techniques, but relies heavily upon suggestion, both to induce emotional expressions and to guide their resolution. The closest parallel to Janov's Primal Therapy is Mesmer's Magnetic Therapy. Both therapies sometimes achieved amazing emotional releases and testimonies of benefits, but neither therapy sustained the changes that patients were provoked to perform. (pp. 398–399)

Drug treatment methods.   Many health professionals believe that Americans live in an overmedicated society. In her survey of the extent to which Americans rely on drugs, Muller (1972) cited overmedication as "one source of reduced human welfare" (p. 488). While the overmedication thesis is applicable to many of the medications currently available (such as antibiotics), it is particularly applicable to psychotropic medication. Pharmaceutical houses that manufacture psychotropic drugs have tried in their advertising to "mystify" their wares and confuse medical problems with existential or social ones (cf. Lennard et al., 1970). One study of adults admitted to *general* medical and surgical wards in Boston-area hospitals (Greenblatt, Shader, and Koch-Weber, 1975) revealed that as many as one in five had a history of psychotropic use, *with the majority of this group reporting that they had been taking such medication for a year or more*. It has been estimated that almost 90 percent of all nonorganic, chronic psychiatric inpatients are on some psychopharmacological maintenance therapy (Lentz, Paul, and Calhoun, 1971). As reported by Gottlieb, Nappi, and Strain (1978) in a recent issue of the *American Journal of Psychiatry*, more than 20 percent of all adult Americans who are not confined to institutions receive at least one prescription for a psychotropic drug annually. Estimates of the large quantities of aspirin, tranquilizers, antidepressants, alcohol, marijuana, and related drugs used in this country suggest, as Carstairs (1969) has observed, that when people are unhappy they have a tendency to believe that something is wrong with them—and that a pill can relieve it.

The enthusiastic endorsement of psychotropic medication by health professionals as well as the public brings with it a responsibility on the part of doctors to be familiar with the physiology, pharmacology, and side effects of the drugs they prescribe. Yet there is suggestive evidence that medical training programs today are not providing that needed familiarity. In one study (Gottlieb et al., 1978), medical students, medical house staff, and psychiatrists at an urban teaching hospital were administered a questionnaire designed to test their knowledge of three commonly prescribed psychotropic drugs. Psychiatrists did not perform significantly better than the medical students or house staff with respect to their knowledge of diazepam and anxiety, and their knowledge in other areas was deficient.

Generally speaking, legal jeopardy would appear to be a positive function of the number of pills prescribed (cf. Appleton, 1968). Dawidoff (1973b) has cautioned, with respect to the package insert accompanying all prescription drugs, that "when a psychiatrist does not, in every particular, follow the precautions laid down in this literature, the door to malpractice litigation may be open" (p. 699). Appleton (1968) has observed that a psychiatrist seldom does a physical examination before prescribing medication and that "this omission makes him legally vulnerable" (p. 882). Reports of death (Plachta, 1965; Moore and Book, 1970; Hollister and Kosek, 1965; Childers, 1961; Ayd, 1956) and of harmful side effects such as dystonia (Swett, 1975; Ayd, 1961) and tardive dyskinesia (Moline, 1975; Turek et al., 1972; Tikare and Tikare, 1973; Schiele et al., 1973; Thornton and Thornton, 1973; Paulson, 1973) are not uncommon when psychiatric medication is used. In reporting that a single bedtime dose of one medication produced night terrors in three-fourths of his sample, Flemenbaum (1976) commented, "This suggests that we may be unintentionally inflicting additional miseries on patients who come to us for relief of their own suffering" (p. 571). Of course, adding to instead of alleviating suffering can be grounds for a lawsuit. Trent and Muhl (1975) reported that a physician and a drug company were jointly sued in an action involving a case of tardive dyskinesia induced by phenothiazine medication. This suit was settled out of court for $190,000. Two other such suits were in litigation at the time of their writing.

Licensing Laws

"Chaotic" properly describes the current state of affairs with respect to laws regulating the licensure and certification of mental health professionals. Although these remarks of B. E. Bernstein (1978) were addressed primarily to social workers, his observations are of interest to all mental health professionals:

> Many states have statutes providing for a Medical Practices Act and a Basic Science Act. These statutes stipulate that both mental and physical health care should be given professionally only by physicians. Exceptions to this statute are provided for such other professionals as nurses and psychologists practicing under the Psychologists' Certification and Licensing Act. In the state of Texas, the limitation states that anyone who is not a psychologist cannot provide "psychological services" and cannot represent himself as a "psychologist." There is nothing expressed or implied in the limitation, however, concerning an individual's right to engage in counseling. In the absence of a specific legislative act or definite judicial interpretation, however, social workers are cautioned against using exotic self-serving titles or appellations. Each state law must be examined to define the limits of both the treatment itself and the title the professional is permitted to use.
>
> If a social worker were to call himself a therapist and if he were to allow a situation to develop in which substantial harm took place... lawsuits would follow.... (p. 110)

In most jurisdictions, titles such as "therapist," "psychotherapist," "psychoanalyst," "sex therapist," "marriage counselor," "hypnotist," and the like remain totally unregulated by law. This means that anyone can use any one (or more) of these and sundry other titles that imply some psychotherapeutic expertise and act totally within the law in doing so. Members of the public who find their way to these "therapists"—who are, by and large, uneducated, uncredentialed, and unethical,—may be very displeased with the results. It is, of course, bad enough when a client is displeased with the services of a properly credentialled therapist and the entire profession receives a bad name as a result. Unfortunately, the good name of professional therapists is as likely to be sullied by an incompetent, non-credentialled "therapist" as by a fellow professional.

Problems of lax legislation also attend the regulation of the terms "psychologist" and "psychiatrist." There are almost as many different statutes defining what a psychologist is as there are states. (In one state, Missouri, there was no regulation of that title at all until as late as 1977.) A truly staggering amount of variation in training, background, and credentials characterizes those who call themselves "psychologists". As for the title "psychiatrist," any physician—regardless of his training in psychology or psychiatry—is entitled to limit his practice to psychiatry and call himself a psychiatrist. Again, the unfortunate consequence of lax legislation regarding the regulation of such professional titles is the heightened possibility of a patient's being dissatisfied with his therapist and the resultant bad name that attached to the profession as a whole.

Changing Judicial Interpretations

Emotional distress as a compensable injury

A woman in her twenties was stopped by a security guard in a large Brooklyn department store because the guard thought that the woman had been an accessory to a shoplifting. Despite the fact that the woman had no stolen merchandise in her possession, the guard took her to the local police precinct for booking. Subsequently, the woman brought suit for false arrest. At the trial, psychiatric testimony was adduced claiming that the woman was a "seriously ill young lady who has had a tenuous social and psychological equilibrium as a result of the events of October 23, 1972. She will require psychological and financial assistance for some time" (Time, May 31, 1976, pp. 45–46). The jury awarded the woman 1.1 million dollars in damages.

Laws providing for the award of damages to injured parties for having suffered emotional distress as a result of and in addition to physical injuries have existed for some time in most states. Similarly, laws providing for the recovery of damages for the intentional infliction of emotional distress on some party have had a long history. It has only been relatively recently, however, that damages for the infliction of emotional distress as a result of negligence (and in the absence of any physical injuries) have begun to be awarded by the courts. In the case vignette above, the emotional distress caused by a woman's false arrest by a store security guard was worth over one million dollars in the eyes of the jury. However justified, the implications of such decisions for mental health professionals are sobering. What of the disgruntled patient who claims that his therapist caused or aggravated or negligently failed to relieve his emotional distress?

The rights of clients and patients.   In the past, courts seem to have generally acted as if it was the mental health professional and not the judge who knew what was best for clients and patients. Judicial decisions that ran counter to the reigning laissez-faire attitude were in the minority and were considered quite revolutionary when they occurred. For example, two decisions in the early sixties (*In the Matter of the Appeal of Arthur T. Thibadeau, Jr.*, and *In the Matter of Van Allen v. Mc-Cleary*—both cited in Herron et al., 1970) addressed the right of parents to inspect their children's school records. Attorneys for the school boards in both cases argued that there was a need to safeguard psychological test data from misinterpretation and that professional freedom would be compromised if parents were allowed access to the files. The decisions of the court in both of these cases may now be viewed as seminal blows to the authority of mental health professionals. An excerpt from the wording of the decision in *Thibadeau* states the court's view in no uncertain terms:

> Parents should be permitted to inspect the records of their children which would include progress reports, subject grades, intelligence quotients, test achievement scores, medical records, psychological and psychiatric reports, selective guidance notes and the evaluations of students by educators. (cited in Herron et al., 1970, p. 244)

In recent years the courts have challenged the authority of mental health professionals in the schools, hospitals and private-practice consulting rooms with a spate of decisions ostensibly designed to safeguard patients' rights. In an article entitled "Who Decides Admission—Judge or Physician?" attorney/physician Walter Feldman (1978) cited a case in which a Florida court had ordered that a patient be hospitalized but a physician refused to admit the patient. The doctor's refusal to admit the mentally ill patient caused him to be cited for contempt of court. Even though the doctor was eventually acquitted of the charge, his acquittal "cost him close to $15,000 in addition to time, energy, frustration, and embarrassment" (p. 8). Presumably, the court had attempted to protect the patient's "right to treatment" regardless of whether the doctor or even the patient felt that treatment was indicated.

More typically, courts have attempted to protect the patient's right to treatment by providing involuntary patients with lawyers who are appointed to seek the patient's release—a duty that is deemed to be in the patient's best interest (Stone, 1977). Right-to-treatment rulings as well as right-to-refuse-treatment rulings have greatly complicated an already complex legal picture, as have other legal doctrines, such as those calling for "least restrictive alternatives." Informed consent to treatment, a legal doctrine formerly of primary concern to surgeons, is fast becoming a matter of concern to psychologists and psychiatrists. (A discussion of informed consent appears on pp. 65–69.) Knotty questions concerning how "informed" the consent of a mental patient must be and how therapeutic or counter-therapeutic giving such consent might be defy completely satisfactory answers. Already, legislative restraint on the mental health profession is present to such a degree that the specter of professionals having to give "Miranda-type" warnings to patients is a reality. In Illinois, the recently published report of the Governor's Commission to Revise the Mental Health Code is a frightening portent. As Spadoni (1977) observes:

> Under a controversial provision dealing with admission and discharge requirements, for example, physicians examining involuntary patients would be required to administer a "Miranda-type" warning, i.e., inform the patient that his comments subsequently may be used against him

during commitment hearings. This would, in effect, place a physician in the role of a policeman arresting a criminal, a role that all physicians would consider abhorrent. Another provision would severely limit involuntary hospitalization only to the *physically dangerous person* who presents an *immediate* threat to himself or others. . . .

Other proposed revisions further intrude on the physician's clinical judgment by enumerating detailed restrictions on the use of restraints, seclusion and psychotropic drugs. In addition, seriously-disturbed patients would be permitted to refuse any type of hospital treatment, including medication, unless immediate physical danger is evident. (p. 86)

In Nebraska, a recently filed civil suit intimated that a "right to normalization" had been violated by an institution for the mentally retarded that employed a token economy program. The parties to the suit reached an agreement which, in part, linked token programs with violations of the Thirteenth Amendment: "Many residents are required to engage in non-therapeutic work for tokens or no compensation, thus violating constitutional provisions that prohibit enforced labor except as punishment for criminal acts" (cited in "Litigation," 1976). The agreement provided that all work done, with the exception of personal housekeeping, be compensated with money at the usual and appropriate rate.

The State of Florida recently legislated a Bill of Rights for the retarded which provides for the prohibition of the use of noxious stimuli on patients. The Florida legislation, along with comparable legislation in other states, was probably undertaken in a much-needed spirit of bringing order, procedure, and guidelines to an area that had previously been administered in a rather nonuniform and arbitrary fashion. The danger is that patients' rights legislation designed to improve the plight of patients may hamstring mental health professionals (because of the threat of legal liability) to the extent that quality treatment will be impossible. The Florida legislation, for example, appears to be a legitimate outgrowth of public outrage attendant to the indiscriminate and arbitrary use of noxious stimuli on patients. But what of the use of aversive stimulation within the context of a comprehensive and systematic behavioral treatment program, in which such stimulation has been shown to be of well-documented therapeutic efficacy (cf. Lovaas and Bucher, 1974; Cohen, 1976c)? Mental health professionals need to be concerned about where their liability will begin and end if the rather extreme proposals and rulings being handed down in the area nominally referred to as "patients' rights" continue to be generated at their present pace.

Society's rights.   Where does the psychotherapist's obligation to his patient end and that to society at large begin? According to the 1974 ruling of the California Supreme Court in the landmark *Tarasoff v. the Regents of the University of California* (case 5.24 in Chapter 5), "protective privilege ends where the public peril begins.'' In making its historic ruling, the court stated, in part:

> Our current crowded and computerized society compels the interdependence of its members. In this risk-infested society we can hardly tolerate the further exposure to danger that would result from a concealed knowledge of the therapist that his patient was lethal. If in the exercise of reasonable care the therapist can warn the endangered party or those who can reasonably be expected to notify him, we see no sufficient societal interest that would protect and justify concealment. The containment of such risks lies in the public interest.

The controversy surrounding the implications of *Tarasoff* will be discussed in Chapter 3. Here we point out only that the effect of the California Supreme Court's decision was to place California mental health professionals in a double bind with respect to confidentiality. Specifically, it made *both* the breaching of confidentiality and the failure to breach confidentiality legitimate grounds for litigation.

Tacit Judicial Doctrines.   Charles Hoffman, chairman of the Medical Liability Commission, attributed the malpractice crisis to, among other things, court doctrines which have held medical professionals liable for oral contracts and guaranteed results ("Chairman," 1975). Medical professionals may also be held liable simply because they are usually better able than patients to bear the loss; this rationale for imposing liability is reflected in the holding of a Washington court that found for the plaintiff in a malpractice action against a physician. As cited by Smith (1975) the judge ruled as follows:

> There are many situations in which a careful person is held liable for an entirely reasonable mistake. . . . [I]n some cases the defendant may be held liable, although he is not only charged with no moral wrongdoing, but has not even departed in any way from a reasonable standard of intent or care. . . . There is a strong and growing tendency, where there is blame on neither side, to ask, in view of the exigencies of social justice, who can best bear the loss and hence to shift the loss by creating liability where there has been no fault. (p. 295)

Smith (1975) referred to the type of thinking reflected in the court's decision as "deep pocket jurisprudence." Smith argued that it is just this type of thinking that drives carriers to seek high-priced out-of-court settlements (even when no blame exists), pushes malpractice premiums higher, and eventually drives carriers out of business altogether. Smith went on to observe that "insurers are quick to smell this 'come and get it' odor of deep-pocket jurisprudence and its underlying presuppositions of surplus value ethics and candy mountain economics" (p. 295).

The Attractiveness of Professional Liability
Work for Attorneys

> Toss a beer can out of any college dormitory in America and chances are
> you will hit somebody struggling to get into law school.... If all the
> students now dreaming of law school manage to get in, the country will
> suffer a plague of lawyers by 1984. We already have at least 10 times as
> many lawyers as any rational society can tolerate. (Baker, 1977, p. 12)

Not only are more lawyers than needed being graduated, but many
attorneys practicing certain types of law have been forced to find work in
other areas. The advent of "no-fault" insurance has driven many lawyers
to search for more fertile areas of practice:

> Since the advent of no-fault automobile insurance in October of 1972,
> this writer already has been defending more malpractice cases brought
> by attorneys who would never have started a malpractice case before,
> and who formerly referred those cases to four or five firms of lawyers in
> the state who specialize in plaintiff's malpractice work. I can visualize
> the trend continuing and that there will be more and more spurious
> malpractice cases started simply because the average practicing attorney
> in the State of Michigan cannot distinguish between malpractice and bad
> result. (Cline, 1973, p. 67)

Other lawyers who may have specialized in work dealing with
psychoactive substances may be forced into new areas by decriminaliza-
tion and other modifications of drug laws in their state. Lawyers doing
divorce work may also be out of a job as the country moves towards
granting divorce on simple petition by the couple. The medical malpractice specialty offers itself as a lucrative alternative, especially for the
experienced trial lawyer. Curran (1977) reanalyzed the data for experienced trial lawyers from an extensive U.S. government survey (1970–
1972) on medical malpractice. His analysis indicated that

> this group earned approximately $250 per hour on cases handled, and
> the average gross recovery in cases won by them was $81,000, with a
> median of $25,000. This compared with a national gross recovery of
> $22,000 with a median of $3,000. It seems clear that well known, experi-
> enced trial lawyers of the country do very well when they win. How often
> do they win a recovery? More often than most lawyers think: the plain-
> tiffs' attorneys in the survey reported that they achieved some recovery
> in 79 per cent of their cases. (p. 25)

Closely related to the burgeoning number of lawyers available to
enter the attractive field of malpractice litigation is the fact that such
litigation is also attractive to lawyers' clients, since a contingent fee ar-

rangement is typically worked out. That is, it costs the patient nothing to initiate the suit, and the attorney is only paid contingent on his winning a settlement from the defendant doctor.[5] Both patients and lawyers are well aware that most doctors today—including mental health professionals— typically carry malpractice insurance policies with high upper limits. One insurance industry spokesman has voiced concern as regards the problem of actually encouraging suits by carrying high amounts of professional liability coverage. M. A. Walters, assistant vice-president for government and industry relations of the Insurance Services Office hypothesized that dissatisfied patients are encouraged to sue for very high amounts when they are secure in the knowledge that their doctor has a policy with a high limit ("ISO," 1976). Ms. Walters further commented that in light of decisions against physicians in recent years, it seemed that judges and juries had a tendency to perceive doctors as inordinately or even unfairly rich and were therefore more willing to compensate the "poor, injured patient."

All of the foregoing is not to deny the fact that there are many reality-based complaints. Martin (1975) addressed this point when he commented on the relationship between behavior modification and our increasingly litigious society, noting that one reason for the recent rise in litigation was that

> there are real complaints, real people actually being affected. Many behavior change practitioners like to discuss the field as if it were theoretical, and they view the classroom or professional journals as the preferred forum for debate. But when an individual claims injury, the appropriate forum is a court. Recent legal challenges reflect the nature of our increasingly litigious society, not a plot to stop behavior modification. (p. 7)

The Psychosomatic Society

The medical establishment and the public at large have long acknowledged the well-documented importance of psychological factors in causing and/or aggravating most varieties of disease. At the same time, however, there may be an unwholesome trend on the part of physicians to "write off" too many of their patients' complaints as "psychological." For example, this author is personally acquainted with a dermatologist who, almost as a matter of course, diagnoses many of the cases of dermatitis that he sees in his daily office practice as psychogenic. This doctor will routinely (mis)inform his patients about the advantages of psychotherapy with respect to the treatment of dermatological problems. Perhaps all of

---

[5]Losing plaintiffs are legally required to bear other costs of litigation (filing fees, depositions, court costs, etc.) although in practice attorneys often, somewhat improperly, absorb these costs in the event of a loss.

these cases are psychogenic and perhaps they are not. Perhaps this doctor is merely "passing the buck" to the mental health professional when he cannot effect a cure himself and perhaps he is not. Regardless, what does the patient come away from the dermatologist's office believing? How many dermatologists or other medical specialists say to their patients: "I'm sorry, but the state of medical technology today does not allow me to tell you what is causing your problem. We simply lack the medical sophistication necessary to detect the pathogen." The point here is that an unwarranted expectancy of therapeutic gain has been set up in the medical patient who is referred for psychotherapeutic treatment. When a belief and expectancy that a certain course of therapy will ameliorate a condition exists in the absence of a technology for effecting such cures, the result is dissatisfaction and a sense of being "wronged." Such feelings are the "royal road to the courtroom."

MORE MALPRACTICE OR MORE MALPRACTICE SUITS?

Early articles by lawyers on the subject of malpractice in the mental health profession appeared to have been designed more to dispense information (e.g., Appleman, 1953; Louisell, 1957) than to provide—as most of today's publications do—tips on how to avoid a malpractice suit (e.g., Dawidoff, 1973a, 1973b; Messinger, 1975; Rothblatt and Leroy, 1973). One might say, "If all mental health practitioners provided reasonably high quality service that obviated the necessity of malpractice litigation, no tips would be necessary." But is that really the case? Specifically, is the rise in malpractice litigation in the mental health profession and in the health profession in general symptomatic of a rise in malpractice?

A series of articles published in the *New York Times* (26 January 1976 to 30 January 1976) by Boyce Rensberger and Jane E. Brody explored the extent of the present-day malpractice problem. It was reported that:

- An estimated 16,000 physicians (about 5 percent of the population of practicing doctors) are incompetent to practice medicine owing to reasons such as mental illness, drug addiction, and ignorance or carelessness with regard to medical practice.

- Yet, only about 66 licenses are revoked annually.

- Incompetent doctors treat an estimated 7.5 million patients. In all too many cases, unnecessary surgery is performed, unnecessary (or contraindicated) drugs are prescribed, and unnecessary fatalities occur.

- Unexplained regional differences in medical practice have become a cause for concern. For example, the likelihood of death during one type of operation is five times greater at one hospital than at another; and people in one region of a state have been found to be three to four times as likely to undergo a common surgical procedure as people in another, similar region of the state.

Startling—almost unbelievable—surgical stories were detailed in the series. Instances in which a host of paraphernalia (e.g., tubing, clamps, sponges, forceps, and a thirty-inch-long towel stamped "U. S. Army") were left inside patients were among the milder of the horror stories cited. Three cases of gross malpractice that led to patients' needless deaths included one in which a surgeon removed a woman's kidney without realizing that the woman's other kidney had been removed previously (no x-ray had been taken). In another case, a man who died shortly after a relatively routine operation for replacement of a heart valve was found, after autopsy, to have died from a valve that had been installed backwards. A young New York woman receiving local anesthetic for a tonsillectomy died shortly thereafter—the anesthesia had been injected directly into the carotid artery (which leads directly to the brain). One university-based doctor who has studied the malpractice problem was paraphrased in the *Times* article as saying that the biggest problem in medicine is not the 5 percent of incompetent doctors but the average doctors who, for a variety of reasons, do not render the best medical services they can.

The quality of service given by another group of health care providers, pharmacists, has also come under scrutiny. According to an article published in the *Journal of the American Pharmaceutical Association* ("Pharmacists," 1977), one study of sixty-nine randomly selected pharmacies in the Boston area yielded the following findings:

- None of the pharmacists gave patients the complete advice, instructions, or warnings required by law for the drugs purchased.

- None of the pharmacists packaged and labeled the drug as required by law.

- Only 43 percent of the pharmacies dispensed the lower-costing generic drug rather than the brand-name drug even though the generic name had been given on the prescription. (Here it is relevant to note that the Massachusetts Formulary Law encourages pharmacists to dispense the generic drug under such circumstances.)

- Pharmacies that charged above-average prices did not comply with requirements in above-average fashion. (p. 62)

Although useful in providing insight into the extent of the malpractice problem, studies comparable to those reported in the *Times* and in the pharmaceutical journal only tell part of the story. They are more reflective of public concern with malpractice than of the scientific study of it. They are the product of a zeitgeist of consumerism and cannot legitimately be used to answer the question, "Is there more malpractice?" since they have no standard of comparison—comparable studies were just not done ten, twenty, or thirty years ago.

Suggestive are findings pointing to differential malpractice litigation risks as a function of geographical area. Evidence suggesting that people in certain parts of the country are either harder to satisfy or quicker to sue or both has been presented by the chairman of medicine at Columbia University, Charles A. Ragan (1974, p. 9):

> There are, however, great differences in malpractice risks and, in consequence, in insurance costs in different geographical areas of the United States. The east and west coast are highest, with the exception of the northeast; the south the lowest. A recent law review study showed that despite the difference in risk between North Carolina and California, there was little difference in the way medicine was practiced. In particular, the elements of practice described as defensive medicine—the number of tests ordered—showed no significant variation between the two geographic areas.

Again, studies comparable to the one cited above may not have been done ten, twenty, or thirty years ago. But what are the implications of research suggesting that there exists differential malpractice litigation risks—significant enough to affect insurance rates—as a function of geographical area? Assuming the quality of the health care offered in the different areas is about equal (and there is no reason to assume otherwise), and assuming that other variables (e.g., "number of patients annually treated by adoctor") remain fairly constant or have been statistically accounted for, Ragan's assertion that "in certain areas of this country people are dissatisfied with the medical profession's performance and are willing to go to court to demand recompense" (p. 9) must be given due consideration.

Lashing out at various media "exposés," many doctors have argued that popular articles and official reports that allege a high incidence of unnecessary surgery are one-sided and ill-informed, to say the least. These doctors cogently point out how difficult it is to determine when surgery is truly "unnecessary." In keeping with the spirit of the times, much of the surgery that is performed today as well as many of the lab studies and other procedures ordered are done in the name of a new variety of "preventive medicine"—medicine undertaken to prevent a medical malpractice suit. Doctors have also lashed out at official agencies which have impugned the quality of health care in this country. A 1973 Health, Education and Welfare report critical of health care professionals was attacked by Smith (1975) as a "put-up job designed to lend authenticity to the conclusions, which had been predetermined" (p. 294). Smith went on to condemn the report as one that "missed the significance of its data, and made interpretations and recommendations contrary to the facts contained therein." Perhaps hinting at the role of politics in governmental reporting, he wrote that the project was "funded expensively to secure the signatures rather than the efforts of the eminent participants."

The unprecedented number of federal dollars flowing into numerous health care programs (e.g. Medicare, Medicaid, etc.) carry with them both greater federal regulation and greater scrutiny of health care providers than has ever before been seen in this country. Any apparent rise in malpractice in the health professions could reasonably be seen as analogous to the apparent rise in traffic violations that occurs at a certain location when a police car is placed there; in both cases there may be no real increase in cases, only better reporting. In this context, it would seem naive to assume that any rapidly rising increase in litigation must be directly proportionate to a comparably rising increase in professional misconduct and negligence. Further, it would intuitively seem that the rising number of malpractice suits against health and mental health professionals is attributable to many of the same factors which we have cited as potential generators of even more litigation in the future (e.g., the attractiveness of professional liability work for lawyers, the psychosomatic society, etc.).

Regardless of whether there is more malpractice or simply more malpractice litigation, the undeniable fact is that claims of malpractice against health professionals have soared in recent years. As has been pointed out, the seeming immunity from litigation once enjoyed by mental health professionals has eroded as a result of a number of factors including

- the rise of consumerism
- declining respect for authority in general
- poor economic times
- the potentially lucrative nature of malpractice litigation for attorneys
- increased willingness on the part of psychotherapy patients to disclose and have disclosed details of their treatment.
- the broadening definition of "psychotherapy" and the introduction of more aggressive therapeutic methods
- lax legislation regarding the credentialing of psychotherapists
- changing judicial opinions concerning that which constitutes a compensable injury, and
- changing judicial opinions concerning the duty psychotherapists have to society in general

While reading this or some other book or article on the subject of malpractice some health professionals might at some point think to themselves, "I am a competent, ethical practitioner and I therefore do not have to worry about being sued." Such complacency minimizes the point made in this chapter; professional competency and ethicalness (or the lack thereof) are only two of many variables that may account for involvement in a malpractice suit. In short, competency and ethicalness are not enough; a knowledge of the law is essential. The following chapter is designed to provide an introduction to malpractice law and malpractice litigation.

2

Professional Liability and the Law

An adequate understanding of the concept of malpractice or professional liability begins with a working acquaintance with the law. What follows is a presentation of some rudimentary points about the law and an introduction to malpractice litigation.

THE LAW AND THE COURTS

Constitutional, statutory, and common law. Broadly speaking there are three equally powerful types of law in the United States. *Constitutional law* derives from the federal and various state constitutions. *Statutory law* is enacted by legislative bodies (Congress, state legislatures and administrative agencies). *Common law* (also called "case law" or "judge-made law") is evolved by judges in the course of their interpretations of the innumerable cases and varied situations that come before them which are not specifically covered by statutes. Sandor (1957) has traced the long history of common law:

> The common law originated in the laws of Anglo-Saxon England and old English customs and dates from the Norman Conquest in 1066. Instead of definite fixed rules as found in the Roman law, the common law as it developed was a flexible system that adapted itself to conditions as they arose. When a question arose for which there was no applicable custom or precedent the judges would decide according to their ideas of what constituted right or wrong.
>
> During the reign of Richard Coeur de Lion at the close of the 12th century, it became the practice to keep an official record of the cases decided by the courts of common law. These records were known as the "plea rolls," and they have been maintained in an unbroken series down

to the present day. From the plea rolls, there developed a body of recorded decisions. Such decisions were usually followed as precedents in subsequent similar cases, and there was developed the doctrine of *stare decisis*—that a decision of one of the higher courts has the force of law and is binding in all future cases. One of the most striking features of the English common law is this adherence to precedent. These precedents control the litigated question, and, if the trial court departs from them, it is likely to have its findings set aside by the higher courts. When a novel question, for which there is no precedent, arises in a state court in the United States, then the court will usually look to the precedents of a sister state for a decision on a like question. Ordinarily, however, a given state is bound only by the precedents of its own appellate courts or, on federal questions, by the precedents of the United States Supreme Court. (p. 459)

Criminal and civil law.   The distinction between criminal law and civil law is also important. Criminal law regulates those actions which may be offensive to society in general (e.g., murder, rape, robbery), while civil law regulates those actions which may be offensive to particular individuals under specific conditions (e.g., disputes between individuals pertaining to family property or contracts). Although no private individual can bring a criminal action to trial (it is up to a district attorney's office to do that), individuals can, if they so desire, sometimes institute a civil action in addition to a criminal action that has been initiated by the state. For example, suppose Bill punches Roy in the presence of a police officer. The officer might arrest Bill, and the state might initiate a criminal action against him. Technically, Roy could also bring a civil suit against Bill for violating his right not to be touched in an offensive manner. Whether or not Roy would want to bring the civil suit might depend on whether Roy could afford the cost of retaining an attorney for civil litigation, felt he could prove damages, felt Bill would be able to compensate him for such damages, and whether or not he wanted to expend the time and energy needed to try the case.

The defendants in both criminal and civil proceedings are presumed to be blameless until it is proven that they are blamable. In criminal proceedings, it is said that the defendant is innocent until proven guilty and that guilt must be proven "beyond a reasonable doubt." In civil proceedings, it is said that the defendant has incurred *liability* or legal accountability for his actions if "by the preponderance of the evidence" such liability can be proven. The amount of evidence needed to prove "guilt beyond a reasonable doubt" is considerably more than that needed to constitute a "preponderance of the evidence."

It should also be noted that the "rules of the game" also change as one goes from the criminal to the civil arena. The elements of proof needed to prove criminal assault may be different from the elements of proof needed to prove civil assault. For example, in a civil action the assaulted individual might have to prove that he suffered damages as a result of the assault, while in a criminal action he might not be required to do so.

The court system. The court system is the societal institution through which individuals violating the criminal law are prosecuted and those involved in civil disputes can attempt to resolve their differences. In the United States, there is a federal court system along with individual state court systems. As provided in the Constitution, federal judicial power is vested "in one supreme Court, and in such inferior Courts as the Congress may from time to time ordain and establish." Most of the cases handled by federal courts concern violations of federal laws. Generally, federal courts handle all questions concerning the United States Constitution, all cases of maritime jurisdiction, conflicts between states, conflicts between a state and a nonresident of the state, many of the cases involving suits between citizens of different states, and some bankruptcy proceedings. The Supreme Court has original jurisdiction in cases involving ambassadors, consuls, and comparable foreign dignitaries.

State courts generally handle questions concerning violations of state laws and most questions concerning contracts, wills, personal injuries, and domestic relations. A casual survey of the structure and nomencla-

Figure 1.   The Federal Court System

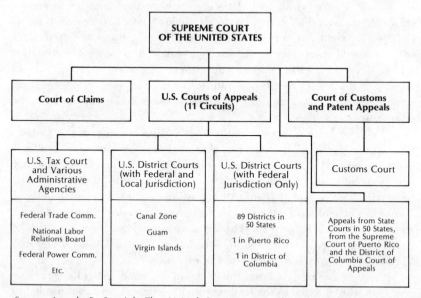

SOURCE: Joseph F. Spaniol, *The United States courts: Their jurisdiction and work* (Washington, D.C.: U.S. Government Printing Office, 1975), a pamphlet prepared for the Committee on the Judiciary, U.S. House of Representatives. Reprinted by permission.

ture of state court systems reveals a bewildering array of names associated with particular functions. Probate court, small claims court, traffic court, and numerous other specialized courts are some of the many cogs in the complex system of state and municipal courts. However, most state court systems have a three-tier system: a trial court, an intermediate court, and a highest court. The intermediate court and the highest court may both be referred to as "appellate courts." In some states the Supreme Court is the highest court, while in others the Court of Appeals is the highest court. Appellate courts rule on questions of law. They are usually made up of panels of three, five, or seven judges, and they have the power to reverse a decision made by a trial court, affirm the trial court's decision, remand the case back to the trial court, or modify the judgment of the trial court. Appellate courts never have juries but come to decisions solely on the basis of the judges' majority ruling.

PROFESSIONAL LIABILITY

If Smith causes hurt to Jones either by intentionally bumping into him in the street or by unintentionally dropping an anvil on his foot, Smith can be held liable for his action. This is so because the law holds each of us responsible for living up to a "standard of care" in our everyday conduct. Given that we all have to exercise at least the same amount of care that the proverbial "average, reasonable person" would exercise under similar circumstances, failing to exercise such care is actionable under law. When the failure to exercise such care is unintentional, the offending act is said to be the result of *negligence*.

Those who present themselves to the public as professionals are—like everyone else—required to conduct themselves with at least as much care as the "average, reasonable person." However, professionals are additionally bound by law to conduct themselves with at least as much care as the "average, reasonable *professional*" in their profession.[1] This means, for example, that services rendered by a psychiatric social worker must be at least as competently and skillfully performed as those of the ordinary psychiatric social worker. Whereas the average person would seldom if every be held liable for someone's suicide, a psychiatric nurse, psychiatrist, clinical psychologist, or some other mental health professional might

---

[1]Legal discussions concerning the tort of negligence frequently make reference to what the "average, reasonable person" would have done under the same or similar circumstances. Analogously, many discussions of professional liability are also couched in such terms as the "average, reasonable professional." However, in the strictest sense, the use of the word "average" as the standard for judging professionals is not quite correct. The law does not assume that one-half of all professionals (those below average) are not up to the standard of care. It should be kept in mind then, that the legal standard is technically not the "average" professional but more like the "ordinary" or "reasonable and prudent" professional.

very well be held liable. This is so because under certain circumstances the courts have held that such professionals have an affirmative duty to prevent suicide. If that duty was breached as a result of the professional's negligent acts or failures to act and if that breach of duty was the cause of the suicide, then *professional liability* would probably exist (and a successful malpractice action would probably result). Professional liability thus includes liability for acts or failures to act in the course of rendering professional services. It is meaningful to talk about professional liability not only with respect to malpractice (i.e., negligence) but also with respect to intentional torts. As such, insurance carriers now refer to their "professional liability insurance" policies rather than their "malpractice insurance" policies—the former term being the more inclusive one.

It should be noted that in some situations it is immaterial whether a party was injured as a result of an intentional or an unintentional tort—all that matters is that the party's injury was causally related to some action by the defendant and that compensation for the injury should be made. In such cases, the doctrine of "strict liability" or "no-fault liability" is said to be applicable. When strict liability is applicable, the defendant will be asked to pay damages regardless of how proper or improper his behavior was. Strict liability has sometimes been invoked by courts in cases involving the torts of defamation (except where the defendant is a news publisher or broadcaster), misrepresentation (when the misrepresentation was neither intentional nor negligent), and invasion of privacy.[2]

THE LIABILITY OF PSYCHOTHERAPISTS

Generally, if a person unintentionally acts in a manner that is in some way "substandard" (i.e., below the level of care that could be expected from any reasonable person under the same or similar circumstances), it is appropriate, in a legal context, to speak of the acts with reference to the tort (see below) of negligence. Similarly, if a professional rendering professional services acts in a manner that is in some way "substandard" (i.e., below the level of care that could be expected from any reasonable person of the same profession in the same or similar circumstances), it is also appropriate to speak of the acts with reference to the tort of negligence, but they are more accurately described as constituting "malpractice" (or professional negligence). If the professional in question is a lawyer, one would speak of legal malpractice; in the case of a doctor, medical malpractice, and so on.

---

[2]This discussion of the complex legal concept of strict liability is necessarily simplistic. Consult Prosser (1971, pp. 492–540) for a more detailed treatment of strict liability in general, and Epstein (1976) for a discussion of the concept with special reference to medical malpractice litigation.

In the circumstance in which the person purporting to be a professional is not really a professional but a quack,[3] the person cannot, technically speaking, be sued for malpractice, though he will be held accountable to the same standard of care (see below) as a bona fide professional acting under the same or similar circumstances. (See *Whipple v. Grandchamp*, 261 Mass. 40; 158 N.E. 270; 57 A.L.R. 974; and *Brown v. Shyne*, 242 N.Y. 176; 151 N.E. 197; 44 A.L.R. 1407.)

Although the applicable statutes vary from state to state, it seems a fair observation that, as regards psychotherapists, it is only mental health professionals (i.e., duly qualified and licensed members of professions in the mental health field) who can be sued for malpractice. Unlicensed, self-proclaimed "therapists," "hypnotists,"[4] and other persons holding themselves out to the public as professionals cannot, generally speaking, be sued for malpractice (in the strict sense of the word) because they are not members of a profession. (See for example *Simpson v. Hubert*, 35 Mich. App. 523; 193 N.W. 2d 68; 70 A.L.R. 3d 108—a case involving a quack dentist.) Quacks can, however, be sued for ordinary negligence, assault, battery, intentional or unintentional causing of emotional distress, and other torts. Reviewing the law in California—a state where there are many nonprofessionals holding themselves out to the public as "therapists"—Marjory Harris (1973) addressed herself to the issue of who could and who could not be sued for malpractice:

> Despite legislative attempts to limit the practice of psychology to certain professionals, a new and unregulated industry has developed to cash in on the growth of interest in psychotherapy and related methods of examining the workings of the human mind. (p. 407)
>
> ... [A]n increasingly liberal attitude on the part of the lay public has encouraged the mushrooming of every conceivable type of "therapy."
>
> ... [T]hose persons who are either licensed or members of professions sanctioned by the state, must follow the standards of care of their professions or they may be subject to either liability for negligence, or loss of license, or criminal penalties. Those people who practice outside the law are either quacks or non-professionals not yet under the state's

---

[3]*Black's Law Dictionary* (Black, 1968) defines a quack as a "pretender to medical skill which he does not possess; one who practices as a physician or surgeon without adequate preparation or due qualification" (p. 1403). For our present purposes, we might substitute "psychotherapeutic" for "medical" and "licensed mental health professional" for "physician or surgeon" in this definition.

[4]Legal regulation of hypnotism—where there is regulation—varies from state to state. In some states, the wording of the law is open-ended and ambiguous. In California the "practice of hypnotism is not prohibited by state law unless such practice constitutes the unauthorized practice of medicine or psychology" (cf. Harris, 1973, p. 408). Hypnosis is sanctioned in that state "for purposes of entertainment, or as an instrument or technique of learning by suggestion or mental adaptation of a skill or of a character trait or projected pattern of behavior."

Figure 2.   Malpractice within the general Schema of the Law

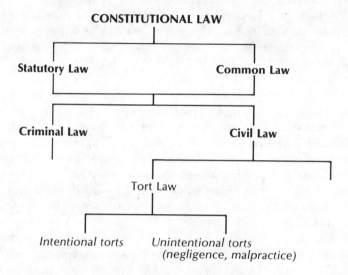

statutory umbrella. Since no standards are established for their reputed
professions, someone injured by their "care" will have to rely on tort
theories other than malpractice....(pp. 408–409)

Strictly speaking, malpractice is a civil offense subsumed under tort
law.[5] A tort is "a harm done to an individual in such a way and of such a
type that the law will order the person who did the harm to pay damages
to the injured party" (Krauskopf and Krauskopf, 1965, p. 227). As
shown in Table 4, torts can be intentional or unintentional. Technically,
malpractice is an unintentional tort (i.e., negligence). However, in this
book we shall employ a broader definition of malpractice—one that is
consistent with both the way the term is colloquially used and the way
insurance companies currently write professional liability policies (see p.
00). Our use of the term malpractice will embrace not only unintentional
(negligent) acts by professionals but also intentional acts such as assault,
battery, and defamation. As per *Corpus Juris Secundum* (1955, p. 1187),
we shall define malpractice as "any unreasonable lack of skill or fidelity
in the performance of professional or fiduciary duties."

Before we proceed with further discussion of the "elements of proof"
(see below) needed for a malpractice suit, we shall clarify the usage of
three terms that will be encountered frequently in our study of malpractice: *fiduciary relations*, *standard of care*, and *damages*.

---

[5]Although lawsuits against mental health professionals have most typically been grounded in
tort theory, suits have been brought under the theory of breach of contract as well. In fact,
some authorities believe that suits against mental health professionals will increasingly be
brought under contract and not tort law (see, for example, "Mal-psychotherapy," Note 4).

Fiduciary relations.   *Black's Law Dictionary* (1968) defines the adjective "fiduciary" as "relating to or founded upon a trust" (p. 753). Fiduciary relations exist between lawyers and clients, guardians and wards, and doctors and patients, to name but a few. According to Black (1968), the fiduciary relation "need not be legal, but may be moral, social, domestic, or merely personal. *Miranovitz v. Gee*, 163 Wis. 246; 157 N.W. 790, 792; *Higgins v. Chicago Title & Trust Co.*, 312 Ill. 11; 143 N.E. 482, 484" (p. 754). As a fiduciary to his client, a psychotherapist is "a person having duty, created by his undertaking, to act primarily for another's benefit in matters connected with such undertaking. *Haluka v. Baker*, 66 Ohio App. 308; 34 N.E.2d 68,70" (p. 753). Because of the nature of this special relationship of trust and confidence, any apparently self-serving acts may be viewed as a breach of fiduciary duty.

Standard of care.   Clients or patients have a right to expect that the services rendered by the professionals they hire will be at least as competently and skillfully performed as those rendered by the ordinary practitioner. As stated by Chief Justice Tindal in the 1832 case of *Lanphier v. Phipus*, a "reasonable degree of care" does not mean an extraordinary degree of care but only a reasonable degree:

> Every person who enters into a learned profession undertakes to bring to it the exercise of a reasonable degree of care and skill; he does not undertake if he is an attorney that at all events you shall gain your case, nor does a surgeon undertake that he will perform a cure, nor does he undertake to use the highest possible skill. There may be persons who have a higher education and greater advantages and competent degree of

TABLE 4.
Breakdown of Intentional and Unintentional Torts*

INTENTIONAL	UNINTENTIONAL (NEGLIGENCE)
Torts to Person	Negligence Based on Duty of Due Care
•Battery	•Breach of duty of due care (malpractice)
•Assault	including special affirmative duties to
•False Imprisonment	prevent harm
Torts to Property	
•Trespass to land	•Duty to prevent suicide
•Trespass to chattels	•Duty to prevent assault to third parties
•Conversion of chattels	
Other	Other
•Intentional or fraudulent	•Negligent misrepresentation
misrepresentation (deceit)	•Negligent causing of emotional distress
•Intentional causing of emotional distress	•Negligent invasion of privacy
•Intentional invasion of privacy	
•Malicious prosecution	
•Abuse of the process of law	

*This listing of torts is not, nor is it meant to be, all-inclusive.

skill, and you will not say whether in this case the injury was occasioned by the want of such skill in the defendant. The question is, whether this injury must be referred to the want of a proper degree of skill and care in the defendant or not.

Malpractice actions always allege that the defendant's conduct fell below some generally accepted or profession-prescribed standard of care.[6] Proving that a defendant's conduct fell below this acceptable level would entail showing that the professional did not possess the same knowledge of the field or did not exercise the same degree of skill as would be expected from a reasonable and prudent professional in his specialty area. Whether or not the standard of care has been met is a matter of fact that the trier of fact (the judge or the jury) must decide on the basis of the evidence (e.g., expert testimony, records, documents) adduced at the trial.

But what constitutes "reasonable professional care"? Defining the precise standard against which the conduct of health professionals should be measured has by no means been a routine matter. In fact, this question could well be the subject of a volume in itself. Should national or local professional organizations define the standard? Should judges and juries (instead of professional organizations) decide the standard, solely on the basis of expert testimony (or even without such testimony)? May a court deem certain practices, even if "accepted" in the profession, to be negligent? Which standard should prevail when there are alternative methods of treatment that could have been used and have been used by a "respectable minority" of practitioners? Must the courts determine professional liability by a plebiscite of the professional community? Should that which is considered to be "customary practice" define the standard of care, or should the standard be what constitutes "accepted" practice? The answers to these and related questions have varied from jurisdiction to jurisdiction.

To focus on just one of the problems attendant to defining a standard of care, consider the "locality rule," which was once in effect in a day when what constituted customary and/or accepted medical practice varied widely from one geographical area to the next. In the past, rural doctors did not have the same training and opportunities for continuing education as doctors in urban medical centers and teaching hospitals. Also, doctors in rural areas may have routinely seen different types of medical problems than city doctors. In those days, courts held doctors to the standard

---

[6]However, as we will see in our discussion of *Helling v. Carey* in Chapter 7, at least one court has assigned liability to a doctor who followed the accepted and customary practice of his profession. Here the court, in essence, deemed the standard of the profession to be too low.

of care of medicine practiced in their local community.[7] However, the rationale of the locality rule has been somewhat weakened by two factors. One is the widespread availability of opportunities for continuing education in the form of journals, professional meetings, etc. The other is the widespread availability of medicines and "miracle drugs," which has had the effect of "equalizing" the kinds of treatments (and diseases) found from locality to locality.

Evidence that modern-day courts are continuing to struggle with the validity of the locality rule comes in the form of decisions—and reversals of decisions—by the highest courts in some states. For example, a sharply divided supreme court of Arkansas in 1975 wrote that contemporary communication avenues had obviated the need for a locality rule in Arkansas. Yet in 1976 that court reversed itself and stated that the locality rule should be applied to determine the applicable standard of care. The court wrote as follows:

> We are not convinced that we have reached the time when the same postgraduate medical education, research, and experience is equally available to all physicians, regardless of the community in which they practice. The opportunities for doctors in small towns, of which we have many, to leave a demanding practice to attend seminars and regional medical meetings cannot be the same as those for doctors practicing in clinics in larger centers. It goes without saying that the physicians in these small towns do not and cannot have the clinical and hospital facilities available in the larger cities where there are large, modern hospitals, and medical centers or the same advantage of observing others who have been trained, or have developed expertise, in the use of new skills, facilities and procedures, of consulting and exchanging views with specialists, other practitioners and drug experts, of utilizing closed circuit television, special radio networks or of studying in extensive medical libraries found in larger centers.

Extended discussions of the various problems attendant to defining a standard of care have appeared elsewhere. (See, for example, King, 1977.) Some of the issues involved, as they specifically relate to mental health professionals, will be briefly discussed in Chapter 7. Suffice it to say here that establishing what should be regarded as an "acceptable level of professional conduct" has been and continues to be a complex problem in law.

Damages. *Black's Law Dictionary* (1968) defines *damage*, in the singular form, as "loss, injury, or deterioration, caused by the negligence,

---

[7]This was particularly true for the general practitioner. In fact, the issue involved has sometimes been referred to as the specialty versus locality rule. Courts tended to hold specialists to national standards and general practitioners to local standards.

design, or accident of one person to another, in respect of the latter's person or property'' (p. 466). In the plural form, *damages* may be considered to be synonymous with "compensation in money for a loss." Persons bringing lawsuits typically specify in their suits the amount of damages they are suing for; that is, they specify the dollar amount (or in rare instances, the specific performance of services) which would make them feel fully compensated for the loss they sustained. Sometimes that dollar amount is simply a matter of arithmetic and sometimes it is most difficult to determine. As an example of the former, suppose Jones contracts to sell Smith 5,000 "mood" rings at $1.00 each, payable when the rings are delivered. Jones subsequently defaults on the contract, stating that he cannot ship the rings because his wife, the shipping clerk, has been in a "bad mood" all week. Smith sues Jones for breach of contract and in the interim buys 5,000 mood rings from White at $1.50 each. When the case of *Smith v. Jones* is heard, the amount of damages claimed by Smith will be at least equal to the dollar amount paid to White ($7,500) minus the price contracted for by Jones ($5,000), or $2,500. Conceivably Jones's breach of contract may have caused Smith even greater financial losses (e.g., the loss of Christmas sales), and that dollar amount (depending on the certainty of the unrealized gains) could be added to the claim.

Up to a point, simple arithmetic can also be used to calculate the dollar amounts to be sued for in medical malpractice cases. For example, suppose that a neurosurgeon's negligence caused a fifty-seven-year-old diamond cutter to lose the use of his thumb. The diamond cutter earned $100,000 annually, and he could have potentially kept on earning that much for the next five years. The malpractice suit against the neurosurgeon would then claim $500,000 in damages. But this dollar amount would only compensate the diamond cutter for his loss of income as a result of the doctor's negligence. What about compensation for the pain and suffering? What about compensation for the emotional distress attendant to losing one's means of earning a livelihood? It can be seen that the question "What price pain and suffering?" is not a question of simple arithmetic. Claims for emotional distress, pain, suffering and the like are part and parcel of medical malpractice litigation, and the dollar amounts asked for in damages—and awarded by juries—are very much matters of subjective judgment.

The damages we have referred to above are technically called *compensatory* damages, since they seek to compensate injured parties for losses suffered. However, litigants may also sue for what are called *punitive* damages. Punitive damages are designed to punish the wrongdoer for the wantonness, recklessness, or heinousness of the acts committed. If the diamond cutter in the above example could prove that the neurosurgeon acted with malice toward him or that he was drunk, reckless, or otherwise irresponsible in the operating room, the court might very well award punitive damages in addition to compensatory damages. (We should note here that many insurers of health service providers specify in their policies that they will pay only compensatory, not punitive damages, and that some states have declared it a violation of public policy for insurers to pay the punitive portion of the damages assessed against the holders of their liability policies.)

MALPRACTICE LITIGATION

In malpractice litigation, as in all civil litigation, the burden of proof is on the plaintiff. It is he who must prove, by the preponderance of the evidence, that the defendant was, in fact, negligent.[8] It is the quality and "weight" of the evidence presented by both sides (i.e., its amount, relevance, credibility, and persuasiveness) that will either establish the plaintiff's case or maintain the defendant's freedom from liability. In legal jargon, one speaks of the "elements of proof" needed to prove that a tort (or a crime) was committed. Basic elements needed to show malpractice or negligence include:

1. action or inaction on the part of the defendant;
2. the existence of a duty of due care;
3. the breaching of a duty of due care;
4. causation in the factual sense;
5. causation in the legal sense; and
6. damages sustained as a result of the defendant's action or inaction.[9]

For example, suppose a psychologist uses the word "moron" to describe a patient in his psychological report, and a malpractice suit results. In order to prove that the psychologist was negligent, it would have to be proved by the preponderance of the evidence that

1. the psychologist did in fact see the patient in question and write the report, using the word "moron" to describe the patient;
2. a duty of due care existed between the psychologist and the plaintiff;
3. the psychologist breached his duty of due care;

---

[8]This is true except for a few rare cases which have been decided on the basis of a doctrine that the negligent act need not be proven; it is sufficient to demonstrate that but for the negligent act, the plaintiff could not have been injured.

[9]The tort of negligence could be reflected by listing only four elements: duty, breach of duty, legal cause, and harm. "Action or inaction" would thereby be collapsed into "breach of duty" and "causation in the factual sense" would be collapsed into "causation in the legal sense" (there can't be legal causation without factual causation). Six elements of the tort are listed here for the benefit of the audience this book is intended for and for the purposes of illustration. The authority on this subject—as well as on most other matters concerning the law of torts—is Prosser (1971).

4. the psychologist was the proximate cause (or "legal cause") of the plaintiff's injuries;[10]

5. the psychologist was the actual cause (or "cause in fact") of the plaintiff's injuries; and

6. the plaintiff suffered damages as a result of the psychologist's action or inaction.

Not infrequently, lawsuits are brought claiming damages as a result of the commission of a number of torts. Conceivably, a plaintiff bringing suit against a psychologist on the grounds of negligence for writing the word "moron" in his psychological report might also claim damages as a result of other torts, such as defamation or invasion of privacy. Again, for the plaintiff to prevail on any of these claims various elements would have to be proven by the preponderance of the evidence. In order to prove defamation, for example, it would have to be proven that

1. the psychologist published his report to a third party;

2. the published matter could be construed as having a defamatory meaning;

3. the published matter was understood as being a reference to the plaintiff;

4. the third party understood the published matter to be defamatory to the plaintiff;

5. the psychologist was the actual cause of the plaintiff's injury;

6. the psychologist was the proximate cause of the plaintiff's injury; and

7. the plaintiff suffered damages as a result of the publication of the report.

Additional elements are needed to prove each of the above elements with respect to each of the two torts cited above. However, listing and analysis of these "elements of the elements" will not be necessary for our purposes.

The Claim Stage

An attempt to collect for alleged malpractice formally begins with the professional's being served with a complaint filed in a local court or a

---

[10]"Proximate cause" or "legal cause" is a relatively complicated legal concept that takes into account the standard of care, the foreseeability of the outcome, the effects of intervening variables, and other factors. It has been defined as "that cause which as a natural and continuous sequence, unbroken by any intervening cause, produces the injury without which it would not have occurred" (*Reder v. Hanson*, 338 F.2d 244). For our purpose, "an action that proximately causes something" shall be equivalent to "a 'substantial factor' in bringing about that outcome." Interested readers are referred to the famous case, *Palsgraf v. Long Island Railroad Company*, 162 N.E. 99, for an expanded discussion of the concept of proximate cause.

letter from the plaintiff's attorney advising him that a suit charging him with negligence has been lodged.[11] The professional will then typically call his insurance company and be told by its representatives to send a copy of the lawyer's letter or complaint and await further instructions. Shortly, the professional will receive insurance company forms inquiring into all conceivable elements of the professional and personal relationship that may have led up to the claim. The diagnosis made and/or treatment provided (with dates), copies of psychological reports, explanations for lapses in treatment, the names of consultants called in to see the patient, copies of written communications to and about the patient—all will be helpful in formulating the professional's defense. Additionally, the professional may be asked to submit a copy of his curriculum vitae and to prepare a statement about his special expertise in the particular area in question. If, for example, the suit involved the misdiagnosis of organic brain damage the investigators would want the facts relating to the professional's formal training and clinical experience in that area. Personal meetings with insurance company representatives and/or lawyers will be required in preparation for a defense.

Under modern "discovery" rules which seek to do away with the old-fashioned "sporting theory of justice" (in which each side springs surprises on the other during the trial), the attorneys for both the plaintiff and the defendant are legally obliged to keep each other abreast of certain information relating to the case so that the two sides can adequately prepare for the trial or enter into an out-of-court settlement. In one malpractice suit against a physician, a plaintiff wished to withold the name of his expert witness for fear that this witness would refuse to testify. The court ruled that the plaintiff was obliged to reveal the name of the witness so that the defense could adequately prepare for the trial (*Klabunde v. Stanley*, 168 N.W.2d 450 [Michigan, 1970]). In many jurisdictions one party may submit to the other written questions called "interrogatories," which are to be answered under oath.

Witnesses may also be asked or subpoenaed to give depositions under oath in the presence of both sides' attorneys and subject to their questions. A legal stenographer will usually record such proceedings verbatim, and the transcript can be adduced as evidence at the trial under certain circumstances. These pretrial "discovery" proceedings do not preclude the possibility of an out-of-court settlement between the parties.

During the pretrial stage a judge may dismiss an action in response to various kinds of motions to dismiss (e.g., lack of capacity to sue or to be sued, failure to state a proper cause of action, or absence of proper procedural or subject-matter jurisdiction). A judge may also issue what is called a *summary judgment* of a case if there is no dispute between the

---

[11]In many instances an attorney may try to get a settlement before filing suit.

parties over any of the material facts, and the decision can be rendered as a matter of law. The judge might also rule that the litigation had not been initiated within the time limit prescribed by the local statute of limitations. A legal action can also end at the pretrial stage if the plaintiff—for whatever reason—withdraws his complaint. Negotiated settlements can be made at any time during the pretrial *or* trial proceedings, right up until the time the court rules on the case.

Most malpractice actions are settled out of court, at the claim stage. The primary obstacle to carrying each case through to trial is the prohibitive cost of such proceedings. The trial lawyers' time in preparing and trying the case, the expert witnesses' time in preparing and giving testimony, and court costs are only some of the initial financial considerations. Insurance companies are aware that plaintiffs will usually settle for substantially less than the amount they are claiming in damages when offered a quick out-of-court settlement. The professional who feels that the charges lodged against him are unjust and that the case should be tried so as to "clear the record" is likely to be discouraged by his insurance company's guiding principle of expediency. Insurance companies sometimes give messages to their defendants such as "settle or go it alone" or "settle or your policy won't be renewed." For example, from the standpoint of the insurance company it is better to settle a claim for $5,000 than to see it through litigation at an estimated cost of $25,000. In some states it is mandatory that the lawyers for the opposing interests meet before the trial judge to discuss the evidence they intend to present at the trial. Such a meeting is designed to explore the possibility of—if not encourage—an out-of-court settlement. Out-of-court settlements do not, in their wording, impute guilt to any party. The settlement merely constitutes an agreement between the plaintiff and the defendant that the suit is being dropped for some unspecified reason. Once all attempts to settle out of court have failed, however, the case reaches the trial stage.

The Trial Stage

Jury selection.   Whereas criminal cases must be tried by a jury, civil cases can be tried either by a jury or by a judge. Without going into great detail on this relatively complicated matter, all parties to civil litigation in federal courts are guaranteed the right to a trial by jury. As for civil cases tried in state courts, all state constitutions have provisions that provide for and/or guarantee the right to a trial by jury under certain conditions (e.g., that the case is a legal case, not an equity case). Generally, in malpractice litigation, jury trials are preferred by attorneys for the plaintiff, the guiding philosophy being that members of the public are more apt to identify and sympathize with the "harmed" patient than with the rich, powerful professional. Juries are selected in different ways in different states, but generally prospective jurors are chosen from county tax assessment rolls or voter registration lists. Most health professionals (as well as others, such as policemen and ministers) can and do obtain exemption from jury duty on the grounds that they are performing an important public service.

From the pool of prospective jurors (sometimes referred to as "veniremen") the attorneys try to select persons who will be sympathetic to (or at least not prejudiced against) their case. In the preliminary examination to determine the competency of prospective jurors (called "voir dire"), lawyers for the opposing interests are usually allowed to reject a certain number of veniremen. When the jury of twelve (and in some jurisdictions fewer than twelve) persons is finally selected, it is given the role of the "trier of fact" in the court proceeding to come. That is, although the judge will decide all questions of law, the jury will decide questions of fact.

Opening statements. The trial begins with attorneys for the plaintiff and the defense making opening statements which present the facts as they see them. They point out what they will attempt to prove as well as how they will attempt to prove it. In malpractice actions (as well as in other lawsuits alleging the tort of negligence), it is incumbent upon the patient/plaintiff to prove by the preponderance of the evidence that a duty to conform to a particular standard of conduct existed, that the professional's conduct lacked the reasonable care and diligence that could be expected under the circumstances, and that some injury resulted from the professional's act of omission or commission. The professional's conduct must be shown to be the direct or "proximate" cause of the injury; that is, it must be shown that had such conduct not taken place the injury would not have occurred. Contrariwise, the attorney for the defendant can be expected to argue that the treatment offered conformed to accepted practice as regards the patient's condition in light of the body of professional knowledge available at the time the treatment was administered, or that the plaintiff had not been damaged, or that the damage resulted from some cause other than the defendant's malpractice.

Because of the nature of mental illness and its treatment, proving that a mental health professional's action was causally related to mental "injury" is no easy matter:

> Besides proving that the psychiatrist has breached the requisite standard of care in some specific detail, the plaintiff must also demonstrate causation and damage. Because the natural pathological development and prognosis of mental disease is not well known, it is frequently difficult to state to a reasonable degree of medical certainty whether the

application or omission of a particular procedure at a specified time caused mental injury to the patient. Thus, it is often difficult for the plaintiff to prove the element of causation. The task is simplified, however, if the alleged negligence in some manner caused or encouraged the patient to sustain or inflict tangible physical injuries upon himself or others. Indeed, this characteristic is typical of almost every successful suit. In this situation, proof of the injuries in addition to proof that ordinary and prudent therapeutic techniques would have prevented the damage may sustain the burden of proof.

The plaintiff who complains of exclusively mental injuries may also have a difficult time proving the element of damages. Not only are his allegations intangible and difficult to demonstrate to the judge and jury, but they also tend to be somewhat speculative because of the state of knowledge about mental illness. Even where improper procedures have been used to institutionalize a person in need of mental care, the courts may absolve physicians from liability by finding that the patient was not injured by receiving the treatment he needed. (Rothblatt and Leroy, 1973, p. 264)

Direct examination and cross-examination. After introductory statements, the plaintiff's attorney calls witnesses whose testimony is known to be favorable to his case. The questioning of witnesses sympathetic to the plaintiff's case by the plaintiff's attorney is called *direct examination*. In most instances, direct examination entails a series of well-rehearsed questions concerning the witnesses' background, special credentials, expertise, and general knowledge of the case. Immediately after direct examination of a witness, *cross-examination* by the opposing attorney begins. During cross-examination, the attorney attempts to call into question the witnesses' credibility, expertise, understanding, recollection, biases, etc. Cross-examination may sometimes entail the attorney's reading from medical textbooks and asking witnesses if they agree or disagree with what is written. In some jurisdictions, the witness must first state that he agrees with the author, accepts the author as an authority, etc. However, in many jurisdictions such agreement is not necessary. The rationale for the latter policy is expressed in the wording of one Missouri court's decision:

Under Missouri law it is proper to cross examine a medical expert by framing a proposition in the exact language of the author and asking the witness whether he agrees to it. Before propounding such a question it is not necessary to ascertain whether the witness agrees with the author. Textbooks on technical subjects may be used in cross examination of an expert witness by reading therefrom and inquiring whether the witness agrees.

We reject the proposition that the expert witness being cross examined must first agree that the text is standard or authoritative. The practical effect of such cross examination would be to give the witness complete control of the cross examination. He need only say that he is not acquainted with the book or its author to prevent its use in testing his qualifications, no matter how eminent or accepted the author may be. The fewer books and authorities the witness knows about or will acknowledge, and the less knowledge he has of what has been written in the field, the more difficult it will be to cross examine him along this line. It gives him full veto power over the cross examiner's efforts.

As we say, it is not necessary that the witness concede that the text is standard or authoritative, although if the witness does so this is sufficient foundation to use the book in cross examination. The party desiring to use the books can also establish their standing by proper voir dire examination of his own expert outside the hearing of the jury, thereby laying the foundation for their use in cross examination at the proper time. There are many standard texts used by practitioners to keep abreast of proper and modern techniques in diagnosis and treatment. We need not fear that such texts are untrustworthy. Such books are not written from a bias in favor of a lawsuit or an individual or by one who is paid a fee to testify; they are written primarily for the writer's profession and his reputation depends on the correctness of his data and validity of his conclusions, all of which he realizes will be subject to careful professional analysis. (*Gridley v. Johnson*, 476 S.W.2d 475 [Missouri, 1972])

As needed, *redirect examination* and *recross examination*, designed to elicit the best possible understanding of the testimony (in a light most favorable to the examining attorney), follows. "Perry Mason" aficionados will know that throughout the proceedings each lawyer has the right to raise legal objections to the manner in which his adversary is acting and to the acceptability of the material that is being introduced as evidence. As the arbiter of questions of law, the judge will either sustain or overrule objections as they are raised. After all of the plaintiff's evidence has been presented, the plaintiff is said "to 'rest'."

After the plaintiff rests.   After the plaintiff has rested, the defense attorney will perfunctorily make a motion to dismiss the claim against his client on the grounds that the plaintiff has failed to make a *prima facie* case. A prima facie case is one that by its nature would allow any reasonable jury to find in favor of the plaintiff if it did not hear any opposing testimony. In essence, the defense is asking the judge to decide whether the preponderance of the evidence adduced up to that point would be enough to find the defendant liable even if no defense were presented. If the judge agrees that a prima facie case has not been established (a relatively rare occurrence, given all the pretrial negotiations that have attempted to stave off a costly court procedure), this means, in essence, that the plaintiff's case has little merit and that he probably has no chance of recovering the damages claimed.[12] After hearing all of the evidence, the trial judge may "direct a verdict" in favor of one of the parties. This relatively rare occurrence takes place when the judge concludes that no reasonable jury could find otherwise than in favor of that party.

If the judge rules that a prima facie case has been established, the defense may either rest and hope to win a more favorable judgment in a higher court or it may proceed with the trial. If the latter course is taken, witnesses for the defendant will be called, to be directly examined by the defendant's attorney and cross-examined by the plaintiff's attorney. Just before closing arguments, the defense attorney may again call for dismissal on the grounds that the preponderance of the evidence does not point to the defendant's liability. The judge may be asked by either the plaintiff or the defendant to direct a verdict or to rule on a question of law.

If the case is to go to the jury, the judge will then give a "charge" to the jury. That is, he will explain what the laws involved are, what the "facts" (in the legal sense) are, which testimony should be ignored, and how to compute the dollar amount of the settlement if the defendant is found to be liable.

The verdict and the appeal.   In most jurisdictions, a jury verdict must be unanimously arrived at, though a simple majority has been deemed acceptable in some jurisdictions. If the jury cannot reach the required number of agreeing votes to constitute a verdict it is called a "hung jury": a mistrial is declared and the case must be retried. If a jury does reach a verdict, the attorney for the losing side may immediately lodge various motions to the trial judge seeking a new trial or a modification or reversal of the verdict. If the judge feels that the jury's findings are contrary to the evidence presented or that the award is too little or too much, he may order a new trial or in some way modify the jury's findings.

At the conclusion of the trial, either side may appeal the final outcome to a higher court, though most appellate courts will only review cases in which there is some question concerning a matter of law, not a matter of fact. Grounds for appeal may include the particulars of the judge's charge to the jury or the admissibility of some evidence. For example, the testimony of one inpatient of a New York State mental hospital who sued the state for unlawful confinement in a camisole was ruled inadmissible on appeal:

> In our opinion the trial court should not have accepted the patient's version of the duration and condition of her confinements. Such ac-

---

[12]Technically, the failure to make out a prima facie case—leading to dismissal—occurs only if the jury cannot reasonably find in the plaintiff's favor. However, if the evidence is so strong as to compel a jury to find for the plaintiff, absent other evidence, then the plaintiff has not only "gotten to the jury" but shifted the burden of going forward with evidence to the defendant who, if he stands silent, will lose.

counts are not supported by the hospital records and, in fact, are in many instances contrary to those records. Moreover, the reliability of the patient's testimony is made extremely suspect by her history of fabrications and exaggeration, whether it be due to a mental illness or be deliberate, and also she is a litigious individual. Accordingly, we can find no support in the instant record for the trial court's conclusion that different restraining devices such as tranquilizers or antidepressants should have been utilized and that physical restraints were improperly utilized. Therefore, the judgment must be reversed and the claim dismissed. (*Morgan v. State*, 337 N.Y.2d 536 [New York, 1972])

A professional who feels that a malpractice suit brought against him has no merit has the option of taking a number of actions, on the advice of legal counsel. Some of these alternative courses of action will be described in Chapter 8.

ETHICS AND THE MENTAL HEALTH PROFESSIONAL

Discussion of important and far-reaching legal concepts must necessarily be accompanied by discussions of ethics; the areas overlap to such a degree that any attempt to segregate them would be hopeless. A constitutional lawyer arguing that capital punishment is "cruel or unusual punishment" may make dispassionate references to legal precedents and adduce "hard" evidence (e.g., statistical data on recidivism, or the number of homicides committed with and without the death penalty in effect) to support his view, but it is unlikely that this lawyer will win his case if the prevailing societal notion is of the moral "rightness" of capital punishment and the justness of the "eye for an eye" axiom. Furthermore, any appeal to the inherent evil in the taking of a human life will run up against such problematic ethical issues as abortion or euthanasia.

Advances in the technology of extrauterine (so-called "test-tube") conception, increasing sophistication in ways of prolonging life through artificial means (e.g., respirators), and progress in other areas of medical science are all sure to be accompanied by legal prescriptions and proscriptions regarding what shall be considered "right," "proper," and "moral" use of the new technology. As questions of death and dying continue to figure prominently in the literature of medical and lay ethics (cf. Cohen, 1976b, 1976c), it is reasonable to expect that parallel questioning will be taking place in lawmaking bodies as well. When should a respirator be turned off, and who should make that decision? What is the definition of "death"? What is the definition of "life"? Are these medical questions, ethical questions, or legal questions? The answer is that they are all three.

A body of law consists of rules governing all persons' conduct for the supposed benefit of society as a whole. A body of ethics consists of principles of "right," "proper," or "good" conduct. Owing to the subjectivity inherent in developing legal and ethical principles, what should and should not be law and what should and should not be considered ethical are very often matters of controversy.

A rapidly growing number of legal/ethical issues face mental health professionals today (cf. Bersoff, 1975; Foster, 1975; Jurow and Mariano, 1972; Roston, 1975; Shah, 1969, 1970a, 1970b; Slovenko, 1973). Consider the following situation:

> *You are relaxing at home watching the evening news on television. A story comes on about a series of gruesome, "Son of Sam"-type murders. An official appeal from the local Police Department is read by the announcer: "Would any psychologist, psychiatrist, or other mental health professional in the area who might have any knowledge concerning the identity of this murderer please contact us before more innocent victims are murdered." New clues about the murderer's identity are revealed in the broadcast, and suddenly you swallow deeply and nearly spill your beer as you feel for the end table. You strongly suspect that the murderer is or has been a patient of yours. What do you do? Do you call the patient or the police? At what point—if any—is loyalty to the patient sacrificed in the interest of society at large?*

Just as high government officials may be faced with dilemmas of divided loyalties (cf. Cohen, 1973), so may mental health professionals be thrust into situations in which the rights of the individual and of society both deserve protection but it is "difficult to serve the best interests of both" (Wiskoff, 1960, p. 656). In Chapter 3 this most difficult question of the limits of patient–therapist confidentiality is broached, along with related contemporary legal/ethical questions, such as "When is a patient's 'informed consent' really 'informed'?" Chapter 3 concludes with a discussion of ethical/legal issues in psychodiagnosis and psychological research. In Chapter 4 the frequently discussed and important issue of control is examined.

3
Current Issues in Ethics

Recently, when I submitted an application to rent an apartment in New York City, the rental agent ran an ordinary credit check. He found my credit in good order and I got the apartment. Subsequently, when I applied for a New York bank's credit card, I was turned down with a letter that stated that the refusal was based on data obtained from a company called T.R.W. Many phone calls and letters later, I obtained from T.R.W. a credit record that they were keeping on me. The credit record had an entry on it which was listed as an "inquiry" from a company I had never heard of. Although T.R.W. never did identify who the company was, I was able to find out that the company was affiliated with the rental agent. In other words, the bank had denied me a credit card on the basis of information from T.R.W. when the only information T.R.W. had was that a rental agent had made an inquiry about my credit. Many weeks later—no thanks to T.R.W.—I finally did get my credit card.

A person's credit rating, the amount of money he has in the bank, and related financial matters are very personal bits of information which most people would like to keep private. Recognizing the extent to which such information is safeguarded from others, some psychologists have quipped that if Freud were alive today he would be writing about money rather than sex. Capitalizing on most persons' need to keep such information private and on other persons' needs to have access to that information, private corporations have been quick to enter the "information business" and to build it into a multimillion-dollar-a-year operation. As information technology progresses and more and more information is stored on more and more people, the already knotty questions concerning what information should be released to whom and under what conditions will become all the more complex. When private corporations are involved in the storage and distribution of such sensitive material, citizens can only hope and trust that governmental regulations and corporate ethics will supercede the corporate temptation to sell whatever is available to the highest bidder. But what about the government itself? And what about individual mental health professionals—our primary point of focus. What of the information *they* collect and store?

The federal government has acknowledged that it maintains over 6,700 computer data banks that store information on millions of persons. Quite understandably, there is a great need for such governmental record keeping. The problem is that existing policies and regulations that attempt to balance the legitimate, lawful, and ethical need for access to such records against the potential misuse of the information they contain are woefully inadequate. The problem with respect to the government's handling of health records, for example, has been well documented in a 1977 federal report issued by the National Bureau of Standards. The report disclosed that the lack of uniformity in states' regulations governing the confidentiality of health records has led to generally careless practices in disseminating such material. In one case vignette cited in the report, a psychiatrist noted on one patient's group health insurance form that the patient was schizophrenic and that she had attempted suicide. The psychiatrist's report went from the insurance company back to the personnel office of the patient's company. On coming into work one day, the patient learned from a fellow employee that her psychiatrist had diagnosed her as schizophrenic. (The psychiatrist had not told this to the patient, owing to the delicacy of her condition.) The woman also found that many people at work knew of her previous suicide attempt.

How typical or atypical such stories are is a matter of conjecture. It is a fact, however, that with third-party payments for medical expenses comes third-party knowledge of (previously confidential) doctor–patient communications (cf. Grossman, 1971), including information pertinent to diagnosis, prognosis, history, and all aspects of treatment. The psychiatrist in the above vignette was certainly not at fault, as he only filled out an insurance form that provided for reimbursement of his fee to his patient. Clearly, psychiatrists and other mental health professionals cannot be held liable for the misdeeds of third-party agents who misuse the information with which they are entrusted. But what about the misuse of confidential information by mental health professionals themselves. What constitutes a misuse? Is revelation of confidential material ever justified? These are some of the questions we will touch on in our discussion of privacy, privilege, confidentiality, and the duty to warn.

PRIVACY, PRIVILEGE, CONFIDENTIALITY, AND THE DUTY TO WARN

In the inaugural issue of *Professional Psychology* Saleem Shah (1969) began a three-part article designed to clarify the definition and usage of the terms privacy, privileged communication, and confidentiality. Shah struggled with the definition of privacy calling it "a complex and still evolving concept which has yet to be fully developed in regard to its precise legal boundaries." After Ruebhausen and Brim (1965) Shah wrote that "the concept of privacy recognizes the freedom of the individual to pick and choose for himself the time, circumstances, and particularly the extent to which he wishes to share with or withhold from others his attitudes, beliefs, behavior, and opinions" (p. 57). Shedding additional light on the definitional problem is the observation that "privacy" is a multidimensional concept:

> "Privacy" is an evolving concept; there is not and may never be an agreed upon definition applicable to all situations. "Privacy" has many dimensions: an anthropological one, a psychological one, a social one, a political one, a legal dimension. "Privacy" can be referred to in spheres or zones: medical privacy, marital privacy, administrative privacy, financial privacy, among others. (Knerr, Note 5)

Courts have ruled that a person has a right to privacy; a right to be "let alone" (see for example *Gallela v. Onassis*, 353 F. Supp. 196). An individual has a constitutional right to privacy when it comes to information that may be self-incriminating; by "taking the 5th" (i.e. by asserting the right to avoid self-incrimination as provided in the fifth amendment of the Constitution) an individual can legally refuse to answer certain questions put to him in a legal proceeding. The withheld information is said to be *privileged* information. As a matter of public policy (not constitutional right) state statutes have provided for a kind of extension of the individual's right to keep certain information private; the right to have kept private communications made to someone with whom the communicater shares a special relationship (e.g., an attorney–client relationship). Statutes provide that attorney–client communication is *privileged communication;* when a lawyer and client meet the information the client gives to the lawyer is privileged information. In court, the lawyer may only disclose privileged information at the request of his client (in fact, under ordinary circumstances, the lawyer *must* disclose privileged information at the request of his client as the privilege belongs to the client not the lawyer). The law provides for privileged communication between an attorney and client in order to allow a client to tell his lawyer everything without fear of reprisal. Safeguarding an individual's right to privacy with respect to consultations with his attorney is thought to serve a greater public interest than insistence that courts have access to *all* information relevant to a particular case.

The right of privileged communication enjoyed by persons in an attorney–client relationship has been extended in most jurisdictions to individuals in numerous other relationships that are comparably "intimate." Thus, husbands and wives may be legally viewed as "extensions" of one another and their communications have been held to be privileged. Also privileged are communications between priest and penitent, doctor and patient, and psychologist and client (as illustrated by the excerpt below from Section 7611, Article 153 of the New York State Education Law):

> The confidential relations and communications between a psychologist registered under provisions of this Act and his client are placed on the same basis as those provided by law between attorney and client, and nothing in this article shall be construed to require any such privileged communication to be disclosed.

Persons consulting professionals expect that the information they impart will not be disclosed improperly—in the courtroom or elsewhere. Patients expect that their doctors will not discuss medical histories over cocktails or peruse personality profiles in crowded buses or trains. This lay expectation of a professional obligation to maintain confidentially resulted primarily from assurances physicians have made to the public via medical codes of ethics. Other professional organizations (e.g., the American Psychological Association) have promulgated their own codes of ethics which similarly provide for professional–client confidentiality as a standard of conduct. It is true as Shah (1969; 1970a) has noted, that "confidentiality relates to matters of professional ethics" though it is also true that "[c]ase law, statutes, and licensing regulations in many states have given this standard of conduct legal status as well. For example, a practitioner is civilly liable for breach of confidentiality" (Swoboda, Elwork, Sales, and Levine, 1978, p. 449; see also *Horne v. Patton*, 287 So.2d 824). Attempting to distinguish "confidentiality" from "privileged communication," Jagim, Wittman and Noll (1978) pointed out that, "[w]hereas confidentiality concerns matters of communication outside the courtroom, privilege protects clients from disclosure in judicial proceedings" (p. 459).

Many mental health professionals confuse the concepts of privileged communication and confidentiality (cf. Swoboda et al., 1978; Jagim et al., 1978) and this confusion is understandable. "Privileged communication" is frequently used interchangeably with "confidential communication" as all privileged communications are confidential (though all confidential communications are not necessarily privileged). Similarly, unauthorized disclosure of privileged information entails a breach of confidentiality though a breach of confidentiality need not necessarily entail disclosure of privileged information. Both privilege and confidentiality may be waived by a competent client. Further, ethical codes provide for the breach of confidentiality under extraordinary circumstances just as the law provides numerous exceptions to rules against disclosure. There is probably a sizable number of mental health professionals who—whatever the legality of so doing—would disclose confidential information only under the most extreme conditions (and even then very reluctantly).Some have argued that a disclosure of confidential doctor-patient communications that has not been authorized by the patient cannot be justified under *any* circumstances. Such an extreme position is in clear violation of the law which holds that privilege is not absolute—that there do exist situations in which the unauthorized disclosure of confidential information is permissable, even mandated. The issues are complex and multifaceted (cf. Curran, 1975; Dubey, 1974; Hollender, 1965; Plaut, 1974; Siegal, 1976; Slawson, 1969; Stern, 1959).

In the course of enumerating exceptions to the rule of privilege, Shah (1969) foreshadowed the dilemma of a legal "duty to warn"; a dilemma now faced by California mental health professionals as a result of the California Supreme Court's decision in *Tarasoff v. Regents of University of California:*

> Since most of the psychologist-client statutes follow the attorney-client model, it is very important to remember that in the latter relationships the privilege does *not* extend to situations in which the legal advice or service sought is in reference to either the client's plans or intentions to commit a crime or fraud. This is sometimes referred to as the "future crime or fraud" exception.
>
> It can readily be seen that were the above exception to apply to the psychologist–client relationship, it would pose very serious problems for psychotherapists. Unlike discussions between attorney and client, communications between an individual and his psychotherapist may often involve disclosures by the client of his thoughts or urges to commit certain criminal acts. Yet, one of the very goals of the therapeutic relationship is to elicit such urges and then to distinguish among ruminative fantasies, more imminent urges, and specific plans to commit anti-social acts. Once such material has been elicited, it may then be handled therapeutically to avoid harm either to the client or to others. (Shah, 1969, pp. 64–65)

In the landmark case of *Tarasoff* (Case 5.24 in Chapter 5) the decision of the California Supreme Court "created a situation in which acceptance of a patient into therapy imposes on the therapist the duty to care for both the patient and any potential victims of the patient's dangerous actions" (Gurevitz, 1977, p. 290). The facts of the *Tarasoff* case were as follows:

> *Prosenjit Poddar, a voluntary outpatient of a university hospital, told his therapist, a psychologist, that he intended to kill an unnamed (but readily identifiable) young woman after she returned from vacationing in Brazil. That young woman was*

Tatiana Tarasoff. Poddar's therapist conferred with the doctor who had initially examined the patient and with the Assistant to the Director of the Department of Psychiatry. It was concluded that Poddar should be hospitalized for observation.

The therapist orally informed two campus policemen of the doctors' decision and then wrote a letter[1] to the Chief of Police asking for help in apprehending Poddar. Poddar was taken into custody and questioned by the police. The police officers found Poddar to be rational and they freed him upon his promise that he would not go near Tatiana. Subsequently, the hospital's Director of Psychiatry asked the police to return the therapist's letter and ordered all copies of that letter as well as the therapist's notes on the case to be destroyed. The director did not order that Poddar be placed in a treatment and evaluation facility.

After his release from custody, Poddar sought out and killed Tatiana Tarasoff. Tatiana's parents brought suit against the Regents of the University of California, the doctors at the hospital, and the campus police claiming that the defendants negligently let the patient free without warning their daughter of her peril. The question of law before the court was whether or not a legal duty to warn Tatiana Tarasoff of the potential danger existed. The defense argued that the opportunity for candid, confidential communication was essential to psychotherapy. If doctors were required to warn all threatened persons of possible danger, then the doctor–patient trust would be violated.

The Supreme Court of California found in favor of the plaintiffs, ruling that "protective privilege ends where the public peril begins." The court ruled that just as a doctor has a legal duty to isolate an individual who has a contagious disease and just as a doctor has a legal duty to warn a patient taking medication that will impair his ability to drive, operate machinery, etc., so a psychotherapist has a legal duty to take reasonable care to warn endangered persons of the potentially harmful acts of patients. (My summary; see *Tarasoff v. Regents of University of California*, 118 Cal. Rptr. 129; 529 P.2d 553 [California, 1974])[2]

The momentous decision in *Tarasoff* legally compels therapists to breach confidentiality when "public peril begins." But when does public peril begin? No clear guidelines for the breaching of confidentiality currently exist, though there are hints of such guidelines in professional

---

[1]See Appendix, p. 307.
[2]The majority opinion in *Tarasoff* was written by Justice Tobriner, and a dissenting opinion was filed by Justice Clark. The entire unedited transcript of these two opinions appears in the Appendix to this book.

codes of ethics. For example, the "loophole" in the Hippocratic Oath that hints that disclosure is appropriate under some circumstances is the sentence "whatsoever I see or hear in my attendance on the sick, which ought not to be noised abroad, I will keep silence thereon." The American Medical Association is equally unclear in its code of ethics about what "ought not to be noised abroad," saying, "Confidence . . . should never be revealed unless the law requires it or if necessary to protect the welfare of individuals or the community." The American Psychological Association's code of ethics states that safeguarding information about an individual that has been obtained in the course of professional practice, teaching, or research is a "primary obligation" of psychologists and that such information is not to be communicated to others unless certain conditions are met. One of the conditions in which revelation of confidential material is deemed appropriate is "after most careful deliberation and when there is clear and imminent danger to an individual or to society."

A limited polling of a sample of mental health professionals on specific issues concerning the ethics of breaching patient confidentiality was undertaken in 1956. Two psychiatrists, Ralph Little and Edward Strecker, sent a ten-item questionnaire to sixty-seven of their Philadelphia colleagues, asking such questions as the following:

> What is your ethical responsibility when a patient relates to you he has committed murder, and then forbids you to notify the police on the basis that his communications to you are secret?
> What is your ethical responsibility when a patient tells you her husband is ill and is planning to kill her, and you have reason to believe this is true, but she will not permit commitment or help from the police, and forbids you to interfere?

Of the forty-two colleagues who responded to the questionnaire, the data from four had to be eliminated because the responses were too general. In answer to the first question, thirty of the thirty-eight responding psychiatrists "felt they would deny the patient's request for privileged communication, and do something" (p. 457). In answer to the second question, "twenty-five individuals expressed responsibility for taking some action" (p. 457), which ranged from reporting to legal authorities to consulting with a colleague to refusing treatment if the patient did not accept help. If this small, geographically segregated sample of psychiatrists is in any way representative of the thinking of psychiatrists and mental health professionals today, then it can be concluded that the "moot questions in psychiatric ethics" discussed by Little and Strecker (1956, p. 459) remain moot.

A more recent survey (Jagim et al., 1978) examined the attitudes and knowledge of North Dakota mental health professionals as regards confidentiality, privacy and disclosure of information to third parties. A total of 100 questionnaires were sent out to psychologists, psychiatrists, social workers and others and 64 were returned and used in the data analysis. It was found that over half of the respondents indicated that they would breach confidentiality under certain circumstances (e.g., danger to third parties and/or statutory requirement to disclose information). Jagim et al. hypothesized that this attitude toward disclosure may have reflected "concern for third party or societal interests" or "merely [the respondents'] feeling that they ought to comply with laws requiring disclosure" (p. 463). Exactly why the respondents expressed this sentiment was seen as a problem for future research.

As courts mandate the disclosure of privileged information (as in the *Tarasoff* decision), professionals attempt to safeguard the right of privileged communication all the more strongly. Psychiatrist Howard Gurevitz, for example, speaking at the American Psychiatric Association's convention in 1976, said of the *Tarasoff* decision:

> It is with a sense of despair that one reads the opinion and recognizes that the increasing manifest violence in our world today has persuaded one of our nation's most distinguished courts to create standards of practice and procedures that ally the psychotherapist more with the goal of protecting society than with that of healing patients. It is not that psychiatrists reject the need to counterbalance these functions; in fact, most psychiatrists attempt to fulfill both responsibilities. However, we have done so with procedures that have not mandated us to routinely perform a duty that is counter to our powers of prescience.

Psychologist/attorney Donald Bersoff (1976) warned that "therapists may find themselves in insolvable conflicts as they attempt to reconcile their own personal morality and training regarding confidentiality, the vague remedies of their professional codes of ethics . . . and the developing legal requirements that demand . . . balancing between client and public interests" (p. 272). Also questioning the ramifications of *Tarasoff* was psychologist A. Kovacs (Note 6), who, speaking at the 1976 American Psychological Association convention, wondered aloud whether civil disobedience might be the proper course of action for mental health professionals to take in response to such decisions.

In defense of *Tarasoff*, Harris (1973) argued that

> . . . a duty to warn is sufficiently limited so as not to cause undue hardship to either the therapist or patient. It does not require extraordinary effort on the therapist's part, nor does it violate the spirit of the psychotherapist–patient privilege. That privilege is not absolute, and must be weighed against the public interest in safety.
>
> In response to the confidentiality argument, there are already several analogous situations. For example, physicians are required to report cases of venereal disease to public health authorities. Statutes provide for keeping such reports confidential.

Another argument in favor of a limited duty to warn is that it might protect the patient himself from carrying out bad impulses and thereby exacerbating his condition. Furthermore, it can be argued that, by voluntarily accepting outpatient treatment, the patient is not confined and, in exchange for this freedom, should be willing to allow limited disclosure.

Enforcement of a limited duty to warn should not cause any burden to either the therapist, the patient, or the court. (pp. 433–434)

The issue of what constitutes a therapist's "justified infringement" on his patient's right to privacy—of whether breaching confidentiality is ever permissible—is likely to be with us, then, for a long time to come. And fortunately, though we do not have any firm guidelines on what constitutes a justified infringement, it seems not as difficult to recognize an *un*justified infringement when we see one. Certainly mental health professionals would do well to employ the "least drastic means" test when considering a breach of confidentiality. Furthermore, any such breach should, if possible, be undertaken only with the knowing, intelligent, and voluntary—that is to say, informed—consent of the patient. (See below and in Chapter 7 for a discussion of informed consent.) Above all, therapists must never lose sight of the fact that they are privy to the most private and sensitive thoughts, hopes, and fears of their clientele. With that privilege comes the great responsibility of not only dealing with that information therapeutically but fiercely protecting its confidentiality.

INFORMED CONSENT

The term "informed consent" has been used in the psychological literature in at least three ways. Perhaps its most common usage has been in the context of pretreatment disclosure of possible risks and benefits attendant to a contemplated treatment. A second and related use of "informed consent" has to do with psychological research. Here the term is used to denote the subject's voluntary participation in an experiment in which the procedures, possible outcomes, and risks have been fully explained in advance. A third use of the term has to do with a patient or research subject's waiver of confidentiality. Just as patients can at any time request their doctors to release information to a third party so experimental subjects may ask that the results be released to a third party. Occasionally mental health professionals disagree with their patients' judgments concerning the release of otherwise confidential information. In such cases the professional is questioning his patient's capacity to make a rational and truly *informed* decision. Another version of this third use of the term comes into play when the treating professional advises the patient to waive his right to have information kept confidential but the patient refuses to do so.

Informed Consent and Treatment

The story of the first electroshock treatment by Italian psychiatrist Ugo Cerletti is a study of the problems inherent in obtaining "informed consent" to treatment. As related by Impastato (1960), most of the medical researchers experimenting with electricity in the 1930s were "timid and feared causing death, irreversible brain changes and epileptic states" (p. 1113) when it came to using electricity on humans. In Impastato's words, "Cerletti was the least fearful" and he "experimented on many pigs which were placed at his disposal at the slaughter house in Rome." The rest is history:

> Now came the search for Rome's first patient. For obvious reasons this was not a simple matter. Then, luckily, a patient from North Italy was admitted to the clinic who was a catatonic schizophrenic and who spoke an incomprehensible gibberish. He was unable to give his name or to state anything about himself. No one could identify him. Dr. Cerletti decided he should be the historic patient. Following adequate preparations the first treatment was given in 1938. Present were Cerletti, Bini, Longhi, Accornero, Kalinowsky and Fleischer. The patient was brought in, the machine was set at 1/10 of a second and 70 volts and the shock given. Naturally, the low dosage resulted in a petit mal reaction. After the electric spasm, which lasted a fraction of a second, the patient burst out into song. The Professor suggested that another treatment with a higher voltage be given. The staff objected. They stated that if another treatment were given the patient would probably die and wanted further treatment postponed until the morrow. The Professor knew what that meant. He decided to go ahead right then and there, but before he could say so the patient suddenly sat up and pontifically proclaimed, no longer in a jargon, but in clear Italian: "Non una seconda! Mortifera!" (Not again, it will kill me). This made the Professor think and swallow, but his courage was not lost. He gave the order to proceed at a higher voltage and a longer time: and the first electroconvulsion in man ensued. Thus was born EST out of one man and over the objection of his assistants. (pp. 1113–1114)

Applying present legal and ethical standards to this fascinating account of the administration of an experimental treatment, it seems reasonable to infer that the patient was in no physical or mental condition to give "informed consent." However, after the first shock was passed and the patient suddenly protested in clear Italian, "Non una seconda! Mortifera!" it is questionable whether Cerletti was on sound legal or ethical ground in proceeding to apply a second shock at a higher voltage and for a longer time. As was recently pointed out by Martin (1975), "Consent is becoming a more important element in much judicial thinking, and courts will look at all conditions to determine whether consent is really informed and voluntary'' (p. 5). In the present instance, the patient was neither "really informed" nor given voluntary choice. Another argument that could be made is that the patient's condition "improved" so dramatically after the first treatment (i.e., he appeared to become rational) that the justification for the second treatment was unclear. Impastato's account also does not tell us whether the patient did in fact die or exactly what the outcome was.

If Cerletti's patient had had a spouse or next of kin, present standards would demand that the informed consent be obtained from them. But here another interesting legal/ethical question about "informed consent" arises. The doctors themselves were dealing with a multitude of unknown factors and really did not know what to expect. Therefore, what could the next of kin (even if there were next of kin) have been told? Of Cerletti's experiments with pigs? That the method had never before been used on humans? What? The question of how much information has to be imparted before a consent can reasonably be assumed to be "informed" is very much a matter of concern to modern-day practitioners:

> The psychiatrist faces a dilemma in communicating the risks of shock treatment to his patient. Flat statements that shock therapy is safe may subject the psychiatrist to liability for breach of warranty. Disclosure of all risks may frighten some patients into nonconsent. . . .(Krouner, 1975, p. 408)
>
> Given that a patient's consent must be obtained, the next logical question which arises is to what extent does informed consent require that risks be disclosed fully? The answer to the degree of disclosure question given by the Supreme Court of New Mexico and the District of Columbia Court of Appeals is that a reasonable psychiatrist should never make statements that shock treatment is "perfectly safe," and should disclose the most likely risks in the treament unless the psychiatrist has a good medical reason for *not* disclosing the risks. (p. 409)

As will be seen in Chapter 7, the courts have begun to invoke a "reasonable man" test in assigning liability in litigation involving informed consent to treatment. In cases where there has been reason to doubt that the consequences of a treatment were fully explained or that the patient understood that explanation, some courts have asked whether the proverbial "reasonable man" would have consented to treatment under the same or similar circumstances. But regardless how reasonable the "reasonable man" test appears to be, some doctors have expressed infuriation at the lengths to which professionals are being compelled to go in order to ensure that their patients' consents are informed.[3]

---

[3]An article by Ravitch (1974), "Informed Consent—Descent to Absurdity," is a humorous but strident attack on how the courts have applied this legal doctrine.

Informed Consent and Research

Like the issues attendant to obtaining informed consent for treatment, the issues pertaining to informed consent for experimental work are complex. As Davidson (1969) has pointed out:

> Getting the patient's consent to the use of a placebo or an experimental drug is a scientific absurdity, although it may be legally necessary. If the patient is told that he is being experimented with, he may refuse to be a guinea pig. And if he is told that he is receiving a placebo, he may either refuse to participate or show unreliable results. (p. 238)

The reader interested in pursuing questions regarding informed consent in research is referred to an authoritative review of federal and state laws pertaining to experimentation with human subjects (Hershey and Miller, 1976).

Informed Consent and the Waiver of Confidentiality

With regard to the third type of informed consent—that involving a patient's insistence on breaking or refusal to break confidentiality—West (1969) has pointed out that psychiatric patients seldom know what is in their charts and therefore can never really give truly "informed" consent. Furthermore, remarks West, "such a breach of confidentiality may impair public confidence in the psychiatrist and the profession because the assurance shall have been belied that psychotherapeutic communications are forever inviolate" (p. 228).

An issue that is inevitably raised as regards the decision-making ability and judgment of persons diagnosed as mentally ill is competency. (A person may simultaneously be considered legally competent for some purposes but not for others; simply being diagnosed as mentally ill is not sufficient grounds to be declared "incompetent.") Problems in determining competency in various circumstances have been discussed elsewhere (Roth, Meisel, and Lidz, 1977). Here it will be pointed out that as the psychiatric patient may not be in the best position to consent to treatment or to consent to be an experimental subject, so the patient may not always have the best perspective on questions of confidentiality. For example, a patient who exhibits paranoid symptomatology at the outset of treatment may be reluctant if not resistant about having any information regarding his treatment revealed to anyone for any reason. However, after treatment such a patient's perspective on the waiver of confidentiality for some specified purpose may be quite different.

The problems attendant to the legal doctrine of informed consent get even knottier when temporal, geographical, and other factors are taken into consideration:

What constitutes a valid consent today may not remain so tomorrow; what constitutes a valid consent in one jurisdiction may not be an accurate representation of the law in a neighboring jurisdiction; and what constitutes a valid consent in one branch of medicine may be a less than wholly accurate guide to a valid consent in another branch of medicine. (Meisel, Roth, and Lidz, 1977, p. 288)

PSYCHIATRIC DIAGNOSIS

Although the subject of diagnosis in almost all other medical specialties does not readily invite discussion of ethical issues, psychiatric diagnoses almost inevitably do. One of the primary reasons for this is that the definition of what is psychopathological is not only temporally and culturally relative but is also a function of the life experiences of the person making the diagnosis. The arbitrariness and unreliability of the diagnosis of psychopathology as well as the potentially harmful consequences of misdiagnosis are driven home in such "horror stories" as this vignette cited by Kittrie (1973, pp. 83–84):

> Mrs. Anna Duzynski was a recent Polish emigrant; neither she nor her husband had learned to speak English. They were living on the northwest side of Chicago when on October 5, 1960, Mrs. Duzynski discovered that $380 in cash was missing from their apartment. Suspecting that the money had been stolen by the janitor, who was in possession of a spare key, Mrs. Duzynski rushed to his flat and demanded the return of the stolen money. The janitor called the police, complaining that both Mr. and Mrs. Duzynski were insane and should be put in a mental institution. Without further examination, the police seized both Anna and her husband, Michael, and took them in handcuffs to the Cook County Mental Health Clinic. At the clinic the Duzynskis were unable to answer any of the questions directed to them in English. Pursuant to lax commitment procedures, the Duzynskis were pronounced mentally ill and were committed to the Chicago State Hospital. Six weeks later, Michael Duzynski still knew less about why he had been denied his freedom than he had when thrown into a Nazi concentration camp in World War II. Finally, in complete desperation, he hanged himself. The very next day, the hospital officials released Anna Duzynski.

Because mental health professionals—unlike other health professionals—sometimes treat individuals who do not want to be treated, the potential for abuse and the need for careful monitoring are made all the more salient. Because courts delegate to mental health professionals the awesome duty of advising them on such questions as whose insanity defense is legitimate, who is "competent" to stand trial, who should retain child custody, or who should be civilly committed, concern over such diagnoses can understandably become a matter of great social and not merely clinical significance. As we move into an era in which greater emphasis is being placed on prevention, new questions arise. For example, if a person is evaluated by a mental health professional as a high suicide risk, should that person be preventively (i.e., involuntarily) confined, and for how long? At what point would such activities undertaken in the name of prevention become veritable detention?

It can be seen that closely related to the ethics of psychiatric diagnosis are the ethics of involuntary hospitalization. The view that mental illness is a myth and that involuntary psychiatric hospitalization should be abolished has come into vogue in recent years. However, opponents of that view have pointed out that to abolish the psychiatric hospital would, in essence, turn the whole world into a hospital—a solution that seems worse than the problem it attempts to deal with. Serban and Gidynski (1974) argued that while the law expects discharged psychotic patients to assume responsibility for their actions and their post-treatment care, few such patients actually do so. They cited data indicating that

> schizophrenic patients, stemming primarily from the lowest socio-economic levels, show generalized resistance towards following through on outpatient remedial care, and have a dropout rate for aftercare of about 75 per cent. The lack of awareness of the schizophrenic patient in need of treatment can be further inferred from the fact that, on the average, only 3.9 per cent of the patients requiring hospitalization are self-admitting, the rest consisting of referrals by family, police, and other social agencies. (p. 1977)

There is little question but that attacks on the unreliability of psychiatric diagnosis and the potentially ruinous consequences of such diagnoses have some validity. But in considering the potential for abuse inherent in the diagnostic process, the need for *some* kind of classificatory framework for treatment and research purposes must also be considered. As with other ethical issues in the mental health profession, then, those surrounding the use of psychiatric diagnosis are extremely complex and resistant to facile solution.

Homosexuality: Diagnosis and treatment.   In the revised *Diagnostic and Statistical Manual of Mental Disorders* (DSM–II) of the American Psychiatric Association, diagnosis #302.0 is homosexuality. This diagnosis is a sexual deviation under the more general heading of "Personality Disorders and Certain Other Non-Psychotic Mental Disorders." According to the manual, sexual deviates are "... individuals whose sexual interests are directed primarily toward objects other than people of the opposite sex, toward sexual acts not usually associated with coitus, or toward coitus performed under bizarre circumstances as in necrophilia, pedophilia, sexual sadism and fetishism" (American Psychiatric Association, 1968, p. 44). After numerous meetings of the American Psychiatric Association's Nomenclature Committee, a vote of that association's Trustees in late 1973, and a vote of the general membership in 1974, homosexuality was declared to be a "sexual orientation disturbance" applicable to individuals disturbed about their sexual orientation.

In an article entitled "Homosexuality; The Ethical Challenge," Gerald C. Davison (1976) proposed that it is widespread societal prejudice that motivates homosexuals to want to change their sexual orientations. Davison argued that psychotherapists should "stop trying to change homosexual orientations" (p. 161). One comment on this article reflected not only impatience with the view expressed by Davison but also concern over the use of the word "unethical" as a scare word:

> Davison's (1976) thesis is simple. He assumes that homosexuality is a normal sexual mode in the wide spectrum of human sexuality and that the psychological problems noted among homosexuals directly derive from societal prejudices. He suggests, therefore, that it is unethical for clinicians to cooperate with homosexuals who wish to change their sexual direction.
>
> The central argument on which his assumptions are based is by now well worn. It comes down to whether homosexuality is, in fact, normal or is the consequence of and an expression of psychopathology. If, as Davison thinks, homosexuality is normal, then patients who seek a change in sexual orientation should be dissuaded. If, as I think, homosexuality is pathological, the failure to develop prophylactic programs or provide therapeutic services for people who wish to become heterosexual would be a grave error. I am not inclined to use the term "unethical." It is a scare word, an accusation really, that implies dubious therapeutic intentions. (Bieber, 1976, p. 163)

Is homosexuality an "ethical challenge" in the sense that Davison is using the term? Or is the invocation of ethics here a "scare word," as Bieber argues? These are questions that the mental health profession—as well as lawmakers and society in general—must resolve.

ETHICAL ISSUES IN PSYCHOLOGICAL RESEARCH

On July 12, 1974, the National Commission for the Protection of Human Subjects of Biomedical and Behavioral Research was created by Congress. By early December of that year, all eleven members of the commission had been sworn in. Considering the varied backgrounds and views of the members of the commission, skeptics at the time it was created, such as Ingelfinger (1975), wondered if "the diverse elements of the Commission really can reach a consensus, or will eternal ethical verities be decided by six-to-five votes?" The Commission dealt with numerous complex issues in ethics surrounding research with human subjects. Included among the ten reports it issued before its term expired in October of 1978 were documents on the use of prisoners and persons "institutionalized as mentally infirm" as experimental subjects.[4] Some of the Commission's recommendations have already become law. For example, it is now illegal to use prisoners as subjects in research that is not relevant to prisoners. This means that behavioral and medical researchers may design experiments to answer questions like "What are the effects of incarceration?" but they may not use a population of prisoners to answer questions like "What is the effect of this new drug in humans?" Recently Congress provided for a new commission with a four year term of office (The President's Commission for the Study of Ethical Problems in Medicine and Biomedical and Behavioral Research) though at the time of press this Commission was not a functioning reality.

Sales and Grisso (1978) observed that "[l]aws that regulate and shape the activities of professional psychologists are increasing in number as well as in scope and complexity." These authors urged psychologists to stay abreast of legal developments not only "to ensure that one's own practice is maintained within the bounds of the law" but "to understand existing and proposed federal and state laws, even scrutinize the wording of such laws, to ensure that appropriate professional viewpoints and concerns are heard within federal and state legislatures" (p. 363). This caution is—or should be—of special interest to researchers in the behavioral sciences. Consider for example the fate of the profession's prohibition against breach of confidentiality with respect to research data in the light of recent judicial actions. Charles R. Knerr (Note 5) focused on the origin and resolution of incidents in recent years in which scholarly researchers were subpoenaed by governmental authorities to reveal confidential research data. In one such incident, the researcher refused to comply with the subpoena and after being found in contempt of court, was imprisoned for eight days. Under what specific conditions is it ethically appropriate to breach confidentiality and reveal information obtained in the course of research? How can the potential for inadvertent misuse of confidential research information be minimized (cf. Roskam, 1979)? Should certain types of research data be treated legally as privileged communication? If so, which types of research data? These are questions that remain to be answered.

In recent years the use of deception in behavioral research has come

---

[4]All of the Commission's reports, including titles such as *The Belmont Report: Ethical Principles and Guidelines for the Protection of Human Subjects of Research* (1978) are available from the Superintendent of Documents, Government Printing Office, Washington, D.C. 20402.

under ethical/legal attack. It is well known that some of the most oft-cited behavioral laboratory findings have included elements of deception which were indispensable to the design. For example, in the Milgram study of obedience, the Asch study on conformity, Darley and Latane's work on altruism, the Sherifs' work on cooperation, and numerous other studies concerning attribution, aggression, and level of arousal, deception was a necessary element if "true" reactions were to be obtained. The valuable fund of knowledge gained from such basic research could not have been accrued had methods which have been proposed as alternatives to deception (e.g., role playing) been used. Should deception have a place in medical/behavioral research? Do placeboes have a future? What kind of experiments do and do not justify deception and who should decide?

Professional and judicial views with regard to these and related ethical issues in psychological research remain very much unresolved and in a state of flux. One psychologist (Gergen, 1973) published a paper stating, in essence, that ethical principles should be established by experimentation and that "if subjects remain unaffected by variations along these dimensions, then the establishment of the principles becomes highly questionable" (p. 907). Strong reaction to Gergen's proposal came from Johnson (1974), who argued that it is a "basic contravention of human rights and dignity to argue that we can set aside the possible effects of research procedures on humans until they are demonstrated to be harmful" (p. 470). Waterman (1974) also questioned Gergen's proposed methodology as well as the logic of his view:

> Rights belong to individuals, not to collectives. When a violation of rights occurs, it is some individual who suffers, not some abstract grouping. By continually referring to "subjects" as if they were an undifferentiated group, Gergen obscures the fact that each participant is a distinct individual entitled to the full protection of his rights. Even if no statistically significant effects of violating an ethical principle can be identified, the failure to adhere to the principle could still entail the violation of the personal rights of individual research subjects.

Rivlin (1974) discussed the problems inherent in social experimentation in terms of five kinds of dilemmas: design, implementation, evaluation, timing, and moral dilemmas. She cautioned that if great care is not taken in each of these areas, social experimentation may one day be banned altogether. Watchdog ethics committees have been created in most universities as arbitrators of ethical dilemmas facing behavioral science researchers. But who will watch over the watchdogs? And who is to say how much deception or manipulation is justified and for what purposes? The multifaceted professional and legal issues concerning psychological research have only recently begun to be more clearly defined.

4
The Issue of Control

Man's increasing power to control other men has raised many important questions concerning "ethics," "values," "freedom," and "power," to name but a few areas. The main problem at this stage, however, is to sift out the important issues from the trivial and to derive workable answers. (Ulrich, Stachnik, and Mabry, 1966, p. 300)

If one issue in ethics could be singled out as being most important to daily practice in the mental health profession, perhaps it would be the issue of control. Amidst an unprecedented public interest in human rights, heated controversies concerning the issue of behavioral control in state institutions, hospitals, prisons, schools, and various outpatient and inpatient settings continue to fill scientific journals, the popular press, and the electronic media. In the years to come the complexity of the already knotty questions being asked is likely to increase with advances in behavioral technology.

One of the most scholarly debates on the issue of control as it relates to behavioral science featured two highly esteemed psychologists, B. F. Skinner and Carl Rogers, arguing opposing viewpoints. In this chapter, we will use the now classic Rogers/Skinner debate as a point of departure from which to discuss other control-related controversies.

ROGERS AND SKINNER AND THE ISSUE OF CONTROL

How much control can or should a therapist exert over his client? What is the place of values in behavioral science? These are some of the issues that Carl Rogers and B. F. Skinner debated in their now classic symposium on control (Rogers and Skinner, 1956). Skinner argued that behavior, examined scientifically, has its roots in prior causation. He went on to say that Rogerian therapists conducted therapy in a so-called nondirective manner because of the reinforcement value such an approach to therapy holds for the therapist: "A therapist relinquishes control because he can thus help his client more effectively" (p. 1065). But Skinner goes further in questioning the rationale of the Rogerian approach to treatment:

> What evidence is there that a client ever becomes truly *self*-directing? What evidence is there that he ever makes a truly *inner* choice of ideal or goal? Even though the therapist does not do the choosing, even though he encourages "self-actualization"—he is not out of control as long as he holds himself ready to step in when occasion demands—when, for example, the client chooses the goal of becoming a more accomplished liar or murdering his boss. But supposing the therapist does withdraw completely or is no longer necessary—what about all the other forces acting upon the client? Is the self-chosen goal independent of his early ethical and religious training? of the folk-wisdom of his group? of the opinions and attitudes of others who are important to him? Surely not. The therapeutic situation is only a small part of the world of the client. From the therapist's point of view it may appear to be possible to relinquish control. But the control passes, not to a "self," but to forces in other parts of the client's world. The solution of the therapist's problem of power cannot be *our* solution, for we must consider *all* the forces acting upon the individual. (p. 1065)

Rogers conceded that behavior has its roots in prior causation, but he took issue with Skinner on what the role of personal choice in behavioral science should be:

> Behavior, when it is examined scientifically, is surely best understood as determined by prior causation. This is one great fact of science. But responsible personal choice, which is the most essential element in being a person, which is the core experience in psychotherapy, which exists prior to any scientific endeavor, is an equally prominent fact in our lives. To deny the experience of responsible choice is, to me, as restrictive a view as to deny the possibility of a behavioral science. That these two important elements of our experience appear to be in contradiction has perhaps the same significance as the contradiction between the wave theory and the corpuscular theory of light, both of which can be shown to be true, even though incompatible. We cannot profitably deny our subjective life, any more than we can deny the objective description of that life. (p. 1064)

The symposium participants extended their arguments to the broader issue of values in science. For Skinner, the role of values in science is that of reinforcers: "An organism can be reinforced—can be made to 'choose'—almost any given state of affairs" (p. 1064). For Rogers, the place of values in science is not as clear, since he holds that individual freedom of choice is part and parcel of science. Rogers struggled with the question saying that scientific endeavors are carried out in pursuit of some value which "always and necessarily lies outside the scope of scientific effort which it sets in motion" and that "I wish to make it clear that I am not saying that values cannot be included as a subject of science" (p. 1062).

Addressing himself to the place of values in applied science, Byrne (1974) cogently argued that the application of science can never be value-free:

> With the application of scientific knowledge, value judgments must be made. Should thousands of men, women, and children be destroyed in order to hasten the end of a war? Is it right to fluoridate a town's water supply over the protests of a frightened minority in order to aid in the prevention of dental cavities? Is it right to pass a compulsory sterilization law in order to decrease the incidence of schizophrenia in the population? Is it right to use subliminal messages flashed on a movie screen in order to increase the sales of a particular product? Is it right to design neighborhoods in such a way that interpersonal contacts are increased and personal isolation is decreased? These decisions are different from those usually required of scientists; there are no generally accepted criteria for moral concepts such as "right." (pp. 13–14)

What about the place of values in applied *behavioral* science? Can a therapist who holds one set of values effectively treat—should he treat—a person who does not share those values? This was one of the questions raised by Cohen and Smith's "Socially Reinforced Obsessing: Etiology of a Disorder in a Christian Scientist" (1976), a question we shall now examine.

THE COHEN AND SMITH CONTROVERSY

> A 28-year-old mother and housewife was referred for treatment for a variety of complaints, the keystone of which was her obsession with disease. As an adolescent she was introduced to Christian Science. During the next decade she had a number of experiences that either reinforced or challenged her beliefs in the efficacy of prayer and the validity of "thought cures." As crises mounted in her life she began thinking about disease to an obsessive degree. In spite of the fact that she recognized these thoughts to be unrealistic and much of her associated behavior to be irrational, she was incapable of resisting either the thinking or the overt behavior. Individual psychotherapy, employing a variety of modes, was quite effective in dealing with her difficulties. (Abstract of Cohen and Smith, 1976)

The case study of the patient ("Mary"), cited in the journal abstract above, suggested that one woman's obsessive disorder may have been causally related to her contact with Christian Science. The article precipitated a storm of controversy revolving around the issue of control. Invited comments on the article by Perry London (1976) and Seymour Halleck (1976) were addressed to the issue of therapists imposing their value systems on patients. Eleven months later, a restatement of the latter's point that "it would seem that the ethical issues could be minimized . . . if the consumer could be adequately forewarned of the possible consequences of treatment" (p. 1168) appeared in the form of a comment by Coyne (1976) that nominally had to do with the issue of informed consent. In December 1977 the views of a representative of the Christian Science church were published (Stokes, 1977), along with the views of two academicians who described themselves as "especially attuned to this problem through serving on the faculty of an APA-approved clinical program that is partially oriented toward training psychologists who will be sensitive to such issues and dynamics" (McLemore and Court, 1977, p. 1172). They considered the case to constitute an important milestone:

> Cohen and Smith (1976) recently reported a case study that crashed through the barrier of a long-established taboo. . . . That this case report is of signal importance in bringing an important ethical issue to the fore, and that the Editor was commendably bold in publishing it, is to be seen in the fact that this appears to be the first time an American Psychological Association (APA) journal has published a clinical case history explicitly highlighting the possible role of religion in the etiology of a particular person's mental disorder. (p. 1172)

The comments on "Socially Reinforced Obsessing" by London (1976), Halleck (1976), Coyne (1976), Stokes (1977), and McLemore and Court (1977) all seem to be addressed to the question of whether or not a person with strong religious beliefs should be accepted into therapy. Unfortunately, each of these commentators and the editors of the *Journal of Consulting and Clinical Psychology* apparently failed to recognize that Mary had been well into treatment before she elected to reveal that she was a Christian Scientist:

> Around the 15th session, Mary reluctantly brought up her involvement with Christian Science (which she had previously avoided mentioning), and a probable basis for her obsessive behavior became clear. (Cohen and Smith, 1976, p. 144)

Furthermore, London (1976) confused the arbitrariness-of-psychopathology question with the etiological one and generalized from the case study to say that Cohen and Smith (1976) were attempting to prove that "religion can make you crazy." With insufficient regard to this patient's history, Halleck (1976) asked, "Did the treatment of a highly religious person succeed at the expense of her abandoning her religious convictions?" (p. 146). Coyne's (1976) comment, entitled "The Place of Informed Consent in Ethical Dilemmas," not only compounded previously made errors but regrettably failed to acknowledge the complexity involved in defining what is meant by "informed consent" as that term can be used in applied psychological settings. Thus, Coyne compared the case of Mary to that of a surgeon obtaining consent before an operation or a lawyer obtaining consent before initiating legal action; but only a clairvoyant could possibly have been able to forewarn a patient of the possibility of the modification of her religious beliefs fifteen weeks before she elected to reveal those beliefs.

The somewhat sensational issue of "mental health professionals using their therapy techniques to change religious belief systems of clients without the knowledge or consent of the client" (Stokes, 1977, p. 1164) was raised by a representative of the Christian Science church, who expressed regret that Cohen and Smith (1976) had read "exactly the same misconception" into Christian Science teachings as had (in his view) the patient. The crux of Cohen's (1977b) reply to Stokes emphasized the integrity and sovereignty of science and religion:

> To ask whether the most useful healing to be sought "is always of one phase or another of the individual's alienation from God" or "classical Freudian to encounter group and screaming therapy" (Stokes, 1977, p. 1165) is to illegitimately pit religion against science—two different systems (each with numerous subsystems) with vastly different sets of rules concerning what constitutes acceptable evidence and proof. And although psychologists have some tentative notions about the kinds of therapy that are most likely to be helpful to some patients under some conditions, we are a long way from a "universal cure." Generally, psychotherapists try to understand presenting problems by integrating data (e.g., the constructs most salient to the patient, environmental factors, etc.) into a diagnostic/therapeutic schema that makes the most sense to them. Stokes confuses Cohen and Smith's attempted understanding of Mary with "reading exactly the same misconception into its religious teachings" and seems not to allow that psychotherapists—like all mortals—can only have a relatively limited acquaintance with the numerous areas that they might want to know more about. Therapists can, however, view the treatment of Christian Scientists, lapsed Catholics, communist FBI agents, and palmist/psychologists as opportunities to learn more about Christian Science, Catholicism, the FBI, and palmistry.
>
> I wish to state as emphatically as possible that I have the utmost respect for pious persons of all faiths who live their lives with exemplary love and regard for their fellow human beings. Although the intermingling of religion with science is not to be encouraged, such enmeshment is

bound to occur from time to time. When dilemmas are raised by such overlapping and conflicting interests, I believe that the solution that sides with life, human welfare, and physical/mental well-being must be sought. I fully appreciate that the latter statement may raise more questions than it answers, but it is the best I can do short of a philosophical treatise. (pp. 1169–70)[1]

Seemingly oblivious to the fact that Mary's therapy was undertaken on account of her problematic behavior and not her problematic religion, McLemore and Court (1977) took up the cudgels against Cohen and Smith (1976), London (1976), and Halleck (1976) and all those who would—from McLemore and Court's perspective—deprive people of their Constitutional right to freedom of religion. Hence London is attacked for being unaware of "the implications of his recommendations for civil liberties" (McLemore and Court, 1977, p. 1174), and Halleck, we are told "misconstrued the ethical question" and raised an ethical question that was "not an ethical question at all" (p. 1174). Early on in their comment McLemore and Court (p. 1172) write that the case of Mary "raises an ethics question that ought to confront every psychotherapist. How should the therapist relate to the religious values of the patient when these values seem to play an important part in the psychopathology?" However, later on these authors seem to backtrack a bit when they cite as the "central ethical question" the "rightness or wrongness of such treatment" (p. 1174).

By some unknown logic, McLemore and Court (1977, p. 1174) come to the conclusion that publishing a case study is prima facie evidence that Cohen and Smith had not been neutral—as if neutrality were at issue. I have pointed out elsewhere that "the myth of therapeutic neutrality has been recognized at least since the days when Rogerians started referring to their treatment as 'client centered' as opposed to 'nondirective' " (Cohen, 1977b, p. 1167). However, to acknowledge that the notion of therapeutic neutrality is a myth is not to deny that psychotherapists do, to varying degrees, attempt to let their patients make decisions for themselves:

> At the time of the Christian Science "revelation," I, "wishing to remain neutral with respect to any resolution of Mary's division of loyalty," let her decide what she wanted to do without overtly applying encouragement or discouragement toward any choice. *Of course* my tacit offer to remain her therapist conveyed my willingness to help her through her disabling obsessions even at the cost of possible infringement on religious beliefs, beliefs that had fostered "a spiral of ever increasing ambiva-

---

[1]Incidentally, the courts have disposed of litigation that pitted medical science against religion on similar grounds (of the priority of "life, human welfare, and physical/mental well-being"). (See, for example, Case 6.48.)

lence" (Cohen & Smith, 1976, p. 144). Fifteen weeks prior to the revelation, the patient had acted decisively to seek out values that she could live with. She had, in effect, greatly minimized the relevance of the principle of neutrality that was alluded to. (Cohen, 1977b, p. 1167)

An extended discussion of McLemore and Court's comments need not be made here. Suffice it to say that these authors inappropriately generalized from the single case when they wrote or implied that Cohan and Smith

1. had been "casually stripping persons . . . of 'bizarre' religious orientations" (p. 1172);

2. were trying to say, à la London, that religious beliefs cause religious neurosis (p. 1173); and

3. were trying to say that "behavioral control initiated in a psychological treatment program is therapeutic while self-administration, utilizing religious belief, is harmful" (p. 1174).[2]

The issues raised by Cohen (1977b; Cohen and Smith, 1976) were further discussed in a symposium on religion and psychotherapy at the American Psychological Association Convention in late August 1978. In his introductory address entitled "When Worlds Collide: Psychotherapy and Religion," Clinton McLemore (Note 7) reiterated his belief that the publication of Cohen and Smith (1976) was a significant event in the American psychology literature. Symposium participant Albert Ellis (Note 8) argued that religion and the belief in an Almighty Being can be used as a crutch by some persons and as a means by which self-pity and lack of initiative can be perpetuated. In such instances, what would an ethical psychotherapist do? Should the patient be referred for treatment to a member of the clergy? Under what conditions, if any, should a patient be referred for pastoral counseling? These were only some of the questions raised during the course of the meeting for which none of the participants had completely satisfactory answers. My own contribution to the symposium (Note 9) focused on the problem of control by psychotherapists and the inadequacy of the legal doctrine of informed consent as a solution to that problem. The following is an excerpt from that speech:

Increasing individual and governmental concern for the sanctity of human rights has led to a general concern with the issue of control that is perhaps unprecedented. Control at the hands of governments that wall

---

[2]McLemore and Court also found it regrettable that Mary's spouse was not in therapy along with his wife. Although it was not stated in the original article, let it be stated here for the record that numerous attempts were made to have Mary's husband come in for treatment, but he was totally resistant to the idea.

people in, silence dissent and/or prohibit emigration; control at the hands of advertisers flashing subliminal messages to unsuspecting viewers; control at the hands of corporations, schools, and other agencies and institutions that have attempted to enforce behavior and dress codes and other regulations that may be viewed as infringements on individual liberty. These are but a few of the many areas in which the issue of control has been a matter of heated public debate.

The idea of control at the hands of mental health professionals is particularly threatening, perhaps because the methods are most unabashed and the consequences most immediate and dramatic. Whether it is control at the hands of a psychiatrist administering a dose of electroshock therapy (or some other, less obtrusive psychopharmacological agent), control at the hands of a shock-stick wielding paraprofessional in a state institution, or control by a psychologist doing talking therapy with a highly religious person (or any other person for that matter), the very idea of one individual imposing or attempting to impose his will or influence on another person is generally considered to be repugnant and untenable. Perhaps this sentiment was most succinctly expressed by the United States Supreme Court in its decision in *Stanley v. Georgia*. In part, that decision read as follows:

> Our whole constitutional heritage rebels at the thought of giving government the power to control men's minds. . . . Whatever the power of the state to control dissemination of ideas inimical to public morality, it cannot constitutionally premise legislation on the desirability of controlling a person's private thoughts.[3]

As eloquent as the Supreme Court statement is, it fails to allow that all of us, with greater and lesser degrees of success, attempt to influence one another. Teachers, parents, stockbrokers, judges, psychologists, and persistent life insurance salesmen are only some of the more obvious examples of citizens who make it their daily business to influence others' private thoughts (or at least try their hardest to do so). Certainly the justices of the Supreme Court in their decisions influence the private thoughts (and behavior) of millions of people. But like Rogerians who have stopped referring to their therapy as non-directive and analysts who have stopped referring to psychoanalysis as non-judgmental, the Supreme Court may one day acknowledge that some degree of control and the attempt to impose one's values on another is very much an activity of daily living. Once this Skinnerian fact of life is acknowledged, the pertinent question then becomes "How much control is acceptable, by whom, for what purposes, and under what conditions?"

Currently, the legal panacea to the dilemma of control has been the doctrine of informed consent. If a controllee is informed by the controller of all the pros and cons of a controlling procedure (and of all the available alternatives to that procedure), if he understands all of the information that is conveyed to him, and if on that basis he gives his

---

[3]*Stanley v. Georgia* (394 U.S. 557, 22 L. Ed. 542, 89 S. Ct. 1243) involved an issue of control by the state.

consent to be controlled, then the control will generally be seen as legally permissible. But this seemingly pat legal solution to the problem of control is complicated as is, and even more complicated when ethical considerations come into play. . . .

Recently, a forum for the discussion of the issue of informed consent to treatment evolved in the *Journal of Consulting and Clinical Psychology* after the publication of Cohen and Smith's, "Socially Reinforced Obsessing; Etiology of a Disorder in a Christian Scientist." As reported in that case study, a sometime Christian Scientist named Mary presented with obsessive symptomatology which appeared to be related to and exacerbated by her religious involvements. In his comment on the case study, Seymour Halleck asked, "Did the treatment of a highly religious person succeed at the expense of her abandoning her religious beliefs?" Halleck went on to caution that "it would seem that the ethical issues could be minimized. . . if the consumer could be adequately forewarned of possible consequences of treatment."

In an article that restated Halleck's position, James C. Coyne argued that, like surgeons preparing to operate and lawyers preparing to litigate, psychotherapists preparing to do therapy must forewarn their clients of possible consequences and obtain their fully informed consent. In using the Cohen and Smith article as a point of departure from which to talk about preparation for surgery and litigation, Coyne overlooked the fact that Mary had been seen in treatment for fifteen weeks before she revealed her Christian Science background. It is, of course, impossible to forewarn a patient of the possibility of the modification of her religious beliefs fifteen weeks before the patient elects to reveal those beliefs. Still, Coyne's article raises some questions. Should therapists be obliged [i.e., other than in the usual course of obtaining demographic data] to delve into their clients' religious beliefs before beginning a course of treatment? If so, should physicians be required to delve into the religious beliefs of their patients before prescribing birth control pills? Should pharmacists be obligated to carefully question a suspected Catholic customer before selling him contraceptives?

I would agree that patients' informed consent to psychotherapeutic treatment should be ethically, if not legally, mandated. However, I have grave doubts about how theory can be put into practice in this context. There will be exceedingly difficult questions to be answered. Who should be informed of what under what conditions? How much information is necessary to make a consent fully informed? Which patients, by virtue of their mental states, are incompetent to give consent? Perhaps the most basic question concerns the incapability of psychotherapists to predict changes in their patients' lives that were not targeted for change when therapy was begun. Some academicians may pontificate on the notion that clinicians have been "naively anti-ecological" in that they haven't anticipated the effects of therapeutic intervention in areas of their patients' lives that were not targeted for change. But most clinician/scholars will candidly admit that they cannot begin to predict all of the life changes that will take place in their patients as a result of psychotherapy. We don't need one-shot surveys or laboratory analogue studies to tell us that there is often a ripple effect during a course of treatment. Read the work of Albert Ellis or Carl Rogers or any other clinician/scholar to begin to appreciate the myriad changes that take place in clients after a course of psychotherapy. Not all of the changes that take place were targeted for change when therapy was begun. The point here is that when it comes to the remarkably complex field of human relations, how precise or accurate can a therapist be in forecasting to his clients possible outcomes?[4] In this context, the analogy of the singularly complex enterprise of psychotherapy to surgery and litigation seems particularly ill-chosen and inappropriate.

The case study of Mary was indeed a rather unique set of circumstances in the psychological literature. Christian Scientists typically do not go to medical doctors or psychologists with their problems—they go to Christian Science practitioners. Mary was a patient who *voluntarily* sought a form of treatment which, by its very nature, tended to compromise her religious beliefs. It can be seen now that the answer to Halleck's question, "Did the treatment of a highly religious person succeed at the expense of her abandoning her religious beliefs?" is "No, she had abandoned them beforehand as evidenced by her voluntary desire to receive treatment." As I have pointed out elsewhere, this patient appeared to be seeking out values she could live with. "But can a Christian Scientist be effectively treated in psychotherapy by a non–Christian Scientist?" asks one of the commentators. Two questions in reply: "Can a Jew be effectively treated by a non-Jew? Can a Democrat be treated by a Republican?" My answer to all three questions: Yes, Yes, and Yes. . . .

Judicious use of the principles of informed consent may just be the answer to the difficult questions attendant to the issue of control in psychotherapy. However, whether truly informed consent to treatment is more a reality or an ideal remains to be seen. Once we, as psychotherapists, are alerted to our handicap in being able to provide the warning for a fully informed consent to take place, we are more apt to be sensitive to the issue of control. With sensitivity to that issue we can take on the treatment of clients of varied religious persuasions and, where appropriate, help those clients to make their religion work for and not against them.

BEHAVIOR MODIFICATION AND THE ISSUE OF CONTROL

For the general public (and for too many mental health professionals), the term "behavior modification" has unfortunately come to conjure

---

[4]Also relevant in this context are Freud's (1913, p. 350) thoughts on the "selective capacity of . . . analysis" cited herein on page 262.

up visions of involuntary M&M's, electric shock, deprivation, and the like. In sensational and graphically portrayed books and movies (such as *A Clockwork Orange*), the theoretical rationale behind behavioral techniques, the modestness of the goals, and the scholarly consideration of the inefficacy of alternative treatment interventions tend to be entirely overlooked or lost sight of.

Although behavioral techniques have been criticized on numerous grounds (see, for example, Breger and McGaugh, 1965), those criticisms focusing on the ethics of behavioral intervention will be of primary interest to us here. It should be noted from the outset that treatment approaches that have been described as "behavioral" run the gamut from the most "orthodox" methods suggested by principles of operant learning to other methods which have empirically been shown to be of value. Accordingly, criticism on ethical or humanistic grounds (e.g., "Behavior therapists disregard the organism in their stimulus–response formulations") becomes substantially less valid as one moves from treatment approaches based on the teachings of B. F. Skinner to the multimodal behavioral treatment of, say, Arnold Lazarus (1973). And while all clinicians practicing behavior therapy—or any other therapy, for that matter (Roston and Sherrer, 1973)—attempt to influence or control their patients, the issue of control has somehow become singularly linked to behavior modification. Perhaps this is so because among their colleagues in the mental health profession, it is the behaviorists whose controlling techniques tend to be the least subtle and the most overt.

Writing in the American Psychiatric Association's journal *Hospital and Community Psychiatry*, Lucero, Vail, and Scherber (1968) examined moral and ethical issues in operant conditioning, posing such questions as "How much can we justify in the name of 'reshaping'?" and "Is deprivation ever justified?" The authors argued that operant methods such as shock, restraints, seclusion, deprivation, and punishment can be "dehumanizing and can at times lead to a total loss of human values" (p. 53). They reported that as a result of a workshop for staff members of the Minnesota State Hospital, guidelines for operant conditioning programs in Minnesota were devised. These guidelines provided that 1) aversive reinforcement was never to be used in general programs for groups of patients, but could be used in "unusual individual cases" under certain conditions; 2) deprivation of expected goods or services or of free movement was never to be used; 3) positive reinforcement was the only conditioning technique to be used; and 4) all new therapy techniques would be reviewed by a medical policy committee and would be administered only by thoroughly trained personnel.

The Lucero, Vail, and Scherber article stirred up a storm of protest. Miron (1968) aptly pointed out that many programs administered in the name of "operant conditioning" are not really operant conditioning programs at all—the use of physical restraints and prolonged seclusion have traditionally been "desperate measures" resorted to by overwhelmed staff. Other points made by Miron included the following:

- Shock-sticks produce a shock generated from flashlight batteries that, although painful, is not much more painful than some injections and is less brutal than electroconvulsive therapy and psychosurgery—the ethics of which Lucero, Vail, and Scherber did not question.

- The purpose of seclusion is not to punish but rather to provide a "time out" period to allow a tantrum to run its course without accidental reinforcement.

- In their attack on the use of deprivation in the context of a token economy system, the workshop participants ignored the fact that we all live under a similar economic system. According to the workshop standards, hundreds of successful token treatment programs would arbitrarily be declared "unethical."

- It is questionable that deprivation in and of itself reduces patients to a subhuman level, as punishment and deprivation are standard techniques in child-rearing practices; objections should not be raised toward the techniques but to the degree of sophistication with which they are carried out.

- The real deprivation with which we should be concerned is the deliberate deprivation of potential benefit to a patient when the alternative clearly amounts to a life sentence in a mental institution and in some cases a life spent in physical restraints.

- The most important aspect of all operant conditioning programs is the use of positive reinforcement.

- Tender loving care, indiscriminately or incorrectly applied (as it too often is) by well-intentioned but naive staff and relatives, reinforces undesirable behavior and too often leaves appropriate behavior unnoticed or ignored.

- According to the standards of the article, psychoanalysis might be prohibited in Minnesota.

Cahoon (1968) questioned Lucero et al.'s argument that certain methods can be in and of themselves labeled unjustified and undesirable. Cahoon also pointed out that deprivation as reflected in the behavior therapy literature includes procedures such as limiting and then systematically reintroducing food intake, cigarette smoking, and television viewing and that "making a patient 'earn' his cigarettes in order to 'buy' better mental health seems to be a good bargain." Lucero et al.'s incorrect usage of the terms "aversive reinforcement" and "deprivation" as well as other data suggested to Cahoon that behavior therapy "in the acceptable professional sense" was not being practiced in Minnesota.

In their comment on Lucero et al., Bragg and Wagner (1968) addressed themselves to the questionable efficacy of nondeprivational contingencies in a hospital setting. They argued that, whether the staff or the patients are aware of it, behavior is shaped by operant techniques anyway and that clearly defining such behavioral contingencies might result in shorter periods of hospitalization.

Ball (1968) tackled Lucero et al. head-on, declaring that their pronouncements resolved nothing and served only to delay discussion of critical issues. Ball noted that all treatments carry with them responsibilities in using them, but this doesn't mean that professionals should shrink from the opportunity of using them. Four questions raised and subsequently discussed by Ball were as follows (my summary):

1. *Are not operant conditioners "playing God" by defining goals of personal and social development for patients?*

   No. The goals of operant conditioning programs are modest (involving activities of daily living) and moreover are (more so than with other therapeutic approaches) open and explicit.

2. *Might some staff members use the behavior control possibilities provided by operant conditioning to justify their repressively punitive, prison-like management of patients?*

   No, because the goals of a systematic, professionally administered operant conditioning program are stated in terms of patient gain, not staff convenience. Such a program determines whether it is the needs of the patient or the staff that are being met by monitoring patient progress with open records and occasional demonstrations of patients' proficiency.

3. *Isn't operant conditioning a form of mechanistic "animal training" that denies the patient's integrity?*

   Operant conditioning is oriented towards learning and growth. At times one must begin teaching "mechanistically" in order for the individual to learn and to achieve a sense of satisfaction and hopefulness, in the hope of setting off a chain reaction of positive emotional experiences for the patient and his or her loved ones.

4. *Are we not depriving the patient of the opportunity of making choices, of exercising free will?*

   No. Patients on token economy wards are given the opportunity to make choices and exercise free will—probably even more than the typical institutionalized mental patient.[5] The only thing token economy patients are being deprived of is their regressive status in life.

---

[5] A provocative discussion of token economies from a legal perspective appears in Wexler (1973).

"That a high-level technology," Ball concluded, "calls for a high level of humanism must not deter us from the task of developing both capabilities" (p. 232).

In their rebuttal to all of the criticism that their article engendered, Lucero and Vail (1968) called the responses of Miron, Bragg and Wagner, Ball, and Cahoon "naive" and claimed that they "missed the point." But a careful reading of Lucero and Vail's reply clearly shows that it is *they* who are naive and "miss the point." For example, although all of the discussants touched on the careful, regimented, and systematic nature of operant conditioning programs, Lucero and Vail insisted on creating straw-man issues by stating that "no one is going to be walking around on his own cognizance in any Minnesota state hospital bearing an electric cattle-prod or whip or any similar engine or device" (p. 233). Moreover, as Miron (1970) stated in a final rejoinder, Lucero et al. were not consistent in demanding that the burden of proof with respect to morally questionable procedures be borne by those administering such procedures. Thus, one of the articles criticized by Lucero et al. had described the indiscriminate use of electroconvulsive treatment. As pointed out by Miron (1970):

> . . . by some obscure reasoning, they interpreted this program as a typical example of operant conditioning, apparently because deprivation was used—after the ECT had failed. They seem to equate all use of deprivation with operant conditioning. Nevertheless, I do not understand the ethical criteria of a workshop which faces the opposite direction when 250 patients are given innumerable convulsive shocks, with minimal clinical justification, and then becomes excessively concerned over the ethics of deprivation, as mild as it was! One is forced to conclude that had the ECT been successful, the question of ethics would never have been raised, since deprivation would not have been used. (pp. 357–358)

The ethical issue raised by Lucero, Vail, and Scherber was viewed by Miron (1968) as spurious:

> The ethical considerations in operant conditioning are no different from those involved in any other form of therapy: to aim for the maximum benefit to the patient and to society, giving careful consideration to cases where the two may conflict.
>
> If the ethical problems of operant conditioning seem more acute than for other therapies, it is because, for the most part, the skillful use of operant conditioning often modifies behavior much more effectively than do the traditional therapies. Because the techniques are novel to the medical profession at large and are almost always designed and implemented by nonmedical personnel, staff members of medical institu-

tions are less likely to be familiar with the procedures and are thus more likely to raise questions of ethics. (p. 226)

SEXUAL CONTACT AND THE ISSUE OF CONTROL

In his controversial book detailing accounts of sexual intimacy between patients and therapists, Martin Shepard (1971) acknowledged that patients in psychotherapy are "far more open to the suggestions of a therapist than they would be to those of a man on the street." The vulnerability and trustfulness of the patient in psychotherapy have been recognized by laws which view the psychotherapist–patient relationship to be fiduciary in nature. How many therapists breach their fiduciary duty by converting their patients' "openness to suggestion" into sexual intimacy? What factors are responsible for such encounters? Can such encounters be beneficial to patients? Are such encounters necessarily unethical? These are some of the questions to be raised in any discussion of sexual contact as it bears on the issue of control.

How Many Therapists Become Intimate with Patients?

For understandable reasons, the full extent of erotic or sexual contact (let us call such contacts "close encounters") between patients and health professionals will never be known. In an oft-cited study of the problem, Kardener, Fuller, and Mensh (1973) surveyed a random sample of 1,000 physicians' attitudes toward erotic contact with patients. A total of 46 per cent of the doctors, representing five medical specialties (gynecology, surgery, internal medicine, general practice, and psychiatry) returned the investigators' anonymous questionnaire. Kardener et al. reported that from 5 to 7.2 per cent of the sampled physicians had engaged in sexual intercourse with their patients. Focusing on the data for psychiatrists ($n=114$), 5 per cent reported that they had had sexual intercourse with their patients and an additional 5 per cent reported that they had indulged in erotic practices short of sexual intercourse.

Using a questionnaire similar to that of Kardener et al., a study by Perry (1976) was designed to determine if beliefs and practices regarding physical contact varied as a function of gender of the physician. Perry mailed her questionnaire to a random sample of 500 female physicians, half in New York and half in California. Approximately one-third of the physicians responded ($n=164$) and there were 156 usable questionnaires. The four medical specialties that were best represented were pediatrics, psychiatry, general practice, and internal medicine, though responses from a total of seventeen medical specialties were received. Generally, the women sampled by Perry tended to be younger than the male physicians sampled by Kardener et al. As a group, more of the female physicians tended to be single than the male physicians. As compared with Kardener et al.'s sample, Perry's sample included more women who had been in practice for one to ten years, fewer who had been in practice for eleven to fifteen years, and approximately the same number for more than fifteen years. Keeping in mind the differences between the two studies, Perry's conclusions were as follows:

> Half of the female physicians believed in nonerotic touching; 2% believed in erotic touching. By comparison, the previous study (1) revealed that fewer male physicians believed in nonerotic touching. However, more male than female physicians believed and engaged in erotic touching. Fewer women than men attempted to treat sexual problems in their practice. More younger women than older women touched patients. Female physicians' attitudes toward touching were not related to the sex of the patient, area of specialty, marital status, or geographical location. . . .
>
> Physicians have definite and sometimes opposing viewpoints regarding nonerotic and erotic involvement with their patients. Male physicians do not believe in erotic involvement but in practice do become involved, while female physicians consistently oppose erotic involvement. (Perry, 1976, p. 840)

In a nationwide survey of 703 licensed psychologists (347 males, 310 females, and 9 undeclared) who responded to a questionnaire that was similar to the one used by Kardener et al., it was found that 5.5 per cent of the male respondents and .6 per cent of the female respondents had reportedly had sexual intercourse with their patients (Holroyd and Brodsky, 1977). Of those who acknowledged that they had had sexual intercourse once, 80 per cent had repeated it. Similarly, Butler (1975) reported in her unpublished doctoral dissertation that of the therapists in her sample who had been sexually involved with one patient, 75 per cent reported that they had gotten sexually involved with at least one other patient. In a published study, Butler and a colleague at the California School of Professional Psychology in Los Angeles estimated—without citing sources—that "one in five therapists would be intimate with his patients" (Butler and Zelen, 1977, p. 139). Exactly how these researchers arrived at this estimate is unclear, as there is no data cited or presented in the article to support it.

Though the available data is by no means definitive, it seems fair to estimate that approximately 5 per cent of all psychiatrists and psychologists in private practice have engaged in sexual intercourse with their patients, and perhaps as many as 10 per cent of all psychiatrists and psychologists have engaged in some form of sexual contact.

What Factors Are Responsible for Close Encounters?

As pointed out in Chapter 1, the range of what is done in the name of "therapy" is rapidly broadening. Psychotherapy has gone from being simply "talking therapy" to talking, feeling, touching, screaming (etc.) therapy. Analogously, the role of the therapist has changed from one that could be described as that of a "mirror" reflecting patients' hopes, fears, and concerns to one that allows for a feeling, acting person who experiences, reacts to, and shares[6] feelings with his patients. This is as true for the behavior therapist who rides elevators with his elevator-phobic patient as it is for the organizer of a nude group marathon. The immediate problem stemming from this societally endorsed "liberation" of the therapist from the mirror role is that which typically accompanies any form of liberation, namely, limit setting. Where is the line to be drawn on all of the feeling, touching, experiencing, and sharing, and who is to draw it?

In his consideration of the factors that led to the seduction of psychotherapy patients, Dahlberg (1970) wrote that "these aging men, some in a depressive and needy period, somehow let themselves be convinced by their patients' fantasies that they might recapture their youth." Marmor (1976) delineated two overlapping categories of factors that contributed to what we are calling close encounters. Situational factors included the nature of the psychotherapy arrangement itself, the aloneness in the office, the baring of highly personal thoughts and feelings, and the therapist's own libidinal needs. Among the characterological factors cited by Marmor were countertransferential needs:

> Most psychotherapists, male *and* female, are motivated to some degree in their choice of profession by a psychological need to be a helping figure, a need which is gratified by the dependent expectations of their patients. Thus, just as the female patient often reacts to the therapist in the transference as a wise, protective, and loving father-surrogate, the therapist's countertransference needs may lead him to respond as a loving and affectionate "parent" to his emotionally deprived "child"....
>
> Others... have used other excuses to mask their own counter-transference needs, excuses such as wanting to help patients overcome their sexual inhibitions, or their feelings of inadequacy, or their "fears of intimacy," or their "rejection of their femininity," or their orgasmic difficulties. Although the immediate impulses behind these rationalizations are usually erotic and situational, there are often characterological features involved that are nonerotic in nature, especially where such

---

[6]Psychologist/humorist Harold Greenwald (Note 10) has quipped that it is impossible to be licensed in California without using the word "share."

behavior tends to be repetitive. One such pattern is an unconscious hostility to women with a sadistic need to exploit, humiliate, and ultimately reject them. Another is the well-known Don Juan complex, a reaction formation against inner feelings of masculine inadequacy or pseudohomosexual fears. (pp. 321–322)

Respondents to the Butler and Zelen (1977) study openly acknowledged their own vulnerability to and need for sexual contact with their patients:

> The data revealed that the therapists' own personal needs and motivations overwhelmingly contributed to the sexual contact, and that the therapists acknowledged their needs as a factor in this sexual behavior (although not necessarily at that time). Ninety percent reported having been "vulnerable," "needy," and/or "lonely" when the sexual contact occurred. These high-need states were related to unsatisfying marriages, recent separations and/or divorces. One might assume the therapists shifted their source of gratification to their patients during these vulnerable or needy periods of time. (p. 142)

Butler and Zelen's data and interpretations should be read cautiously, however, in light of the extreme limitations of their sampling methodology.

Are Close Encounters Beneficial to Patients?

Lief (1978) has argued that "it would be detrimental to humanistic medicine for all affectionate 'touching' to be rigorously avoided, yet practitioners have to be careful not to go beyond rather obvious limits, and to be particularly scrupulous with those patients who may be prone to misinterpret such behaviors" (p. 57). Unfortunately, there are no "rather obvious limits" for those practitioners who have an ample supply of legitimate-sounding rationales for engaging in therapist–patient sexual intercourse. Forty-five percent of the therapists in the Butler and Zelen (1977) sample rationalized their conduct with statements like "The patient needed the assurance that she was an attractive and desirable woman" (p. 143). In a more extensive survey of psychologists' opinions on this matter, only 9 per cent responded to the question "Under what circumstances might . . . erotic behavior be utilized in treatment?" (Holroyd and Brodsky, 1977); among those who responded, the answers ran the gamut from "Almost anything could conceivably be used in treatment" to more specific notions about how such behavior might be useful for therapists treating sexual problems, how it might help to develop "mutual positive regard," and how it might promote patient personality growth by enhancement of the patient's self-concept or broadening of his or her experiences. Less than 3 per cent of the psychologists sampled indicated that patient–therapist sexual involvement might be beneficial:

> The comments could be grouped under vague benefits ("the possibility of positive results exists"), specific purposes ("if a person were crippled by inferiority feelings based on the conviction of being unacceptable to anyone for anything; if one is having severe doubts of sexual identity, and if a person truly does not know the mechanics of sexual intercourse"), and the belief that erotic contact and/or intercourse are not outside the boundaries of the therapy relationship ("nor should psychotherapy per se exclude the obvious, i.e., the need/desire to touch, stimulate, and explore the boundaries of contact and intimacy"; "the use of sexual energy, up to and including actual intercourse between therapist and client, can have considerable healing effect for the client"). (Holroyd and Brodsky, 1977, p. 849)

The thesis of McCartney (1966) was that some patients needed to work out their transference-related problems by doing more than talking about them. On this ground, McCartney condoned as therapeutic therapist/patient nudity, touching, and intercourse. McCartney advised therapists who pursued the latter course of action that they might have to "remain objective and yet react sexually appropriately in order to lead the immature person into full maturity."

But how objective can a therapist be with his pants down? Masters and Johnson (1966) have observed that "It's damn hard to be in bed and be objective at the same time." In the Holroyd and Brodsky (1977) study, the few respondents who indicated that erotic contact might be helpful qualified their remarks by noting "the danger of losing objectivity, the requirement that the therapist must not be personally needy, and the importance of erotic contact serving primarily the needs of the client" (pp. 848–849). One study that reviewed and analyzed the effects of intercourse between therapists and patients found that in 47 per cent of the cases negative effects were reported, in 32 per cent mixed effects were reported, and in 21 per cent positive effects were reported either for the patient or for the therapist (Taylor and Wagner, 1976).

Marmor (1976) observed that "most erotic breaches of the therapist–patient relationship occur with women who are physically attractive, almost never with the aged, the infirm, or the ugly, thus giving the lie to the oft-heard rationalization on the part of such therapists that they were acting in the interest of the patient!" (pp. 320–321). He cautioned that "when a therapist lends reality to a patient's erotized fantasies of transference love, he fosters a serious confusion between reality and fantasy in the patient, with inevitably antitherapeutic results" (Marmor, 1976, pp. 322–323).

Are Close Encounters Unethical?

Ethical issues seldom have clear and straightforward solutions. Yet therapist–patient sex has been considered wrong virtually since the time that psychotherapy, in the formal sense, was conceived. One analyst in Freud's circle, Sandor Ferenczi, rationalized his kissing and hugging of patients by saying that he was, in essence, providing emotional restitution for the love and support that the patient did not receive as a child (Marmor, 1976). Ferenczi was strongly reprimanded for this by Freud, who warned that the same rationalization might lead others to take further liberties with patients.

In 1973, the American Psychiatric Association straightforwardly stated that sexual contact between therapists and patients was unethical. Four years later, in its revision of its Code of Ethics, the American Psychological Association (1977) made a similar statement. The overall position of the American Psychological Association was stated in paragraph *a* of Principle 6: Welfare of the Consumer.

> Psychologists are continually cognizant of their own needs and of their inherently powerful position *vis à vis* clients, in order to avoid exploiting their trust and dependency. Psychologists make every effort to avoid dual relationships with clients and/or relationships which might impair their professional judgment or increase the risk of client exploitation. Examples of such dual relationships include treating employees, supervisees, close friends or relatives. Sexual intimacies with clients are unethical.

Another side to the issue of control. It is true that patients come trustingly to psychotherapists and to some extent place themselves in the psychotherapist's hands. Therapists who exploit their patients by manipulating them into sexual involvement do so out of their own psychopathological needs and in violation of what are widely accepted standards of right and proper behavior for therapists. Yet there is another side to the issue of control in relation to sexual contact.

If the fact that therapist–patient sex is unethical has been sufficiently popularized in the mass media, why do patients continue to allow themselves to be exploited by therapists (assuming that patients in therapy are not raped)? It does seem to be a reasonable assumption that denunciations of therapist–patient sexual involvement by professional organizations and more sensationalized accounts of such activities in the media have reached the vast majority of the psychotherapy-consuming public. And yet therapist–patient sex continues to be a problem. Why?

Of the patients who have heard or read about the unsavory aspects of therapist–patient sex, perhaps some don't believe it, some don't care to believe it, and some don't care. Some patients might believe that it is unethical for *other* therapists to engage in such behavior but not for theirs, because he knows what he is doing. For some who are fully aware of the taboo against it, the very idea of therapist–patient sex may represent a tremendously exciting and stimulating prospect in an otherwise dull and miserable existence. For others, it may well represent the ultimate "conquering" of a significant and heretofore unattainable love object. Conversely, therapist–patient sex may be an expression of hostility against the therapist or against some figure the therapist represents. Marmor (1976) discussed the possibility of an eroticized transference as an element in therapist–patient sex: "A . . . factor is the degree of seductiveness or flirtatiousness exhibited by the patient, including the way she dresses and displays her physical attributes and actually reaches out for or invites physical closeness' (p. 321). It is again emphasized that the therapist who responds to such cues does so out of his own vulnerability and/or his own nonprofessional desires. However, the question of interest in the present context is "Who is controlling whom?"

The case of Roy v. Hartogs. A detailed account of plaintiff Ms. Julie Roy's relationship with defendant Dr. Renatus Hartogs is presented in her book *Betrayal* (Freeman and Roy, 1976), written with a professional writer (who had previously written a book with Dr. Hartogs on Lee Harvey Oswald and Jack Ruby). This relationship deserves examination in the context of the issues of control under discussion (my summary):

In March 1969, on the advice of a female psychologist, Julie Roy began therapy with psychiatrist Renatus Hartogs on a twice-weekly basis. According to Ms. Roy, by July 1969, after many exhortations to do so by Dr. Hartogs, the two were having sexual intercourse regularly as a part of "therapy." At the trial Hartogs denied ever having had sex with this or any other patient and based his defense on the following points: 1) Ms. Roy was a psychotic (paranoid schizophrenic) individual with a hatred of men and had initiated this legal action maliciously; 2) When Ms. Roy was asked if Hartogs had any gross abnormalities in his genital area, she had replied "No," though pictures supplied to the court graphically showed such an abnormality (a tumor); 3) Hartogs testified that he had been unable to have sex since 1965 because of the tumor (after a court-initiated urological examination indicated that Hartogs was able to have sex, he said that he was able to have an erection but that it was too painful to engage in sexual intercourse); 4) Hartogs presented as evidence photographs of the couch on which Roy alleged that they had had intercourse, arguing that the couch was too small for such activity; 5) Although Roy alleged that Hartogs had taken her to the movies and out to eat at a restaurant, he flatly denied this (in fact, Roy's allegations in this regard were never substantiated).

An expert witness testified that the tumor Hartogs had was one that could be drained by Hartogs himself. When drained the tumor would not readily be identifiable as an abnormality to the untrained eye. Also during the course of the proceedings the plaintiff attempted to admit into evidence—the judge disallowed it—the testimony of other women who claimed that Hartogs had attempted to have sexual intercourse with them in the guise of psychotherapy. At the end of the nine-day trial, the judge's charge to the jury emphasized that it was the jury's responsibility to decide whether Julie Roy's charges against Dr. Hartogs were fact or fantasy. The question each of the six jurors were charged with answering "Yes" or "No" to was "Did the defendant, Dr. Hartogs, a psychiatrist, induce the plaintiff, Julie Roy, to have sexual intercourse with him while she was his patient, and did he, in fact, have such intercourse with her?" The jury deliberated for a little over two hours and reached a verdict of "Yes," with five of the jurors agreeing and one (the forewoman) voting "No."

When arguments about monetary damages were made, Roy's lawyers asked for $250,000 in compensatory damages and $1 million in punitive damages. Hartogs's lawyer argued against payment of any damages to Roy on the grounds that no damage had been done, since the woman had been paranoid at the beginning of the affair and was paranoid at the end of it. In his charge to the jury concerning damages, the judge emphasized that the question at issue was whether or not Roy's condition had been aggravated by Hartogs's "treatment." In less than two hours the jury returned a verdict of $250,000 in compensatory damages and $100,000 in punitive damages. Subsequently, the trial judge reduced the compensatory damages to $50,000 writing in a twenty-three-page opinion that it had not been proven that permanent emotional damage had resulted from Hartogs's treatment. Hartogs appealed the trial court's decision in the Appellate term of the Supreme Court of New York, and that Court totally eliminated the punitive damages and reduced the compensatory damages to $25,000.

In the interest of a balanced presentation it is important to note that Dr. Hartogs's claims concerning the severity of Ms. Roy's condition, the hostility she harbored toward her father, and the malicious basis of the lawsuit as a result of displaced hostility find some support in the text of *Betrayal*. In that book we learn that Roy wore the same dress for months and that she was troubled by suicidal ideation and bisexuality. As regards the possibly vindictive nature of the lawsuit, there are statements in Roy's book that will cause mental health professionals to wonder whether it was in fact Hartogs by whom the plaintiff was betrayed or her father:

> She realized her experience with Dr. Hartogs had reawakened the feeling she had suffered when her father had abandoned her. Perhaps the trial did bring a certain feeling of revenge, she thought, a revenge she really wanted to inflict on the most important man in her life—her father. (p. 260)
>
> ... she laughed over a sketch a television artist was drawing of Dr. Hartogs; no cameras were allowed in court.... if she could draw her own sketch of Dr. Hartogs, she thought, he would come out looking like Rasputin, with strange, messianic eyes. (p. 235)

The two vignettes reprinted above—one clearly linking her hatred of Hartogs to her father and the other betraying her "messianic" perception of her doctor—persisted even at the trial. Hartogs's contention that Roy was out to destroy him—that she had, in fact, threatened to murder him—was also substantiated in her book: "At one time she had been very serious about killing Dr. Hartogs, then herself" (p. 259). Whether or not Hartogs had indeed sexually exploited his patient was a matter for the jury to decide, and they answered that question affirmatively. Whether or not Hartogs (or any other clinician) could be exploited by a patient is a matter that merits consideration by mental health professionals. Current mental hygiene laws in New York and other states have been viewed by some mental health professionals as unrealistic with respect to the suppositions they make concerning the competencies of psychotic patients (see Serban and Gidynski, 1974). According to research psychiatrist George Serban of New York University Medical School, inadequacies exist in right-to-treatment laws as they affect the patient–therapist relationship: "On the one hand, the right-to-treatment law in New York assumes that any patient, even the psychotic patient, is aware and knowledgeable enough to accept or refuse any form of treatment; on the other hand, the implication of Roy v. Hartogs is that the patient was not aware of the nature of the 'treatment'—a 'treatment' which was pursued on a regular basis for thirteen months" (Serban, personal communication).

Like most other mental health professionals, Serban sees no place for any form of sexual activity between patients and therapists. However, Serban points out that legal/ethical dilemmas remain unresolved with respect to the controversial treatment of patients with sexual dysfunction; treatment that includes patient–therapist or patient–surrogate sexual intercourse as an integral component of the treatment. Serban cautions that "any distortion of the therapeutic relationship for the personal gain of the therapist should be considered a breach of the doctor–patient relationship and dealt with by the appropriate authorities. Patients must be fully informed of the nature and possible outcomes of the treatment (e.g., one possible outcome might be the disruption of the patient's existing or previous emotional ties)." Serban argues that terms like "sex therapy," "sex therapist," "surrogate," and related terms associated with the therapy techniques of Masters and Johnson will need to be better defined legally before patient–therapist sexual activity can legitimately constitute the basis of a malpractice suit.

What Can Be Done about Close Encounters?

Regardless of whether what we have called "close encounters" are a matter of the patient controlling the therapist or vice versa, the problem involved can no longer be downplayed or merely treated as a complicating feature of treatment. (See, e.g., Voth, 1972; Siassi and Thomas, 1973.) Blanket declarations by professional organizations citing patient–therapist sexual involvement as unethical is a fine first step but much more needs to be done; more specific legal and ethical guidelines to reduce ambiguity and to close gaping loopholes are needed. For example, is it legally or ethically permissible for doctor and patient, counselor and counselee, or sensitivity trainer and trainee to engage in sexual intercourse "outside" of their working relationship? Indeed, can an "outside" of such a working relationship exist? What about the situation where the sensitivity trainer happens to be a psychiatrist?

Consider the case of psychiatrist Martin Shepard who had his license to practice medicine revoked by the New York State Board of Regents on the grounds of sexual misconduct with patients. On the basis of material contained in an autobiographical book (originally published in 1972 with the title *A Psychiatrist's Head* and subsequently re-published with the title *Memoirs of a Defrocked Psychoanalyst*) Shepard was indicted for cohabiting with patients. In an interview on NBC's *Tomorrow* program (aired February 22, 1979) Dr. Shepard denied that he had ever engaged in sexual relations with a patient. The host of that talk show, Tom Snyder, asked Shepard if he had written anything in the book "that would make people tend to think" that he had been intimate with a patient:

> *Shepard:* Um... well, it depends. You know, it depends. I think that there are some people who might think that. But the people who would think that are the people who think that every person who sees somebody, and they know they're a doctor, that person is a patient of theirs. I mean that was the charge of the State. At that point I wrote about a lot of experimenting I had in one summer, really, a summer where my marriage broke up and lots of other things were going on. I mean that was part of it but it certainly wasn't the whole book.
>
> I was at that time working with, uh, in a center in New York that was modeled after Esalen in California. We're doing a lot of groups.

We never considered it for the treatment of sick people. The brochure—it was a place called Anthos [?]—it said, "this isn't for the treatment of sick people, these are retreats in the country, a weekend, a workshop." And I was the only physician working there—I wasn't even the director of it—but I was a doctor working there and other people leading groups were college dropouts and dentists and an advertising man; a lot of skillful people who didn't have the credentials. And, um, people would sign up for a weekend and that would be it. And in some of those groups I was intimate with some people. And I wrote about that in the book—

Snyder: [Responding to the phrase, "I was intimate with some people"] But not in the professional sense. You weren't counseling them at the time—

Shepard: I wasn't counseling them, I—they never said they considered me their doctor, I never considered them patients of mine but I was there as a group facilitator or a group leader or whatever. So the State, in its ultimate wisdom, decided that since I was a group leader and I had credentials after my name, all these people must have thought of me as a doctor. And, uh, therefore if I were writing about intimacies with them, I was taking advantage of a doctor–patient relationship. When I had the hearings, I brought in one person who was one of the characters in the book and she said, "Look, this man, I never considered him a doctor, and he wasn't a doctor"—that was the one person that the State never asked any questions of. And I brought in a letter from another character in the book who was a psychotherapist herself also saying she was not a patient of mine (she's a psychotherapist, she went up, her husband was a doctor)—had nothing to do with the doctor–patient relationship. They wouldn't admit that as evidence because they thought that was only a written word; it was hearsay. And I would say to the chairman of the hearing panel, I'd say, "But a book is hearsay. Where are your people accusing me?"

It was no good. I mean it was a Catch-22 where people were out to make an example of me. And I think it had to do with, uh, some ways people—there may have been souls who feel they have to safeguard morality in general. And anytime that sex rears its pretty or ugly head they want to make an example.

Some may feel that under the circumstances described above the revocation of Shepard's license was justified. Others may argue that such a punishment was unjustifiably harsh and that less extreme action could have been taken. Clearly, more specific professional guidelines are needed. Perhaps what professional organizations and state licensing boards need to do first is to specify in terms as unambiguous as possible exactly what actions by whom and under what conditions shall be considered to be ethically unacceptable and/or legally actionable. Second, some equitable procedure for enforcing the guidelines as well as for the lodging and the answering of complaints must be devised. Peer and/or citizen

review of claims against professionals seems desirable. The range of punitive and/or rehabilitative sanctions applied against offending professionals
needs to be innovatively broadened. For example, calls for the enforcement of the professional code of ethics through insurance proscription
have been made (Asher, 1976) and eventually enacted. (For example,
in the professional liability insurance policy offered to psychologists by
American Home Insurance, the carrier assumes no responsibility for the
sexual misconduct of the insured person; the insurance company may
provide a lawyer to defend the psychologist against a complaint of sexual
misconduct, but it will not pay damages in the event that such charges are
proved.) In addition to disciplining their colleagues, concerned mental
health professionals and organizations must work to clearly convey to the
public their sense of the unethicalness and impropriety of sexual contact
between therapists and patients. The problem of "close encounters" will
hopefully be less of a problem in the future as a result of the efforts of a
concerned professional community (e.g., Masters and Johnson, 1970;
Marmor, 1972, 1976; Demac, 1975; Finney, 1975; Macklin, 1976; Davidson, 1977; Lief, 1978), and an informed public.

ETHICS, LAW, AND THE MENTAL HEALTH PROFESSIONAL

In their *Professional Psychology* article entitled "Malpractice:
What's New?" Roston and Sherrer (1973) cited the decision of a federal
court in *United States v. Simon et al.* (425 F.2d 796), which held that
professionals may be held liable for acts a jury considers detrimental to
the public interest *whether or not* professional organization guidelines
had been adhered to. The court rejected the argument that compliance
with established standards was a valid defense, holding that such compliance was "persuasive but not conclusive" evidence. Roston and Sherrer commented on the implication of the *Simon* decision:

> The thrust of that decision was that unless ethical and professional
> standards promulgated by professional associations afford adequate
> safeguards to members of the general public, said standards afford little
> or no protection to the professional from either criminal prosecution or
> civil (malpractice) action.
>   The lesson to be learned from the *Simon et al.* decision is that
> ethical or professional standards adopted by various professions will be
> given less than conclusive weight unless standards and ethics are spelled
> out with a sufficient degree of specificity and validity to be of clear value
> to the professional in his day-to-day activities. Highly embellished lan-
> guage to the effect that in his practice a professional shall always use
> "mature judgment" based on his education and experience is ineffec-
> tual. With the weight of the *Simon et al.* decision on the books, profes-

sional societies should periodically update and improve their ethical and professional codes of conduct. Further, professional societies should encourage legislatures to translate the most valid and accepted aspects of those codes into legal statutes. (pp. 271–272)

The need for sober, well-informed, and well-focused discussion of current ethical/legal issues attendant to the delivery of mental health services is critical. The welter of ethical/legal problems—only touched on in these two chapters—begs ordering. Today, activities that are legal and considered to be ethical in California may be illegal and considered ethically improper in Nebraska. What is considered legal is not necessarily ethical. For example, suppose a patient gives his informed consent to engage in sexual intercourse with his therapist; such behavior on the part of the therapist would probably be held to be within the law, though it would hardly be considered ethically appropriate. Other problems attaching to the use of the doctrine of informed consent as the panacean solution to the problem of control were discussed in this chapter.

Working closely with responsible public representatives, professional organizations need to formulate specific professional guidelines and then disseminate those guidelines to members of the profession and the public. Until such guidelines are prepared, mental health professionals must practice within the relatively nonspecific guidelines of their professional organizations, monitor and participate in lawmaking activity in this area, and remain responsive to an internalized code of ethics that is in the finest traditions of the profession.

MALPRACTICE
LITIGATION

In our introduction to the area of malpractice we have examined some
of the evidence which suggests that the number of claims against mental
health professionals will be rising in the near future. We have looked at
the anatomy of a malpractice suit and at how some of the ethical and legal
issues involved in mental health practice are interrelated. We now turn
our attention to malpractice litigation itself. The following two chapters
contain vignettes of cases and claims brought against health professionals
and institutions. In Chapter 5 most of the defendants named in the suits
were involved in the delivery of mental health services. In Chapter 6 a
sampling of suits against other health professionals is presented. Both
chapters illustrate how a wide range of legal principles have been applied
and interpreted by the courts.

The cases presented in Chapters 5 and 6 were culled from appellate
court reporters, law review articles, articles in scientific journals, and
conversations with practicing attorneys. In some instances the details
presented by the source were sketchy, and that lack of detail is reflected
in the case vignette as it is presented herein. Some of the cases were in the
claim stage, or still in litigation, or in the process of being appealed at the
time of this writing. Where a claim was settled through a private agreement and not a public proceeding, the reference "Citation Withheld"
appears. Citations were also withheld from some of the case vignettes at
the request and the discretion of the attorney who supplied the case
material. Some of the cases (e.g., 5.67, 5.91, 5.94, 5.108, 5.109, and
5.115) are not malpractice proceedings—not even by our broad definition
of malpractice (see p. 40)—but have been included here for their interest
value to mental health professionals. None of the case material should be
construed as constituting a definitive statement of the law.

5

Cases Involving Mental Health Professionals

The claims and litigated cases in this chapter have been arbitrarily grouped according to the following overlapping categories of interest:

- Suicide or Attempted Suicide (5.1–5.23)
- Assault and/or Battery by Patient (5.24–5.43)
- Assault and/or Battery by Therapist (5.44–5.46)
- False Imprisonment (5.47–5.54)
- Treatment with Medication (5.55–5.57)
- Electroshock Therapy (5.58–5.66)
- Breach of Confidentiality (5.67–5.74)
- Defamation (5.75–5.80)
- Sexual Improprieties (5.81–5.91)
- Violation of Civil Rights (5.92–5.100)
- General Diagnosis and Treatment (5.101–5.123)

A discussion of some of the legal and ethical issues raised by these cases and claims will appear in Part IV of this book.

SUICIDE OR ATTEMPTED SUICIDE

5.1 BAKER v. UNITED STATES
226 F. Supp. 129 (Iowa, 1964)

Kenneth Baker, age 61, had been referred to the Veterans Administration (V.A.) Hospital by his attending physician, Dr. C. E.

Schrock. Dr. Schrock's note accompanying the application for admission indicated that Mr. Baker had exhibited progressive symptoms of depression over the prior three months and that "suicidal content" was evident. According to the patient's wife, at the time of the patient's admission to the V.A. Hospital she had conferred with Dr. James Kennedy who was then acting Chief of the Neuropsychiatric Service. Mrs. Baker testified that she advised Dr. Kennedy that[1]

> ... there was a suicidal tendency on the part of her husband and told him about finding a gun her husband had hid in one of the buildings on the farm about three weeks before. Dr. Kennedy interviewed the patient for an hour to an hour and a half, visited with the patient's wife and brother, examined the admitting certificate above referred to, and advised the patient's wife that the patient would be admitted provided certain financial data concerning the patient was furnished (the doctor requested this data for the purpose of confirming that the patient's belief as to his state of poverty was in fact a delusion and completely unfounded). This data was furnished the next day and Dr. Kennedy then ordered his admission to Ward 10E, an open ward, because as the doctor testified "in my opinion he did not present himself as a suicidal risk." The patient remained on this open ward on the 10th floor for the next three days and had free access to go to the 3rd floor for meals, to the canteen, and to go outside. On August 27, 1960, the patient left the ward on the 10th floor voluntarily and went to the grounds immediately outside the hospital building. At about 7:30 p. m., the patient jumped into a window well 13 feet deep in an obvious suicide attempt. He suffered scalp wounds, fractures of the left clavicle, the 8th, 9th and 10th ribs, and the left transverse processes of the 3rd, 4th and 5th lumbar vertebral bodies. About six hours later the patient suffered an occlusion of the left carotid artery. Thereafter the patient suffered a complete paralysis of his right side. On April 19, 1961, the patient was removed to Restopia, a private nursing home, where he now remains. The patient is completely and permanently disabled both mentally and physically and requires constant nursing attendance.

Mrs. Baker brought suit against the United States, seeking $100,000 in damages for injuries sustained by her husband and $25,000 in damages for loss of consortorium. The complaint specifically charged the V.A. staff with negligence in failing to

> (1) maintain sufficient physical restriction over said patient; (2) maintain proper supervision over said patient; (3) exercise ordinary and due care for said patient in his existing mental and physical condition; (4) properly diagnose the patient's illness and mental condition and to

---

[1]The text that follows was excerpted from the court reporter. Liberal use of quotations from court reporters has been made throughout this book in order to provide readers with both the content and "tone" of the judicial record. These excerpts have not been edited and will therefore vary in terms of the referencing style employed.

reasonably determine that he was in such condition that he might be reasonably expected to commit suicide if not properly supervised and restrained; (5) heed the information and warning from the patient's attending physician and family regarding his condition; and in (6) maintaining a deep pit or window well uncovered in close proximity to the area provided for mental patients and freely accessible to them.

The court rendered judgment for the United States, holding that the evidence was sufficient to establish that the acting chief of the neuropsychiatric service exercised the proper standard of care. No evidence was found to indicate that the hospital employees failed to carry out the orders of Dr. Kennedy or any other physician. Neither was there any evidence indicating an appreciable change in the patient's condition (over the course of time he spent in the V.A. hospital) which might have required action on the part of the hospital employees not covered by Dr. Kennedy's instructions. With regard to the hazard of the window well and the issues of the requisite standard of care, the court concluded as follows:

> ... The window well into which the patient leaped was enclosed by a heavy mesh wire fence which was at least three feet high. This was not a case of the patient falling into the window well but the injury was caused by a deliberate leap of the patient over the fence into the window well.
>
> Although it may have been better practice to cover the window well the Court finds that under the evidence in this case the defendant was not negligent in failing to close the window well with a suitable covering.
>
> The negligence, if any, which was the proximate cause of the patient's injuries arises out of the failure of Dr. Kennedy to properly diagnose the patient as a sufficient suicide risk so as to require closer supervision than was furnished by the immediate assignment of the patient to an open ward. A closed ward on the 9th floor was available to which patients were assigned when close supervision was deemed advisable. The issues are: What standard of care was required of the hospital and its staff? Was that standard of care violated in assigning the patient to an open ward?
>
> [5, 6] There appear to be no Iowa cases involving the standard of care required of mental hospitals toward their patients. But it appears generally, that the care required of a hospital includes giving such care to a patient as the hospital knew or in the exercise of reasonable care should have known was required. This duty is measured by the degree of care, skill and diligence customarily exercised by hospitals generally in the community. A hospital is not an insurer of a patient's safety and is not required to guard against that which a reasonable person under the circumstances would not anticipate....
>
> The standard of care required of mental hospitals in other jurisdictions follow these same general standards. Mounds Park Hospital v. Von Eye, 245 F.2d 756, 70 A.L.R.2d 335 (8 Cir. 1957). It is particularly recognized in the treatment of mental patients that diagnosis is not an exact science. Diagnosis with absolute precision and certainty is impossible. Further the objective is treatment not merely incarcera-

tion. Treatment requires the restoration of confidence in the patient. This in turn requires that restrictions be kept at a minimum. Risks must be taken or the case left as hopeless. See Fahey v. United States, 153 F.Supp. 878, 885 (S.D.N.Y.1957), reversed on other grounds, 2 Cir., 219 F.2d 445; Mills v. Society of New York Hospital, 242 App.Div. 245, 274 N.Y.S. 233, 270 N.Y. 594, 1 N.E.2d 346 (1936). The standard of care which stresses close observation, restriction and restraint has fallen in disrepute in modern hospitals and this policy is being reversed with excellent results. See, Perr, Suicide Responsibility of Hospital and Psychiatrist, 9 Cleveland-Marshall L.Rev. 427. This trend in the treatment and care of the mentally ill is reflected in regulations promulgated by the Administration of Veterans Affairs pursuant to the authority granted in 38 U.S.C.A. § 621:

> *Treatment and care of the Mentally Ill.* The policy of the V. A. is to allow each psychiatric patient the maximum independence that his condition permits and to administer the hospital so as to allow as normal a life as possible for the patient. All medically accepted therapeutic facilities will be available to each patient as required and if necessary such facilities will be made available by transfer to appropriate hospital.

The difficulty lies in the application of the foregoing policy. Each case must rest on its specific facts. The assignment of the patient to an open ward by Dr. Kennedy is the critical issue before this court. Was the doctor negligent?

... [T]he Court finds that Dr. Kennedy exercised the proper standard of care required under the circumstances. Calculated risks of necessity must be taken if the modern and enlightened treatment of the mentally ill is to be pursued intelligently and rationally. Neither the hospital nor the doctor are insurers of the patient's health and safety. They can only be required to use that degree of knowledge, skill, care and attention exercised by others in like circumstances.

5.2   MEIER V. ROSS GENERAL HOSPITAL
69 Cal.2d 420; 71 Cal. Rptr. 903; 445 P.2d 519 (California, 1968)

The widow and children of the deceased patient, Kurt Meier, brought a wrongful death action against Ross General Hospital and Dr. James M. Stubblebine, director of the hospital's psychiatric wing, after the patient had committed suicide while in the hospital. The family had brought the patient to this hospital after the patient had attempted suicide by cutting his wrists. As stated in the published record of the case, the policy on the psychiatric wing at Ross General was "open door":

> The hospital had adopted the "open door" policy for its psychiatric patients. This method of treatment de-emphasizes physical restraint by providing a "homelike" atmosphere in the hospital. The patients are free to move about and even to leave the hospital if they are so inclined. No mechanical security devices are regularly used; the doors are not locked; the windows are not barred.

The policy rests upon the premise that freedom of movement and personal responsibility of patients, even potential suicides, improve the process of their rehabilitation and reduce possible emotional stress. The proponents of the "open door" policy concede, however, that the lessening of physical security exposes a potentially suicidal patient to greater risk. They assert that no amount of security or physical restraint short of rendering the patient unconscious can effectively prevent suicide. Nevertheless, recognizing the risk of suicide in certain patients, the proponents of "open door" therapy normally employ larger staffs to facilitate surveillance and administer chemotherapy to those patients whose symptomatic restlessness and agitation indicate severe depression which may lead to suicide.

Approximately one week after the wrist-slashing incident, the patient committed suicide by jumping head first out of the open window on his second-floor room. The plaintiffs offered evidence which tended to show that secured windows should not have been incompatible with the open door policy. The defendants offered expert testimony stating that the operation of the psychiatric facility at the hospital, including the openable window, conformed with accepted hospital and medical standards.

The trial court found in favor of the defendant hospital and doctor. On appeal to the California Supreme Court the plaintiffs won a reversal and a remand for a new trial. Writing the opinion of the court, Justice Tobriner held as follows:

> If those charged with the care and treatment of a mentally disturbed patient know of facts from which they could reasonably conclude that the patient would be likely to harm himself in the absence of preclusive measures, then they must use reasonable care under the circumstances to prevent such harm. (*Wood v. Samaritan Institution* (1945) 26 Cal.2d 847, 853, 161 P.2d 556.) Even in the absence of expert testimony which describes the probability that the death or injury resulted from negligence, the jury may competently decide that defendant more probably than not breached his duty of care when the evidence supports a conclusion that the cause of the accident (here, the openable window) was not inextricably connected with a course of treatment involving the exercise of medical judgment beyond the common knowledge of laymen.
>
> [5] Finally, we conclude that we must reverse the judgment and remand for a new trial because the jury's verdict may have been based on the erroneous instruction; prejudice appears from the probability of a determinative application of an erroneous instruction, and this court should not speculate upon the actual basis of the verdict.

5.3 GREGORY V. ROBINSON
338 S.W.2d 88 (Missouri, 1960)

A patient who was considered to be at risk of committing suicide was placed on an open ward because, it was argued, the potential therapeutic benefits of being on an open ward outweighed the risk of suicide for this patient. The patient did subsequently commit suicide. The court found in favor of the defendant and held that the potential value of the open ward did seem to outweigh the risk of suicide.

5.4   KENT V. WHITAKER
58 Wash.2d 569; 364 P.2d 556 (Washington, 1961)

A patient hospitalized for attempting to commit suicide did commit suicide by strangling herself with plastic tubing while alone in a hospital room. The treating psychiatrist was found to be liable for $10,000 for not exercising reasonable care to prevent the patient from committing suicide.

5.5   HUNT V. KING HOSPITAL
481 P.2d 593 (Washington, 1971)

A twenty-year-old man was forcibly taken to a private hospital with handcuffs on his wrists and ankles and a belt around his knees. Hospital authorities were informed of the man's history of drug abuse. The patient's father told one of the doctors that his son would make every effort to escape, but the doctor assured the father of the hospital's security. The patient was taken to the fifth-floor, locked psychiatric ward of the hospital. Four days after admission, the patient darted to a utility room (that was usually locked) and jumped out of the unscreened window, sustaining serious injuries. Suit was brought against the hospital by the patient's father, and the hospital was found to be negligent in its assessment of the patient's needs and in providing for those needs.

5.6   FATUCK V. HILLSIDE HOSPITAL
45 A.D.2d 708; 356 N.Y.S.2d 105 (New York, 1974)

A patient with a long history of emotional problems and at least one indication of suicidal intent escaped from a psychiatric hospital and committed suicide. The hospital was held to be liable for the death of the patient because it had failed to provide fifteen-minute checks on the patient, as had been ordered by the doctor.

5.7   COHEN V. STATE
382 N.Y.S.2d 128 (New York, 1976)

A hospital was held liable for the death of a patient who was considered to be at high risk of committing suicide when that patient was allowed off the ward and did commit suicide.

5.8   PIETRUCHA v. GRANT HOSPITAL
       447 F.2d 1029 (Illinois, 1971)

A patient who had recently attempted suicide was admitted to the psychiatric ward of the defendant hospital and placed in a four-bed room. Despite the fact that the staff had been warned about the patient's extreme depression and suicidal tendencies, the patient had hanged himself with a belt by 3:30 the next morning. The widow brought suit against the hospital. All testimony for the plaintiff said that the belt used in the hanging had belonged to the patient. However, the hospital nurses denied this, stating that the patient's belt had been removed when he entered the hospital. The hospital defense amounted to the claim that the patient appeared to have voluntarily brought about his own death. The court ruled in favor of the plaintiff, noting that

> [t]he hospital held itself out as rendering the kind of psychiatric service the plaintiff sought for the decedent and accordingly it had the affirmative duty to protect the decedent against his own action.

5.9   DINNERSTEIN v. UNITED STATES
       486 F.2d 34 (Connecticut, 1973)

A veteran jumped to his death from the seventh-floor, unsecured lavatory window in a Veterans Administration hospital. For six years prior to the suicide, he had had recurrent periods of depression, for which he had voluntarily hospitalized himself. A year earlier, he had run his car into a bridge in what he described as a suicidal gesture (though he did little damage to either himself or his auto). Under the coaxing of his private psychiatrist, the patient had had himself admitted to the VA hospital for protection against possible suicide for a period of some three weeks. Subsequently, the patient's private psychiatrist [Dr. "X"] again recommended VA hospitalization. Two days before the suicide, the patient approached the VA hospital's physician on duty, Dr. "Y," asking for individual psychotherapy. The patient was told that he would not be able to obtain individual therapy but would be able to obtain group therapy. The patient was allegedly further depressed by this and refused to admit himself. However, he did come back the next day, asking for admission. Dr. "Z," handling the admission, diagnosed the patient as "depressive reaction" and was aware of the patient's history. Dr. Z assigned the patient to a seventh-floor ward without any special restrictions of supervision and had antidepressant medication discontinued. Dr. Z subsequently testified that he did not consider the patient to be suicidal and that the medication was discontinued so that the true psychological state of the patient could be better assessed. That evening, the patient complained to Dr. Z that he had become more depressed because of the inadequacy of the group therapy program. Dr. Z did not issue any additional orders regarding supervision of the patient, nor did he order antidepressant medication. At about 3:00 P.M. the next day, the patient leaped to his death. The patient's widow brought suit against the United States for negligence. The trial court found in favor of the plaintiff, stating that

> ... the hospital knew or should have known of the real possibility of a suicide attempt, that it failed to take appropriate measures to guard the deceased against that danger, that it was its duty to do so, and that, having failed to act with due care in the discharge of that duty, the United States is liable to the plaintiff for the losses caused thereby. . . .
>
> At the least, for the first few days of the deceased's admission his movements should have been restricted so that he could be closely watched. As he was assigned to a ward on the seventh floor, measures should have been taken to see that he could not jump from a window. His own denial upon admission of suicidal ideation and even Dr. [X]'s belief that he was not imminently suicidal cannot excuse the complete absence of precautions to insure the safety of a patient with a suicidal gesture in his past, a long history of psychiatric treatment for recurrent and severe depression, [and] previous hospitalization to protect against possible suicide.

The government appealed this case on the grounds that no psychiatric expert had testified that the appropriate standard of medical care had not been met. The appeal was unsuccessful, with the decision again going in favor of the plaintiff:

> From these facts, when combined with a six year history of deepening depression, it was not at all unreasonable for the trial court to conclude that the deceased should have been supervised more closely. This is not to suggest that every potential suicide must be locked in a padded cell. The law and modern psychiatry have now both come to the belated conclusion that an overly restrictive environment can be as destructive as an overly permissive one. But while we must accept some calculated risks in order to insure the patient's legal rights and provide him with the most effective therapy, we must also admit that errors in judgment do occur and that when they do, medical authorities must assume their rightful share of the responsibility. Here, in short, we cannot say the trial court erred in concluding that the hospital staff was negligent in allowing the deceased—an emotional unknown quantity—unrestricted movement on the seventh floor.

5.10 EADY V. ALTER
380 N.Y.S.2d 737 (New York, 1976)

The defendant in this case was found negligent in not providing closer supervision to a suicidal patient who did commit suicide. The court admitted as evidence of the patient's state of mind and potential for self-harm an intern's note which stated that the patient had tried to jump through a window just ten minutes before she did commit suicide.

5.11 CARLING V. STATE
294 N.Y.S.2d 30 (New York, 1968)

A patient who had never before attempted suicide jumped from an unguarded window in a mental institution. Suit was brought to recover for injuries sustained as a result of the fall. The hospital was not found to be liable for the injuries because the patient had not previously exhibited suicidal tendencies.

5.12 HARPER V. CSERR
544 F.2d 1121 (Massachusetts, 1976)

A voluntary patient committed suicide in a state mental institution. The plaintiffs claimed that the patient's right to treatment under the Eighth Amendment had been violated. The court held that the patient's right to treatment had not been violated, but that if the patient was helpless her rights may have been violated by supervision that was so loose that it permitted her to do harm to herself.

5.13 MILTON V. LOUISIANA
293 So.2d 645 (Louisiana, 1974)

A psychiatric patient's death resulted from his wandering away from his dormitory in a state hospital. The patient's next of kin (the plaintiff) argued that hospital authorities knew of the patient's tendency to wander and were negligent in taking precautions against mishaps. The court found in favor of the plaintiff, noting that the hospital was obliged to keep the patient in locked quarters when it could not observe his movements. The court awarded $549 for funeral expenses, $12,000 to the widow, and $5,000 to each of the deceased's fourteen children.

5.14 (Case Cited in Slawson, 1970)

A man was referred to Dr. Knight's Oceanview Sanitorium by his family physician. Dr. Knight interviewed the patient and his wife and was given a history of worry, agitation, and depression, which had worsened over the last six weeks. The patient would frequently stare off into space, and he had not gone to work in the last three days. Dr. Knight recommended immediate hospitalization and entered the following note in the patient's chart: "Patient is obviously suffering from an involutional reaction, depressed type, and will require shock therapy—lab in A.M., treatment to be started in the morning." Dr. Knight did a physical before the shock treatment and wrote in a note that "patient appears depressed, but smiles occasionally . . . and does not seem to have suicidal preoccupations." At 7:50 A.M. the treatment was administered and there were no complications. Dr. Knight's note after treatment said that the patient smiled and seemed to show improvement. A nurse's note written that morning, however, said that the patient "appears very depressed . . . wrings his hands . . . states it isn't worthwhile." Shortly thereafter the nurse noted that the patient asked how long it would take for the medication to take effect. The patient was not in his room when the nurse went to collect the lunch tray. He was found dead in the bathroom with the belt of his bathrobe tied around his neck and attached to the doorknob.

The patient's wife brought suit against Dr. Knight and his staff, claiming that they so "negligently, recklessly and unlawfully did treat, care for and prescribe for the decedent so as to cause [him] to, and he did, die of strangulation." The court found in favor of the plaintiff and awarded her $100,000. The actual settlement was $80,000 after the defendants agreed not to appeal.

5.15 HIRSH v. STATE
8 N.Y.2d 125; 168 N.E.2d 372; 202 N.Y.S.2d 296
(New York, 1960)

Alice Hirsh, as administrator of the Estate of Irving S. Hirsh, deceased, brought suit against the State of New York claiming negligence on the part of the Brooklyn State Hospital staff in failing to prevent Irving, a patient there, from committing suicide. The trial court (Court of Claims) entered a judgment in favor of the plaintiff. The decision of the trial court was affirmed by the Supreme Court, Appellate Division. The state next appealed to New York State's highest court, the Court of Appeals. This court found no evidence to support the claim that there was a lack of reasonable care to protect the patient against himself. Therefore, the court found in favor of the defendant, reversed the previous decision and dismissed the claim. The specific fact situation of the case appeared in the published opinion of Judge Van Voorhis:

> The State appeals from an affirmance of a judgment against it in the Court of Claims based on alleged negligence in failing to prevent plaintiff's intestate from committing suicide while he was a patient at the Brooklyn State Hospital. He had a previous history of mental illness at

other hospitals where he had made two suicidal attempts, one with phenobarbital and the other by hanging. This time he succeeded in accomplishing his aim. He was pronounced dead on September 4, 1953 of barbiturate poisoning. Death was caused by swallowing about a dozen capsules of seconal at night.

Nobody knew where or how this drug was obtained by him nor where he had kept or accumulated these capsules in his room. It was not medicine that was ordinarily used at the Brooklyn State Hospital at this time. He had been assigned to a ward for suicidal patients. Eighty-five patients were in this ward. Decedent was given his meals in the ward where he was confined, which he left only for treatment or for interviews with a psychiatrist. On these occasions he was accompanied by an attendant or a nurse. When medication of any kind was required on this ward, the nurse would unlock and relock the door upon departure, relocking it after her return with the drugs. These medications—not seconal—would be brought to the ward in such amounts as were used immediately, even though this meant repeating the procedure every four hours. Visits from family or friends were supervised, and gifts brought into the ward were checked by an attendant. Patients were allowed a monetary allowance of less than $1 at a time, enough to send for cigarettes or gum but insufficient to bribe anyone to get drugs. Decedent had not recently drawn upon this small allowance. When this patient was admitted to the State Hospital, he was completely examined, his clothes removed and he was furnished with State clothing. The regular practice was for the night shift attendants to put the patient to bed after examining his clothing and bed. He had been put to bed wearing only a pair of shorts so as to prevent his secreting anything potentially dangerous. The regular routine included removal of the mattress and inspection under the bed by the attendants.

[1–3] How he obtained the barbiturates which resulted in his death is a mystery in the record. The burden of proof to establish causal negligence is upon the plaintiff (Morris V. Lake Shore & Michigan Southern Ry. Co., 148 N.Y. 182, 42 N.E. 579). The state could not have provided an employee to watch every move made by this unfortunate man during 24 hours of the day. We are not persuaded that it is evidence of negligence that he was not repeatedly wakened and his bed searched during the night. If institutions for the mentally ill are required to take all of the precautions contended for in this case, and are to be held liable for such delicate mistakes in judgment, patients would be kept in strait jackets or some other form of strict confinement which would hardly be conducive to recovery. No reason is asserted that decedent was not given suitable electric shock treatments, tranquilizers or other treatment designed to mitigate mental depression and self-destructive tendencies. Reasonable care is required to protect such patients against themselves (Martindale v. State of New York, 269 N.Y. 554, 199 N.E. 667; Gries v. Long Island Home, 274 App. Div. 938, 83 N.Y.S.2d 728) but no evidence of lack of it has been shown in this case. An ingenious patient harboring a steady purpose to take his own life cannot always be thwarted.

The judgment appealed from should be reversed and the claim dismissed, without costs.

A dissenting opinion was filed by Judge Froessel:

Upon the findings below, amply supported by the evidence in this record, and in light of the cases herinafter cited, I am of the opinion that the judgment appealed from should be affirmed.

Irving Hirsh, claimant's decedent, died by suicide on September 4, 1953, while a mental patient at Brooklyn State Hospital. Hirsh, when admitted to the hospital on August 21, 1953, had a record of mental illness dating back to 1933, which included numerous attempts at suicide. His suicidal propensities were known to the authorities at Brooklyn State. He had been there previously in 1938–1939. He was returned to Brooklyn State in 1953 as a direct result of two attempts at suicide which occurred during the immediately preceding three weeks. On August 2, 1953 Hirsh, then a patient at the High Point Hospital in Port Chester, New York, attempted suicide "by taking an indeterminate number of pehnobarbitol tablets which he had *secluded in his room*" (emphasis supplied). His second attempt during that period was by hanging.

In view of his record, the examining physician at Brooklyn State noted in his report that Hirsh "need[ed] . . . constant nursing attention". He was placed in the suicidal ward, known as Ward 5. That ward, consisting of several dormitories ranging in size from 2 to 12 beds—decedent's dormitory had 12 beds—was directly supervised by attendants and nurses. There were three tours of duty, or shifts, among the attendants and nurses: the first from 8:00 A.M. to 4:00 P.M.; the second, known as the "evening shift", from 4:00 P.M. to 12:00 midnight; and the third, known as the "night shift", from 12:00 midnight to 8:00 A.M. It was during the evening shift that the patients in Ward 5 were put to bed.

The duties—as generally described at the trial—of the members of the hospital staff who worked on the evening shift were "To observe patients, to help them in their needs, feed, clothe them, to carry out the orders of the physician and the nurses in charge of the service"; and more particularly it was their responsibility to "examine clothing and the beds of the suicidal patients". Those engaged on the night shift, at which time the patients would be sleeping, would "make rounds at frequent intervals" of the various dormitories in Ward 5. Their inspections were of a cursory nature, looking "to see if the patient was all right and in good condition". At 6:00 A.M. the patients would be awakened, and the night shift attendants would see to it that they dressed and were taken to breakfast.

On the morning of Friday, September 4th, the night shift attendant attempted to awaken decedent Hirsh but he failed to respond. A physician was summoned who pronounced Hirsh dead. That physician, Dr. Cohen, testified that Hirsh appeared to be in a "deep sleep". He was clad only in shorts—the bed attire customarily worn by the patients in Ward 5. A search was made of the immediate surroundings, but no containers or boxes were discovered.

An autopsy performed subsequently disclosed that Hirsh died by barbituric poisoning, and claimant's expert testified that the 19 grains found establish that decedent had ingested *12 to 15 second capsules* of the gelatin covered type. When he was found dead at 6:00 A.M., his body was still warm and there was no sign of lividity, indicating that he had expired 1 to 2 hours previously. The quantity of seconal which he had taken was capable of producing death within from 1 to 6 hours. Hence Hirsh could have taken the seconal at any time after 10:00 P.M. on September 3d.

The record does not reveal the method used by decedent to acquire the seconal capsules. That is a subject of some speculation. There was conflicting testimony as to whether seconal was kept at Brooklyn State Hospital. In any event, since visiting days were on Wednesday and Saturday, decedent could not have had visitors on Thursday, the day before he died. None of decedent's relatives remembered at the trial when they last visited him. The trial court, after seeing them and hearing them testify, expressly dismissed any speculation that they might have brought decedent the seconals.

It is obvious, moreover—and the trial court so found—that, regardless of the method used by Hirsh in acquiring the seconals, he managed to keep the *12 to 15 capsules secretly hidden* from the hospital staff for whatever period he had them. The failure of the hospital staff to find the drugs before they could be used by Hirsh for self-destruction was negligence. It is my opinion that this finding of negligence by the Court of Claims, which was affirmed by the Appellate Division, is amply supported by the evidence in this record, and we are precluded from disturbing it.

As previously pointed out, the authorities at Brooklyn State Hospital had abundant knowledge of decedent's suicidal propensities, and in particular, knew that he had attempted suicide on a prior recent occasion by means of ingesting barbiturates which he had *"secluded in his room"*. Previously decided cases make it clear that such knowledge on the part of the hospital authorities merit weighty consideration in determining whether they are negligent in preventing the self-infliction of harm by a mental patient committed to their charge (Martindale v. State of New York, 269 N.Y. 554, 199 N.E. 667; Shattuck v. State of New York, 166 Misc. 271, 2 N.Y.S.2d 353, affirmed 254 App.Div. 926, 5 N.Y.S.2d 812; see, also, Weihs v. State of New York, 267 App.Div. 233, 45 N.Y.S.2d 542; Gries v. Long Island Home, 274 App.Div. 938, 83 N.Y.S.2d 728; Curley v. State of New York, 148 Misc. 336, 265 N.Y.S. 762, affirmed sub nom. Luke v. State of New York, 253 App.Div. 783, 1 N.Y.S.2d 19). "The degree of care to be observed is measured by the patient's physical and mental ills and deficiencies as known to the officers and employees of the institution" (Zajaczkowski v. State of New York, 189 Misc. 299, 302, 71 N.Y.S.2d 261, 263).

Thus, in the Martindale case, supra, for example, the decedent died after escaping the institution by removing a "lug" from a window. The State had notice, in light of a previous attempt of decedent to escape by the same method—namely, removing a "lug" from a window. We affirmed a finding for the claimant on the ground that the State was liable for the negligence of its officers in failing to protect the window, and in failing to provide constant supervision of the patient *after knowledge* of her desire and propensity to escape. Similarly, the Shattuck case, *supra*, involved a mental patient with a known propensity to escape by climbing through an unlocked top portion of a window. The State was held liable for injuries sustained as a result of a *second* escape by the same method. In the case now before us, the authorities at Brooklyn State Hospital—having knowledge of decedent's past attempt at suicide by means of barbiturates "secluded in his room"— failed to take the precautions reasonably necessary to prevent a recurrence of the act.

The standard of care, or procedures, commensurate with the risk to be perceived, which should have been followed by the hospital authorities in this case, were outlined by plaintiff's expert witness at the trial. In view of decedent's "mental history", he stated that proper standards required a "search of personal effects and the immediate surroundings" frequently each day: "I would have instructed my attendants to search Irving from head to foot before they put him to sleep, and to search him several times during the day to examine him several times during the day and to examine his person and every part of his personal effects, and because of these suicidal tendencies I would have reminded and especially alerted the personnel and also the fact that he was a potentially barbiturate suicide, and if I may say so, counsel, I would have alerted them to the fact that they can't be sure that they have checked carefully unless they had searched him repeatedly, and unless they did a thorough, and I mean a thorough searching by means of palpating every part of his body and all of his clothing and—".

In accordance with outlined statement of procedures, which are undisputed, the Court of Claims found that it was the "responsibility" of the *"Evening Shift"* (emphasis supplied) to "examine the patient's clothing and inspect his immediate environs to determine and discover any irregularities that would indicate a suicide attempt." (Finding of Fact No. 11.) These "simple rules" the Court of Claims found were "violated" by the State, particularly in that "The employees of the Evening (4 P.M. to 12 Midnight) shift failed to adequately inspect and examine Hirsh's clothing and bed on September 3rd, 1953" (Finding 12) and "The State's employees failed to adequately care for, supervise and have under surveillance Irving Hirsh on the night of September 3rd–4th, 1953." (Finding 22; see, also, Findings 14, 23, 24.)

Such findings—which the Appellate Division affirmed—are justified in light of the proof in this record that Hirsh consumed *12 to 15* gelatin covered capsules of seconal. Such a quantity of capsules comprises a substantial physical bulk. Had the staff properly palpated his body, checked his clothing, bed and environs as they were duty-bound to do, the seconal would have been uncovered. The situation would be far different if we were dealing in this case with a suicide committed by means of ingestion of a few diminutive pills.

There is also evidence in this record that the staff were never alerted to the fact that decedent was a potential barbiturate suicide, and that he had once attempted such a suicide by means of barbiturates *secluded in his room*—notwithstanding the fact that the hospital authorities knew of this. The five attendants who served on the evening shift on September 3, 1953 did not testify at the trial. They had resigned since Hirsh's death. However, the nurse in charge on that shift was present at the trial and testified as follows:

"Q. Did you have anything to do with searching the environs of the patients to see if they were hiding medication? A. Not unless I had reason to be suspicious.

"Q. Did you at that particular time in September or around September 3rd, 1953 know that Irving Hirsh had at one time attempted suicide by taking an indeterminate amount of phenobarbital? A. I don't recall, I knew at the time—

"Q. Nobody told you about that? A. *No, sir*" (Emphasis supplied.)

One of the attendants on the night shift at the hospital during the time that Hirsh was there testified that he had not been given any special instructions with regard to Hirsh; and when asked if he knew that Hirsh "had attempted suicide by taking barbiturates on a prior date than his date of admission to Brooklyn State", he replied: *"No, I didn't know that."* (Emphasis supplied.)

The majority of the Appellate Division in its opinion for affirmance in this case took note of the fact that decedent Hirsh had consumed 12 to 15 capsules of seconal, and aptly observed that "Each case must be decided on its own merits but the rule is clear (Van Patter v. Charles B. Towns Hospital, 246 N.Y. 646, 159 N.E. 686; Paige v. State of New York, 245 App.Div. 126, 281 N.Y.S. 98; Martindale v. State of New York, 269 N.Y. 554, 199 N.E. 667)"—namely, "that the State is liable for the failure of its hospital personnel to take reasonable and necessary precautions to protect mental patients from self-inflicted injuries."

Such "reasonable and necessary precautions" were not taken by the hospital authorities or staff in this case. It is stated in the majority opinion of this court that it was the regular practice for the *night* shift attendants to put the patient to bed after examining his clothing and bed, which included the removal of the mattress and inspection under the bed by the attendant, although these attendants did not report for duty until midnight. However, the record in this case disclosed only the *duties* of the hospital staff as outlined earlier in this opinion—*not that they were in fact performed.* Indeed, there is absolutely no evidence in this record that these duties were performed or any practice or custom carried out on the morning, afternoon, evening or night of September 3, 1953, the day immediately preceding the fatal early morning hours of September 4th when Hirsh expired from barbituric acid poisoning. The record does contain evidence that the mattress was removed and a search conducted underneath the bed of Hirsh and in that entire area, but that was done only *after* 6 o'clock on the morning of September 4, 1953, *after* the attendants had found Hirsh *dead* in his bed.

Inasmuch as there is ample evidence here in support of the facts found by the Court of Claims, and these findings have been affirmed by the Appellate Division, we have no alternative but to affirm.

5.16 FERNANDEZ v. STATE
45 A.D.2d, 125; 356 N.Y.S.2d, 708 (New York, 1974)

Asbel Fernandez, as Administrator of the Estate of Amina Fernandez, deceased, brought suit against the State of New York to recover for personal injuries sustained by Amina in an attempted suicide while she was a patient in Bronx State Hospital. The Court of Claims entered a judgment in favor of the plaintiff and the state appealed. On appeal, the decision of the lower court was reversed and the claim was dismissed. Amina Fernandez did subsequently commit suicide in Van Etten Hospital, which is not a state-run institution. In his published opinion, Rustice Greenblott detailed the facts of this case and cited *Hirsh* (Case #5.5) as controlling:

Amina Fernandez, a patient at Bronx State Hospital, injured herself in a suicide attempt on August 18, 1970. Decedent had been admitted to Bronx State Hospital on May 28, 1970, after having attempted to cut her throat with a razor. This claim is brought to recover for the alleged negligence of the State in failing to properly observe the patient so as to permit her to injure herself.

The only evidence in the case with the exception of the hospital records was the examination before trial of Dolores Jones, the attendant in charge of Mrs. Fernandez. It reveals that she was assigned to watch the decedent and no other patient. She had been briefed by the physician in charge as to the patient's condition and was told that because of the patient's expressed desire to kill herself, she was to be observed at all times.

The attendant testified that upon receiving her instructions, she went to the patient's bed and sat beside her. While the patient was sleeping, the attendant examined the room for hidden articles and found none. When she awakened, the attendant searched the bed. After dinner, they returned to the room and the patient appeared to fall asleep. Miss Jones then left the room for only five minutes to go to the bathroom. When she returned she observed the decedent emerging from the room, having stabbed herself with a large knife. The trial court, on the basis of this evidence, awarded claimant $5,000 for conscious pain and suffering, the claim for wrongful death having been withdrawn at the trial.

While a suicidal patient must be given close supervision, a five-minute absence while the patient appears to be sleeping cannot afford a reasonable ground for recovery against the State. The decision of the Court of Appeals in Hirsh v. State of New York, 8 N.Y.2d 125, 202 N.Y.S.2d 296, 168 N.E.2d 372, is controlling. In *Hirsh* there was no evidence of how the patient came into possession of a dozen seconal tablets which he used to commit suicide. As the court stated in p. 127, 202 N.Y.S.2d at p. 298, 168 N.E.2d at p. 373:

"The State could not have provided an employee to watch every move made by this unfortunate man during 24 hours of the day. We are not persuaded that it is evidence of negligence that he was not repeatedly wakened and his bed searched during the night. If institutions for the mentally ill are required to take all of the precautions contended for in this case, and are to be held liable for such delicate mistakes in judgment, patients would be kept in strait jackets or some other form of strict confinement which would hardly be conducive to recovery."

Reasonable care is required to protect such patients against themselves (Martindale v. State of New York, 244 App.Div. 877, 281 N.Y.S. 686, affd. 269 N.Y. 554, 199 N.E. 667). In our view, such care was provided in this case, for even if it can be said that the State did assume a duty of continual observation, a five-minute absence when a patient appears to be sleeping and thus incapable of inflicting self-harm does not constitute an act of negligence.

The judgment should be reversed, on the law and the facts, and the claim dismissed, without costs.

5.17 FORDE v. COUNTY OF LOS ANGELES
      64 Cal. App. 3d, 477; 134 Cal. Rptr. 549
      (California, 1976)

Michael Henry Forde was seen by a psychiatrist at Los Angeles County Hospital on August 29 and admitted as an involuntary patient with a diagnosis of acute psychotic reaction. The admitting psychiatrist believed the patient to be a danger to himself and others, and the patient was placed on a locked ward. The following morning, Forde was seen by a second psychiatrist. The second psychiatrist subsequently transferred Forde to an open ward and changed his status from involuntary to voluntary. On September 6, while Forde was supposed to be attending a dance for the patients, he was discovered to have eloped. When a nurse notified a psychiatric resident of the elopement the resident gave the nurse instructions to write the patient a pass until the next morning. Within hours after eloping, Forde jumped off a bridge, sustaining injuries which gave rise to the suit against the County of Los Angeles, the admitting psychiatrist, the second psychiatrist, and the psychiatric resident.

The trial court found in favor of the defendant county and the other defendants on the grounds that the Government Code provided immunity to the defendants in this fact situation. The relevant wording in section 856.2 is as follows:

> Neither a public entity nor a public employee is liable for . . . an injury to, or the wrongful death of an escaping or escaped person who has been confined for mental illness or addiction.

On appeal, the plaintiff contended that the trial court had erred in granting immunity, since Forde had been a voluntary patient at the time and could therefore not "escape" or "elope." However, as reflected in the opinion of Presiding Justice Kaus, the Appellate Court did not agree:

> In 1970, the statute was amended, *inter alia*, to substitute the word "confined," for the word, "committed." "The substitution of 'confined' for 'committed' makes clear that the immunity covers all persons who are confined for mental illness or addiction, whether or not they are 'committed.' " (Law Rev. Commission Comment—1970 Amendment.) Thus, contrary to plaintiff's contention, the immunity conferred by section 856.2 applies whether the mental patient is voluntarily or involuntarily confined.
>
> Plaintiff makes much of the fact that hospital personnel described plaintiff's conduct as an "elopement." Defendants' euphemism does not alter or affect what plaintiff indisputably did. He left the hospital without authorization or without officially signing himself out as a patient.

The plaintiff also charged that the psychiatric resident attempted to cover up the hospital's negligence by having a pass written for the patient after the patient was discovered to be missing. However, here again, the court did not agree:

> Plaintiff also points out that after his absence was noted, a resident ordered that he be given extended leave. That plaintiff's departure was ratified or covered up does not change the undisputed fact that when he left, he was not authorized to do so.

The court also rejected the plaintiff's contention that "escape immunity here would be absurd" and related arguments. The court left the matter of the absurdity of the immunity as a matter for the Legislature. The holding of the trial court was affirmed.

5.18 RUNYON V. REID
510 P.2d 943 (Oklahoma, 1973)

Suit was brought against a psychiatrist who had known that his patient, whom he deemed not at high risk of committing suicide, possessed a lethal amount of barbituates. In holding that the psychiatrist was not liable for the death of the patient, the court found that any reasonably skilled psychiatrist using customary methods would not have viewed the patient as being at high risk of committing suicide.

5.19 JOHNSON V. GRANT HOSPITAL
291 N.E.2d 440 (Ohio, 1972)

An attending physician at a general hospital ordered that his patient's door be kept locked nightly, but did not mention anything about daytime precautions against a suicide attempt. The patient jumped to his death during the day. A suit holding the hospital negligent in not taking adequate precautions to guard against such an incident was decided in favor of the hospital, as it had followed the attending physician's orders. Furthermore, the court ruled that general hospitals could not reasonably be expected to provide the same standard of care for psychiatric patients as psychiatric hospitals, since they are unequipped to do so.

5.20 TISINGER V. WOOLEY
122 Ga. App. 231; 50 S.E.2d 122 (Georgia, 1948)

After a hospitalized patient committed suicide, the psychiatrist who had hospitalized the patient was sued for not selecting a hospital that had adequate facilities to supervise the patient. The doctor was not found to be liable, on the grounds that the hospital had routinely admitted known mental patients in the past.

5.21 Centeno v. City of New York
48 A.D. 2d 812; 369 N.Y.S.2d 710 (New York, 1975)

Soon after release from a psychiatric hospital, the patient committed suicide. The plaintiffs brought suit against the hospital, and an expert witness testified on behalf of the plaintiffs that a defendant doctor's conduct was not in accordance with accepted medical practice. The defendant was not held to be liable for making an honest error in judgment.

5.22 Charouleau v. Charity Hospital of New Orleans
319 So.2d 464 (Louisiana, 1975)

A patient was seen in a public hospital emergency room by a physician who referred the case to psychiatry. While a psychiatric resident was interviewing the patient, the patient took a revolver from her purse and pointed it at the resident. The resident took the gun from the woman, determined it was unloaded, and handed it back to the woman "to establish a rapport." The woman told the resident that she had previously been admitted to this hospital and that she was seeking admission now to rid herself of a drug abuse problem. The resident told the patient that she would not be committed to an institution against her will, and he proceeded within the patient's view to write a note stating that it was his opinion that the woman could benefit from prolonged hospitalization. The resident did not review the patient's chart, which could have been obtained from the records room, and he did not instruct anyone to keep an eye on the patient. He escorted her to the admission desk and instructed her to sit down and wait for the clerk to return. As well as can be determined, the patient took her chart sometime after the resident dropped her off, straying from the admission area. The patient was found dead the following morning in a hospital toilet, from a self-inflicted bullet wound.

The patient's husband brought suit against the resident and the hospital. The case against the resident was settled out of court, but the hospital contended that it could not be held legally culpable as the proximate cause of the patient's death. The plaintiff charged that the hospital negligently had a resident instead of a psychiatrist in the emergency room, that it did not have a procedure for direct admission into psychiatry, that it allowed psychiatric patients to stray before admission, that it did not prevent patients from seeing their own charts, and that it did not have a policy of reviewing the past records of potentially suicidal patients.

The court did not find the defendant hospital culpable, because as a matter of course previous records are not examined in emergency-room treatment, in order to expedite dispositions. The court found the admissions procedure used by the defendant hospital to be much the same as in comparable hospitals and did not find compelling evidence that the hospital was the proximate cause of the patient's death.

5.23 BOGUST V. IVERSON
(Case cited in Parker, 1961)

A dean of students with a doctorate in education counseled a nineteen-year-old girl over a period of six months. Six weeks before the girl committed suicide, the dean had terminated the counseling relationship. The girl's parents brought suit against the dean for improper guidance and failure to inform them of their daughter's intentions so that they could obtain proper psychotherapeutic assistance. The suit also alleged that the dean failed to seek out emergency psychiatric care for the girl on his own. The dean's defense was that because he was an Ed.D., he did not have sufficient training in clinical psychology and psychiatry to be able to judge the girl's suicidal tendencies. The court found in favor of the defendant, noting that no cause-and-effect relationship existed between the girl's suicide and the dean's action; even if the dean had referred her for proper psychiatric treatment or had informed the parents or had not stopped seeing her, the girl might still have committed suicide.

ASSAULT AND/OR BATTERY BY PATIENT

5.24 TARASOFF V. REGENTS OF UNIVERSITY OF CALIFORNIA[2]
118 Cal. Rptr. 129; 529 P.2d 553 (California, 1974)

Tatiana Tarasoff was murdered by Prosenjit Poddar. Poddar had been in therapy with psychologist Dr. Lawrence Moore at the Cowell Memorial Hospital of the University of California at Berkeley. Poddar had made known to Moore his intention to kill an unnamed girl two months prior to the murder. After conferring with

[2]The complete text of the significant decision in this case, including the majority opinion by Justice Tobriner and a dissenting opinion by Justice Clark, appears in the Appendix to this book. Also included in the appendix is an excerpt from Dr. Moore's letter to Police Chief Beall.

psychiatrists Gold and Yandell, Moore had written a letter to campus police chief William Beall requesting the assistance of the police department in securing Poddar's confinement. Dr. Harvey Powelson, the chief of the department of psychiatry at the hospital, asked Beall to return Moore's letter and directed that all copies of the letter and Moore's other notes on the case be destroyed. Powelson also "ordered no action to place Prosenjit Poddar in seventy-two-hour treatment and evaluation facility." After Tatiana was murdered, her parents brought suit against Doctors Moore, Powelson, Gold, and Yandell, Police Chief Beall, four campus police officers, and the Regents of the University of California as the employer of all of the other defendants.

The Supreme Court of California ruled that a psychotherapist has a duty to warn endangered third parties of their peril. The court recognized that many therapy patients make idle threats, and it acknowledged the need for privacy in therapist/patient communications. However, it ruled that screening the idle from the genuine threats was a matter of professional judgment and that the public interest superceded the individual patient's interest under certain conditions. It said:

> First, defendants point out that although therapy patients often express thoughts of violence, they rarely carry out these ideas. Indeed the open and confidential character of psychotherapeutic dialogue encourages patients to voice such thoughts, not as a device to reveal hidden danger, but as part of the process of therapy. Certainly a therapist should not be encouraged routinely to reveal such threats to acquaintances of the patient; such disclosures could seriously disrupt the patient's relationship with his therapist and with the persons threatened. In singling out those few patients whose threats of violence present a serious danger and in weighing against this danger the harm to the patient that might result from revelation, the psychotherapist renders a decision involving a high order of expertise and judgment.
>
> [5] The judgment of the therapist, however, is no more delicate or demanding than the judgment which doctors and professionals must regularly render under accepted rules of responsibility. A professional person is required only to exercise "that reasonable degree of skill, knowledge, and care ordinarily possessed and exercised by members of [his] profession under similar circumstances." (Bardessono v. Michels (1970) 3 Cal.3d 780, 788, 91 Cal. Rptr. 760, 764, 478 P.2d 480, 484.) As a specialist, the psychotherapist, whether doctor or psychologist, would also be "held to that standard of learning and skill normally possessed by such specialist in the same or similar locality under the same or similar circumstances." (Quintal v. Laurel Grove Hospital (1964) 62 Cal.2d 154, 159–160, 41 Cal.Rptr. 577, 580, 397 P.2d 161, 164.) But within that broad range in which professional opinion and judgment may differ respecting the proper course of action, the psychotherapist is free to exercise his own best judgment free from liability; proof, aided by hindsight, that he judged wrongly is insufficient to establish liability.

In other words, the fact that a decision calls for considerable expert skill and judgment means, in effect, that it be tested by a standard of care which takes account of those circumstances; the standard used in measuring professional malpractice does so. But whatever difficulties the courts may encounter in evaluating the expert judgments of other professions, those difficulties cannot justify total exoneration from liability.

Second, defendants argue that free and open communication is essential to psychotherapy (see In re Lifschutz (1970) 2 Cal. 3d 415, 431–432, 85 Cal.Rptr. 829, 467 P.2d 557); that "Unless a patient . . . is assured that . . . information [revealed by him] can and will be held in utmost confidence, he will be reluctant to make the full disclosure upon which diagnosis and treatment . . . depends." (Sen. Committee on the Judiciary, comments on Evid.Code, § 1014.) The giving of a warning, defendants contend, constitutes a breach of trust which entails the revelation of confidential communications.

We recognize the public interest in supporting effective treatment of mental illness and in protecting the rights of patients to privacy (see In re Lifschutz, *supra*, 2 Cal.3d at p. 432, 85 Cal.Rptr. 829, 467 P.2d 557), and the consequent public importance of safeguarding the confidential character of psychotherapeutic communication. Against this interest, however, we must weigh the public interest in safety from violent assault. The Legislature has undertaken the difficult task of balancing the countervailing concerns. In Evidence Code section 1014, it established a broad rule of privilege to protect confidential communications between patient and psychotherapist. In Evidence Code section 1024, however, the Legislature created a specific and limited exception to the psychotherapist–patient privilege: "There is no privilege . . . if the psychotherapist has reasonable cause to believe that the patient is in such mental or emotional condition as to be dangerous to himself or to the person or property of another and that disclosure of the communication is necessary to prevent the threatened danger."

[6] The revelation of a communication under the above circumstances is not a breach of trust or a violation of professional ethics; as stated in the Principles of Medical Ethics of the American Medical Association (1957) section 9; "A physician may not reveal the confidences entrusted to him in the course of medical attendance . . . *unless he is required to do so by law or unless it becomes necessary in order to protect the welfare of the individual or of the community.*" (Emphasis added.) We conclude that the public policy favoring protection of the confidential character of patient–psychotherapist communications must yield in instances in which disclosure is essential to avert danger to others. The protective privilege ends where the public peril begins.

5.25 JOHNSON V. STATE

69 Cal.2d 782; 73 Cal. Rptr. 240 (California, 1968)

The State of California, acting through its placement office in the Youth Authority, placed a sixteen-year-old foster child in the home of foster parents Mr. Floyd N. Johnson and Mrs. Ina Mae Johnson. Subsequently, Mrs. Johnson was physically beaten by the foster child. Mrs. Johnson brought suit against the state alleging that the Youth Authority acted negligently in allowing "a 16 year old boy with homicidal tendencies, and a background of violence and cruelty towards both animals and humans to be placed in the home" without notice of any "dangerous propensities." The defendant State of California argued that it was immune from liability and that it owed no duty of care to the plaintiff. The trial court found in favor of the defendant, and Mrs. Johnson appealed. The Supreme Court of California denied the state immunity in this case and ruled that the defendant did have a duty to warn Mrs. Johnson of her peril:

> At the outset, we can dispose summarily of the contention, not strenu-
> ously pressed by defendant, that the judgment should be affirmed
> because the state owed no duty of care to plaintiff. As the party placing
> the youth with Mrs. Johnson, the state's relationship to plaintiff was
> such that its duty extended to warning of latent, dangerous qualities
> suggested by the parolee's history or character. (Cf. Langley v. Pacific
> Gas & Electric Co. (1953) 41 Cal.2d 655, 661, 262 P.2d 846; Crane v.
> Smith (1943) 23 Cal.2d 288, 296, 144 P.2d 356; Gherna v. Ford Motor
> Co. (1966) 246 Cal.App.2d 639, 650–651, 55 Cal.Rptr. 94; Crane v.
> Sears Roebuck & Co. (1963) 218 Cal.App.2d 855, 859, 32 Cal.Rptr.
> 754; Ellis v. D'Angelo (1953) 116 Cal.App.2d 310, 317, 253 P.2d 675;
> Rest.2d, Torts, § 301(2) (b).) These cases impose a duty upon those
> who create a foreseeable peril, not readily discoverable by endangered
> persons, to warn them of such potential peril. Accordingly, the state
> owed a duty to inform Mrs. Johnson of any matter that its agents knew
> or should have known that might enganger the Johnson family; at a
> minimum, these facts certainly would have included "homicidal ten-
> dencies, and a background of violence and cruelty" as well as the
> youth's criminal record.

The Supreme Court of California reversed the decision of the lower court and found in favor of the plaintiff, Johnson. A dissenting opinion was filed by Justice McComb, who stated that he would affirm the lower court's decision for the same reasons the presiding justice in the Court of Appeal did (see *Johnson v. State of California*, 65 Cal. Rptr. 717)

5.26 MERCHANTS NATIONAL BANK AND TRUST COMPANY OF FARGO V.
UNITED STATES
272 F. Supp. 409 (North Dakota, 1967)

Mrs. Eloise A. Newgard, a woman shown by the evidence to have been "an outstanding registered nurse, a fine woman, a splendid mother and a faithful wife" was shot and killed by her husband, William Bry Newgard, a mental patient on leave from a Veterans Administration hospital. A suit on behalf of the estate of Eloise Newgard was brought by the Merchant's National Bank and Trust

Company (as administrator of the decedent's estate) against the government's agents and employees, who, it was alleged, negligently ignored indications of the seriousness of the patient's condition. An excerpt from the court record provides a graphic behavioral record of Newgard's condition some seven months before he murdered his wife:

> Early in the morning of January 17, 1965, Dr. Mack V. Traynor, a Fargo physician, was called to the Newgard apartment in Fargo, North Dakota, by Newgard's wife, Eloise. She was frantic-voiced and said she needed help. The doctor, promptly responding to the call, found Newgard glassy-eyed and making senseless talk about horses, cattle "and God most of the time." Dr. Traynor felt Newgard was completely psychotic. Earlier that same morning Eloise had telephoned her pastor, Reverend Richard C. Faust, who knew both Newgard and his wife. He, too, came to the apartment. A daughter, Elizabeth, admitted him. Eloise asked for his help. From elsewhere in the apartment Newgard was shouting "get him out." Reverend Faust says that Newgard finally appeared, yelling that he was "the reincarnation of Jesus Christ." He was clad in boxer shorts and T-shirt. Newgard pulled his shorts down, exposed himself and said he was "going to repopulate the world." Newgard accused his wife of unfaithfulness and threatened to kill her. Reverend Faust also understood Newgard to say that the "God of Fire" would repopulate the world.

The court found in favor of the plaintiff and awarded $200,000 as compensatory damages for the wrongful death of a mother who had three minor children. The court found the clinical psychologist who had arranged for the patient to take a leave of absence from the hospital at a nearby ranch to have been negligent in telling the ranch owner that the patient had had a nervous breakdown. The psychologist should have told the ranch owner that the patient was mentally ill, and he should have provided him with specific instructions concerning what he should do if the patient left the ranch.

The psychiatrist who had spoken to Eloise Newgard shortly before her husband's release was also found to be negligent in not taking note of the call and pursuing it further. A second psychiatrist was also found to be negligent for having "ignored and rejected every warning signal" during the course of his treatment of the patient and conferences with the decedent. The court held that if the psychiatrist had "devoted more of his time to Newgard and less . . . to diagnosing Newgard's wife, conceivably she would never have met so tragic and untimely a death."

5.27 SEMLER V. PSYCHIATRIC INSTITUTE OF WASHINGTON, D.C.
538 F.2d 121 (Virginia, 1976)

Helen Semler's daughter, Natalia, was murdered by John Steven Gilreath, a man who had previously pleaded guilty to charges stemming from his abduction of a young girl. A presentencing report indicated that on three previous occasions Gilreath had molested other young girls. The court imposed a twenty-year sentence on Gilreath but suspended it with the usual conditions of probation and the special condition that "he continue to receive treatment at and remain confined in the Psychiatric Institute until released by the Court." Approximately five weeks after Gilreath was given the status and privileges of an outpatient at the Institute (without the permission of the court) Natalia Semler was murdered. Helen Semler, as administratrix of the estate of her daughter, brought suit against Psychiatric Institute of Washington, D.C.

The trial court found in favor of the plaintiff and awarded her a $25,000 judgment, half of which was to be paid by the Institute and half by Gilreath's parole officer. On appeal, the United States Court of Appeals ruled on whether or not the Psychiatric Institute owed a duty of protection to the public (including Natalia Semler) as well as a duty of treatment to Gilreath. The Court of Appeals agreed with the trial court that the defendants did owe a duty to the public. It rejected the defendants' argument that the Institute did not owe the public a duty on the grounds that the court order provided for rehabilitation for Gilreath and that the duty of the defendants extended only to Gilreath and not to Natalia Semler. In his opinion, Circuit Judge Butzner rejected the notion that the tragic event could be construed as an "unavoidable accident," and he alluded to the foreseeability of its happening:

> As we have noted, the Supreme Court of Virginia cautions that an unforeseeable accident is not actionable. *Trimyer v. Norfolk Tallow Co.*, 192 Va. 776, 780, 66 S.E.2d 441, 443 (1951). Therefore, the nature of the appellants' duty depends in large part on the reasonable foreseeability of harm to the public, including the Semler girl, if Gilreath were released from the Institute in violation of the court's order. In this respect, the concepts of duty and proximate cause are related. See Prosser, Law of Torts 244 (4th ed. 1971).
>
> Confinement of criminals frequently is intended to protect the public as well as to punish and rehabilitate the wrongdoer. But we need not rely on this generality to determine the nature of the duty imposed on Gilreath's custodians by the state court's probation order. The order itself discloses that the state trial judge had a dual purpose in placing Gilreath on probation. The judge's willingness to allow Gilreath to continue his private psychiatric treatment shows concern for his welfare. At the same time, the requirement of confinement until release by the court was to protect the public, particularly young girls, from the foreseeable risk of attack.

The court of Appeals held that the Institute breached its duty to protect the public by transferring Gilreath to outpatient status without the approval of the court and that this breach was proximately related to the murder. The probation officer had the responsibility of seeing that Gilreath was not released until court approval for such release was obtained. When the probation officer approved the Institute's transfer of the patient to outpatient status without consulting the court, the probation officer was deemed not to be immune from liability. Under Virginia law, a state employee who exercises discretionary judgment within the scope of his employment is immune from liability for negligence. However, he will be held liable if injury results from negligent performance of a ministerial act.

5.28 HIGGINS V. STATE
24 A.D.2d 147; 265 N.Y.S.2d 254 (New York, 1965)

The plaintiff was injured in a public park by a mental patient who had been permitted to go to the park. Because the plaintiff failed to prove that the hospital staff had been negligent in permitting the patient free access to the park, the defendant prevailed.

5.29 LOGAN V. ST. LUKE'S HOSPITAL
65 Wash.2d 914; 400 P.2d 296 (Washington, 1965)

The defendant hospital was not held liable for the consequences of one patient's wandering into another's room. The therapeutic benefits of the patient's freedom of movement were seen to outweigh the potential harm that could result from his having that freedom.

5.30 DOCTORS HOSPITAL, INC. V. KOVATS
16 Ariz. App. 489; 494 P.2d 389 (Arizona, 1972)

A psychiatric patient slipped out of his restraints (a Posey belt) on five occasions. The next time he slipped out, he hit another patient (the plaintiff) with a chair. The plaintiff's suit alleged the hospital to be negligent in allowing the patient to extricate himself. The court ruled that the hospital was liable, because it had inadequately restrained a patient with a known mental disturbance. Expert testimony was held to be unnecessary in this case.

5.31 UNDERWOOD V. UNITED STATES
356 F.2d 92 (1966)

After committing numerous assaults on his wife, an airman in the United States Air Force was hospitalized and diagnosed to be suffering from a mental illness. Sometime later the patient was released as an outpatient, a status which allowed him to have weapons in his possession. The patient subsequently shot his wife. Suit was brought against the United States, and the plaintiff prevailed in getting a judgment against the defendant.

5.32 CAMERON V. STATE
37 A.D.2d 46; 322 N.Y.S.2d 562; 282 N.E.2d 118 (New York, 1971)

A state hospital released a patient who brutally assaulted an infant. The plaintiff brought suit against the state, claiming negligence in releasing the patient. The court ruled that while the hospital may have been wrong in its decision to release the patient, it had not been negligent, since all usual precautions had been taken and no omission in the usual procedure could causally be related to the plaintiff's injuries.

5.33 JOHNSON V. UNITED STATES
409 F. Supp. 1283 (Florida, 1976)

Under an Army "open door" policy, a psychiatric patient was permitted to leave the hospital. The plaintiff sought to recover for damages incurred by the patient's homicide and suicide while out of the hospital. The defendant was not found to have acted negligently in permitting the patient to leave the hospital.

5.34 DUNN V. STATE
29 N.Y.2d 313; 327 N.Y.S.2d 662 (New York, 1971)

Plaintiff brought suit on account of the death of a motorist who was killed by the reckless driving of an escaped psychiatric patient. Evidence showed that the patient had been inadequately guarded at the state institution. Still, the court did not find the defendant liable, because the hospital's negligence was not deemed to be the proximate cause of death.

5.35 ORMAN V. STATE
37 A.D.2d 674; 322 N.Y.S.2d 914 (New York, 1971)

A psychiatric inpatient was permitted to leave the state hospital to go home on a visit. While away, the patient shot the plaintiff. The defendant was not found to be liable for the plaintiff's injuries, because there was no negligence proved and an honest error in professional judgment is not actionable.

5.36 THALL V. STATE
329 N.Y.S.2d 837 (New York, 1972)

A patient who in the past had been prone to assault women and to attempt to escape from the hospital in which he was confined did

escape and did assault a woman. Because of this patient's prior
history, the defendant state (New York) was found negligent in not
providing tighter security so that the patient would not have been
able to escape.

5.37 HERNANDEZ V. STATE
46 A.D.2d 712; 360 N.Y.S.2d 314 (New York, 1974)

A patient who had tried to escape from the state hospital in
which he was confined on three previous occasions incurred injuries
during an escape attempt. The defendant was not found to be liable
for the injuries, since it was not, in this court's opinion, under a
duty to maintain twenty-four-hour-a-day surveillance of the patient.

5.38 HOMERE V. STATE
370 N.Y.S.2d 246 (New York, 1975)

A patient released from a mental institution committed assault.
The defendant was found liable for the assault because it was held to
be negligent in not carrying out a reevaluation of the patient's mental condition before his release from the institution.

5.39 HARRIS V. STATE OF OHIO
48 O. Misc. 27; 358 N.E.2d 639 (Ohio, 1976)

A mental patient who was released from a state mental institution committed an assault, and a suit was brought against the state.
The court did not find the defendant to be liable, because the patient had been released two years prior to the assault.

5.40 (Citation Withheld)

A man released from a state institution for the criminally insane
murdered his mother and his brother. The father brought suit
against a psychologist fo a little over half a million dollars for damages resulting from the psychologist's part in having his son freed.
(In litigation.)

5.41 (Citation Withheld)

An adolescent patient leaving a psychologist's office struck and
injured the doorman of the building. The doorman suffered some
facial scarring and had four teeth knocked out. The doorman
brought suit against the psychologist in the amount of about
$100,000, claiming that the psychologist should have had enough

prior knowledge to guard against such incidents. The psychologist was found to be free from liability.[3]

5.42 SEALEY v. FINKELSTEIN
206 N.Y.S.2d 512 (New York, 1960)

Doris Sealey was a practical nurse in a nursing home who was allegedly assaulted in one of the rooms by Mrs. Stein, a sixty-two-year-old patient in that home. Sealey brought suit against Rubin Finkelstein, a doctor who had previously treated the patient, and against the patient's daughter, Doris Stein. Sealey sought damages as a result of the defendants' failure to warn her of the patient's "dangerous and vicious propensities." Both defendants, Doris Stein and Dr. Finkelstein, denied knowledge of any such propensities on the part of the patient. The medical co-director of the nursing home testified in a supporting affidavit that the plaintiff's duties included attending to the aged, handicapped, and chronically ill and that varying outbursts and states of agitation were dealt with in the regular course of such duties. The court held that neither defendant was liable for the plaintiff's alleged injuries, since they did not know of the patient's hazardous propensities:

> The keystone of her claim is that the defendants failed to inform her or her employer "as to the *known* existing mental condition of the patient," her "*known* dangerous and vicious and hazardous propensities," and her "*known* dangerous tendencies and disturbed mental condition" (emphasis supplied). But plaintiff has failed to show any facts in support of her claim that the defendants knew of the patient's foregoing alleged propensities.

5.43 BULLOCK v. PARKCHESTER GENERAL HOSPITAL
4 N.Y.2d 894; 174 N.Y.S.2d 471 (New York, 1957)

A practical nurse, hired to care for a cardiac patient, was struck by a telephone and a glass which the patient threw at her. Sedatives and fever were presumed to be the cause of this transient psychotic episode. Named as defendants in the nurse's suit were Parkchester General Hospital (a private hospital), the doctor who had hired her, and the patient. The suit against the patient was dropped, but the plaintiff did recover damages in the lower court from both the doctor and the hospital for their failure to warn her of the patient's psychotic condition and "violent trends and disposi-

---

[3]He was, however, found to be in violation of his building's lease, which did not allow him to maintain a private practice in that apartment, and had to leave the building.

tions." The defendants appealed and the Appellate Division reversed, dismissing the complaint against the hospital but ordering a new trial against the defendant doctor. In a pretrial examination, the doctor had testified that the patient did present a "hazard" both to others in her vicinity and to himself. This admission of prior knowledge precluded the possibility of dismissing the complaint against the doctor: "Were it not for his testimony in the examination before trial as to the patient being a 'hazard' we would be inclined to dismiss the complaint as to him."

ASSAULT AND/OR BATTERY BY THERAPIST

5.44 ABRAHAM V. ZASLOW
(Case cited in "Psychologist faces malpractice," 1972)

The defendant, Dr. Zaslow, was a psychologist practicing in California who employed a technique called "Rage Reduction Therapy" in treating his patients. The therapy involved prolonged physical stimulation of the patient's rib cage. Injuries (contusions, etc.) were claimed by the plaintiff Abraham, and the court found the psychologist liable for the injuries. A judgment in the amount of $170,000 was awarded to the plaintiff.

5.45 HAMMER V. ROSEN
7 N.Y.2d 376; 165 N.E.2d 756; 198 N.Y.S.2d 65 (New York, 1960)

The defendant in this case, Dr. Rosen, was a psychiatrist who had achieved some success in treating schizophrenic patients by acting in a schizophrenic manner at times in the course of the treatment. The patient, a schizophrenic who had been beaten by Dr. Rosen, brought suit against the doctor. Dr. Rosen's defense was that there was no expert testimony supporting the plaintiff's contention that the battery constituted malpractice or improper treatment. The defense did not call any experts to testify on behalf of the propriety of Dr. Rosen's treatment methods and medical judgment. The court found Dr. Rosen liable and held that "the very nature of the acts complained of bespeaks improper treatment and malpractice."

5.46 STOWERS V. WOLODZKO
386 Mich. 119; 191 N.W.2d 355 (Michigan, 1972)

As a result of commitment papers signed by Dr. Wolodzko and Dr. Anthony Smyk, Mrs. Ethel Stowers was involuntarily committed to a private mental hospital. The suit brought by Mrs. Stowers alleged malpractice, assault and battery, and false imprisonment and named Wolodzko, Smyk, and the hospital as defendants. Prior to the trial in circuit court, the suits against Smyk and the hospital were dismissed. At the conclusion of that trial, the judge let only the assault and battery and false imprisonment counts go to the jury. The jury returned a verdict in favor of the plaintiff and awarded her $40,000. The court of appeals upheld the verdict and did not find the jury award to be excessive (*Stowers v. Wolodzko,* 19 Mich. App. 115; 172 N.W.2d 497).

On appeal to the Supreme Court of Michigan, it was ruled that a jury could find the defendant liable for assault and battery for ordering shots and medication administered to Mrs. Stowers against her wishes. In rendering this decision, the court took into account not only the fact that Mrs. Stowers had been committed to a private (and not a state) mental institution, but that the attorney general had clearly stated in a prior case that "any treatment given without consent of the patient, other than that necessary to keep him on the premises and to prevent his injuring himself or others, is given at the peril of the superintendent, and may give rise to liability for assault or for trespass." In its decision that there was sufficient evidence from which a jury could find the defendant to have committed the tort of assault and battery, the supreme court cited the decision of the lower court (the court of appeals):

> The sanctity of one's body is such that a possible absence of pain and suffering in its unwarranted and nonconsensual touching does not eliminate the need for protection from, or compensation for, such touching in the absence of a court order or an emergency. Any submission by plaintiff, no matter how benign, was not voluntary. It was not necessary that she violently resist at every juncture as a prerequisite to recovery for assault and battery if her lack of consent was clearly manifested.

The Supreme Court of Michigan also found that there was sufficient evidence from which a jury could find false imprisonment, since the patient had been held incommunicado at the hospital and "holding a person incommunicado is clearly a restraint of one's freedom, sufficient to allow a jury to find false imprisonment." Expert testimony sympathetic to Wolodzko's argument that mental patients are, as a matter of course, restrained from communicating with the outside world was held to be insufficient:

> Defendant contends that it was proper for him to restrict plaintiff's communication with the outside world. Defendant's witness, Dr. Sidney Bolter, testified that orders restricting communications and visitors are customary in cases of this type. Hence, defendant contends these orders were lawful and could not constitute the basis for an

action of false imprisonment. However, the testimony of Dr. Bolter is not conclusive at this point.

Psychiatry is a relatively new professional discipline and, as with all disciplines, there is a great deal of controversy within the profession as to precisely what methods of treatment should be used. Psychiatrists have a great deal of power over their patients. In the case of a person confined to an institution, this power is virtually unlimited. All professions (including the legal profession) contain unscrupulous individuals who use their position to injure others. The law must provide protection against the torts committed by these individuals. In the case of mental patients, in order to have this protection, they must be able to communicate with the outside world.

FALSE IMPRISONMENT

5.47 BEAUMONT V. SEGAL
283 N.E.2d 858 (Massachusetts, 1972)

After her confinement in a Massachusetts state hospital, the plaintiff named four physicians in an action to recover for malpractice and false imprisonment. Two of the defendants were psychiatrists on the staff of the hospital, one was a psychiatrist in private practice who was a consultant to the hospital, and the fourth physician was the hospital superintendent. The hospital superintendent was additionally sued for assault and battery because of the conduct of his "agents and servants" in the state hospital. At the trial, the judge directed a verdict in favor of the defendants after listening to the plaintiff's lawyer's opening statements. The plaintiff filed an appeal, and the appeals court upheld the defendants' freedom from liability, noting that:

1. There was no ground for recovery for false imprisonment, since the detention of the patient had essentially been conducted in compliance with existing state law.

2. There was no ground for recovery for malpractice, because

the fact that it was determined that the plaintiff could safely be discharged ... is no evidence that her confinement before that date was caused by negligent malpractice on the part of the defendants.... In summary, the opening statement discloses that she was interviewed and examined by at least five different doctors, with the first examination occurring immediately upon her admission to the hospital. She was also interviewed in at least one appearance before a medical staff conference. The opening shows no intention of plaintiff to introduce any expert testimony, by the defendants or other witnesses, from which the negligence of the defendants could be inferred.

3. There was no ground for recovery for assault and battery, because "as hospital superintendent [the defendant] was a public

official and, consequently, not responsible for the misfeasance of his servants and agents under the doctrine of respondeat superior [see Chapter 7, pp. 237–238]."

5.48   CAWTHON V. COFFER
264 So.2d 873 (Florida, 1972)

Two court-appointed psychiatrists were asked to determine the plaintiff's competency; they reported back to the court that, on the basis of their thorough examination, the plaintiff was incompetent. The psychiatrists were subsequently sued on the grounds that they had not made a thorough examination and that the plaintiff was, in fact, competent. It was also charged that the psychiatrists had caused the plaintiff to suffer physical, mental, and financial losses as a result of their lax examination. Consistent with most court rulings pertinent to the liability of court-appointed examiners, the defendants were not found to be liable. The court stated that "a doctor who is appointed by a court for the purpose of making a physical examination to determine mental capacity in an incompetency proceeding should be immune from liability based upon his negligence in making the examination."

5.49   CARPENTER V. CITY OF ROCHESTER
324 N.Y.S.2d 591 (New York, 1971)

A man was arrested and charged with loitering, to which he pleaded "not guilty" in municipal court. The court ordered a psychiatric examination of the man at the request of an assistant district attorney. The court-appointed psychiatrist diagnosed the man as psychotic, and the court ordered the man to a county infirmary for a period not to exceed thirty days, in accordance with New York State law. After fifteen days the man was back in court, and the case was ultimately dismissed on the grounds that the arresting officer did not adequately fill out the proper papers in making the arrest. The man brought suit against the city of Rochester and its agent, the psychiatrist, for defamation, false arrest, false imprisonment, malicious prosecution (groundless institution of legal proceedings), abuse of process, unlawful psychiatric detention, and conspiracy. A summary dismissal of the suit was made on the grounds that the psychiatrist was functioning as a court-appointed officer and therefore was immune from prosecution. The court held that

official functions of the assistant district attorney are privileged and he is protected in their performance by the doctrine of immunity from civil suit. Concomitantly, the functions of the psychiatric examiner who performs the medical screening and evaluation at the request and for the benefit of the Court is also acting in a quasi-judicial capacity and is immune from civil suit arising from the performance of his functions.

5.50 MEZULLO V. MALETZ
331 Mass. 233; 118 N.E.2d 356 (Massachusetts, 1954)

The plaintiff alleged that the defendant physician (1) unlawfully and improperly conspired with her husband to have her committed to an institution for the insane when she was not, in fact, insane; (2) negligently performed a mental examination on her and found her to be insane; and (3) maliciously and in bad faith signed a commitment certificate.

In a previous case in which a plaintiff had lodged similar allegations against a physician, the court had held the defendant physician immune from liability provided that his actions were executed in good faith. The court in *Mezullo*, however, held that a physician who signed a commitment certificate could be held immune from liability—just as a witness could be held immune—even if his actions were *not* executed in good faith:

> But whatever the law may have been formerly on this subject it is now settled that words spoken by a witness in the course of judicial proceedings which are pertinent to the matter in hearing are absolutely privileged, even if uttered maliciously or in bad faith. Laing v. Mitten, 185 Mass. 233, 235, 70 N.E. 128; Sheppard v. Bryant, 191 Mass. 591, 592, 78 N.E. 394. And this is the prevailing view elsewhere. Kintz v. Harringer, 99 Ohio St. 240, 124 N.E. 168, 12 A.L.R. 1247 et seq. and cases there collected. Prosser on Torts, §94. Restatement: Torts, §588. If a physician signing a certificate is entitled to the privilege of a witness . . . then it would follow that he does not lose it on proof of malice or bad faith.

The court in this case further noted that "although the certificate of the examining physicians in a commitment proceeding is intended to, and does in practice, have great weight, a commitment cannot take place without an order from the judge, and a finding by him that the person committed is insane." The court went on to hold (and cited precedents for holding) that a physician who makes false statements attendant to the signing of a commitment certificate should not incur liability: "One who procures the arrest or confinement of another on lawful process is not liable to an action of false imprisonment, although he caused the process to issue by means of false statements. Coupal v. Wash, 106 Mass. 298; Mullen v. Brown, 138 Mass. 114; MacLean v. Naumkeag Trust Co., 268 Mass. 437, 167 N.E. 748; Jordan v. C.I.T. Corp., 302 Mass. 281, 285, 19 N.E. 2d 5. Doggett v. Hooper, 306 Mass. 129, 133, 27 N.E. 2d 737."

The trial court held in favor of the defendant physician, and the Supreme Judicial Court of Massachusetts upheld that ruling.

5.51 BRANDT V. BRANDT
286 Ill. App. 151; 3 N.E.2d 96 (Illinois, 1936)

Mrs. Rose Brandt brought suit against her former husband and a physician, Dr. Freedman, for conspiring to commit her to a mental institution and for malicious prosecution. The complaint alleged that approximately four years before she was arrested "without reasonable or probable cause" and confined in a mental hospital for approximately one-and-a-half months, Mrs. Brandt had won a divorce from her husband, custody of their two children, and a $9,500 alimony settlement (which Mr. Brandt subsequently failed to pay according to the schedule set up by the divorce decree). While court proceedings concerning her husband's nonpayment of alimony were pending, Mrs. Brandt was visited at her home by the defendant, Dr. Freedman, who said he had come to see the two children. Mrs. Brandt testified that she told Freedman that her children weren't sick and that if they were she would call her own doctor. Freedman's account of the incident (as related in the court record) was that he called on Mrs. Brandt at about 9:00 A.M.

> when plaintiff appeared "dressed in an unkept house-apron, in a state of agitation," and in response to his inquiries said she was Mrs. Brandt; that he told her he came to give medical service to the two little sick girls whom he saw through the door unclean and dirty; that with a series of agitated frowns, alternating pallor, and flushing of the face, she said her children were not sick, that when she needed a doctor she would call on him, and in fact would call one that very day; that he persisted that she permit him to enter but she told him to get out, slamming the door in his face. . . .

Other observations of Mrs. Brandt by Freedman led him to believe that Mrs. Brandt was paranoid schizophrenic and that for her own welfare and the welfare of others she should be committed to a hospital. At the trial, Mrs. Brandt's father testified that his daughter was not insane. Also adduced as evidence for the plaintiff was the testimony of a neighbor whom Dr. Freedman had visited at her home. Freedman had asked the neighbor whether she found Mrs. Brandt to be peculiar, and the neighbor had said that she did not. Freedman then asked the neighbor whether Mrs. Brandt neglected her children and the neighbor said, "No, she is a very good mother." When asked by Freedman if she had known that Mrs. Brandt had been examined for insanity the neighbor replied, "I know nothing about that, and I cannot think that Mrs. Brandt was insane.''

The court ruled in favor of the defendants, finding no evidence either for conspiracy or for malicious prosecution:

> The certificates attached to the petition seem to indicate a proceeding in conformity with the statute and a proceeding which was intended to, and in the natural order of things would, give protection to a person whose sanity was questioned. Dr. Freedman, so far as the evidence discloses, had no ulterior motive. He made statements which would seem to have been required by the statute, in the proper exercise of his professional obligations. He was not asked on this trial whether he was employed by his codefendant to make the examination and observations, concerning which he gave his opinion. The statements were in the nature of evidence required by the statute in a proceeding of this kind, and public policy would seem to require that statements of this kind, made in good faith and without ulterior motives, should be entitled to the same privilege as other statements made in connection with court proceedings.
>
> Whatever the evidence thereafter may have disclosed, we think that up to the time plaintiff closed her evidence she had entirely failed to produce any facts from which a conspiracy to have plaintiff unjustly declared insane could be inferred. We do not forget that actual proof of conspiracy cannot in the nature of things usually be made, and that often it must be inferred from proof of the acts of the parties and circumstances in connection therewith. . . . Plaintiff had offered no medical testimony as to her actual mental condition up to the time this order was entered.

5.52 DANIELS V. FINNEY
262 S.W.2d 431 (Texas, 1953)

A psychiatrist prepared commitment papers for the plaintiff solely on the basis of communication with the wife of the plaintiff and a minister. Suit was brought against the psychiatrist for malicious prosecution. The court found in favor of the defendant, noting that while the doctor's actions and his diagnosis of paranoid schizophrenia may not have been entirely appropriate, there was no malice toward the plaintiff. Furthermore, the doctor's diagnosis was not found to be lacking in probable cause.

5.53 KLEBER V. STEVENS
39 Misc.2d 712; 241 N.Y.S.2d 497; 249 N.Y.S.2d 668 (New York, 1964)

A psychiatrist's commitment papers were found to be improper in that they were based on hearsay. The psychiatrist pleaded immunity from liability on the grounds that he was compelled by the court to testify. This motion was denied, and the psychiatrist was judged not as a witness or as an officer of the court but as a medical expert. The trial court awarded the plaintiff $20,000 in damages, an award that was affirmed on appeal.

5.54 WHITREE V. STATE
56 Misc.2d 693; 290 N.Y.S.2d 486 (New York, 1968)

A patient who had been confined to a state hospital in New York for fourteen years brought suit against the state, claiming that he had been falsely imprisoned for twelve of the fourteen years. In finding in favor of the plaintiff, the court remarked on the infrequency with which the plaintiff had been examined and on the lack of depth of those examinations. Additionally, the court noted that the psychiatric records were inadequate and that "the lack of psychiatric care was the primary reason for the inordinate length of this incarceration, with the concomitant side effects of physical injury, moral degradation, and mental anguish." Whitree was awarded $300,000 in damages.

TREATMENT WITH MEDICATION

5.55 HIRSCHBERG V. STATE
398 N.Y.S.2d 470 (New York, 1977)

At 10 A.M. on a mid-November morning Harry Hirschberg swallowed 100 aspirins. At 2 P.M. that afternoon he attempted to jump in front of a school bus. The bus driver took the man to the police. From the police, Hirschberg was seen by a nurse at a nearby hospital and then by his own psychiatrist in a state-run clinic. The psychiatrist transported the patient to a state hospital where instructions were left to give the patient only clear fluids. The patient was admitted by a psychiatric resident who had a license to practice medicine only in the Republic of Yugoslavia. The resident placed the patient on suicide alert and prescribed 100 milligrams of thorazine. The resident did not advise the staff to notify him of any irregular reactions to the medication. At about 11 P.M. that evening the patient died of salicylate poisoning.

A suit brought by Hirschberg's estate charged wrongful death. The court ruled in favor of the plaintiff, holding that the resident did not exhibit the knowledge or skill to provide, "essentially unsupervised, . . . ordinary and reasonable psychiatric medical treatment." The court went on: "The failure to have examined the decedent more thoroughly upon admission, the absence of any attention to the available history, prescribing drugs when only fluids were ordered by a qualified physician, omitting to report decedent's reaction to the medication, failure to call a specialist on internal medicine, the lack of concern for any precautions and the baseless assumption that others had effectively tended to the salicylate poisoning, warrant a finding of mindless professional care and treatment, tantamount to gross negligence."

5.56 SARON V. STATE
24 A.D.2d 771; 263 N.Y.S.2d 591 (New York, 1965)

Plaintiff brought suit claiming that the use of an experimental drug in the treatment of schizophrenia constituted malpractice. An expert witness testified that the alleged injury could have been caused by factors other than the drug. The testimony as to the then known negative consequences of the drug was equivocal. The court ruled in favor of the defendant.

5.57 BELLANDI V. PARK SANITARIUM ASSOCIATION
214 Cal. 472; 6 P.2d 508 (California, 1931)

A violent patient was restrained by knocking him down, applying a tourniquet to his neck, and forcing him to inhale ether. The patient subsequently died, and the hospital was successfully sued for wrongful death on the grounds that this method of restraint was excessive.

ELECTROSHOCK THERAPY

5.58 McDONALD V. MOORE
323 So.2d 635 (Florida, 1976)

A psychiatrist treated a patient for a narcotics addiction problem with medication (methadone) and shock treatments. The psychiatrist neither warned the patient of the possible complications of shock therapy nor administered a muscle relaxant before administering the shock. After the fifth shock treatment, the patient complained of a severe pain in his right shoulder. The psychiatrist minimized the complaint and instructed the patient to return the following day for a sixth treatment. After that treatment, the patient found out that his shoulder had been dislocated and fractured. He brought suit against the psychiatrist. Expert witnesses testifying on behalf of the plaintiff noted that the treating psychiatrist's failure to warn and to administer a muscle relaxant fell below the standard of care. The jury found in favor of the plaintiff and awarded $5,000 in compensatory damages but no punitive damages (as he had requested). Failure to warn of the risk of fracture and failure to administer a muscle relaxant were held to be insufficient to warrant the award of punitive damages.

5.59 STONE V. PROCTOR
259 N.C. 633; 131 S.E.2d 297; 99 A.L.R.2d 593 (North Carolina, 1963)

A psychiatrist was found liable for malpractice for failing to diagnose a fractured vertebra following each of five shock treatments even though the patient complained of back pain following each of the treatments.

5.60 ADAMS V. RICKS
91 Ga. App. 494; 86 S.E.2d 329 (Georgia, 1955)

A doctor was found liable for injuries sustained by the patient when the patient fell out of bed following electroshock therapy. The court held that the doctor did not offer adequate supervision to guard against such injuries.

5.61 MAYNIER V. DePAUL HOSPITAL
336 So.2d 521 (Louisiana, 1976)

The defendant hospital was found liable for injuries sustained by a seventy-two-year-old patient who, after electroshock treatment, fell while being assisted down a flight of stairs. The court held that the hospital should have used a wheelchair to transport the patient through an existing, shorter, and more direct route.

5.62 PETTIS V. LOUISIANA
336 So.2d 521 (Louisiana, 1976)

The court found the defendants liable for failing to determine if fractures had occurred after one electroshock treatment before proceeding to apply another treatment.

5.63 RICE V. MERCY HOSPITAL
318 So.2d 436 (Florida, 1975)

A voluntary patient treated with electroshock therapy claimed that the treatment constituted an assault on his person. The court held that the treatment did not constitute such an assault.

5.64 PRICE V. SHEPPARD
       239 N.W.2d 905 (Minnesota, 1976)

After unsuccessful attempts at voluntary treatment, a mother concerned with her son's drinking and drug problems had him committed to a state institution. Because of an assault on a staff member in the hospital, the patient was subsequently transferred to a more secure setting. The patient was given trials of antidepressants and tranquilizers, but no improvement in his condition was noted. Electroshock therapy was suggested as one possible course of treatment that might be beneficial to the patient. The permission of the patient's mother was sought, and she had her son seen by a consulting psychiatrist for a second opinion. The consultant suggested that the medication be continued for a while, but that if the patient did not respond, electroshock therapy would be advisable.

The patient was kept on the medication for some time longer, though he did not seem to be responding to it. Electroshock therapy was subsequently begun without the consent of either the patient (a minor) or his mother. Twenty electroshock treatments were administered over the course of two months, and the patient was discharged approximately four months after the last treatment. A suit was brought by the mother claiming that the hospital's unauthorized administration of electroshock to her son constituted a violation of her son's right to be free from cruel and unusual punishment as well as his right to privacy.

Despite the fact that the patient had been assaulting hospital staff members and other patients, there was no evidence in the court record to suggest that the electroshock therapy was in any way being used as a method of punishment. The court held that the administration of the shock was done in good faith, without malice, and in accordance with accepted medical practice. Therefore the patient's rights to privacy and to freedom from cruel and unusual punishment had not been violated.

5.65 BROWN V. MOORE
       143 F. Supp. 816; 247 F.2d 711 (Pennsylvania, 1957)

A patient hospitalized in a sanitorium for anxiety neurosis was administered electroshock therapy on the fourth day of hospitalization. About seven hours after the treatment the patient fell down a flight of stairs and immediately claimed that he had broken his neck and was dying. Symptoms that appeared immediately or soon after the fall included paraplegia of the legs, paralysis of one arm, quadriplegia, abdomen distension, inability to defecate, vomiting, and respiratory embarrassment. Four days after the fall, the patient died. The patient's wife brought suit against the sanitorium, charging wrongful death. After trials and appeals in which other issues (e.g., the negligence of the treating psychiatrist) were considered, the final disposition entailed a $60,000 settlement in favor of the plaintiff, including $25,000 in damages for wrongful death and $35,000 in survival action (the latter calculated from the amount of money the deceased would have earned at his job had he survived).

5.66 MITCHELL V. ROBINSON
334 S.W.2d 11 (Missouri, 1960)

A patient who was not informed of the possible complications of electroshock therapy brought suit against the treating psychiatrist when injuries resulted as a result of the treatment. The court held the doctor liable for failing to inform the patient of the possibility of fractures and other possible hazards in treatment.

BREACH OF CONFIDENTIALITY

5.67 BELMONT V. CALIFORNIA STATE PERSONNEL BOARD
111 Cal. Rptr. 607 (California, 1974)

Psychiatric social workers Josephine Belmont and Glenda Pawsey were suspended from their jobs at the Department of Social Welfare for willful disobedience of an order to furnish information to the Department concerning their patients. The Department was installing a computerized record-keeping system to be integrated with county, state, and federal welfare agencies. The information requested had already been in the possession of the Department of Social Welfare; the purpose of the order was to have the social workers prepare it for electronic data processing. After their suspension for five days without pay, Belmont and Pawsey had their case reviewed by the State Personnel Board, and the suspension was upheld. Their complaint was next heard by the California Superior Court, and the court also upheld the Department's order of suspension.

The court of appeals affirmed the decision of the Superior Court. The appellate court held that these social workers' clients were actually clients of the state and its Department of Social Welfare. It denied that psychiatric social workers in such settings have a privilege to refuse to disclose confidential communications between patient and psychotherapist (appellants Belmont and Pawsey worked with emotionally disturbed persons who were receiving public assistance). Excerpts of Associate Justice Elkington's opinion in this case appear below:

> Appellants insist that a special professional relationship exists between themselves and their "clients" entitling them to assume an adversary position toward their employer, the State of California, defending "the rights of their clients." They speak of a social worker's "code of ethics" designed to "protect those clients who come into professional contact with the social worker," to which they owe a higher duty of obedience than to their employer. And they argue that the Department's order tends to "seriously undercut the relationship between the patient and the psychiatric social worker," a relationship which they strongly suggest is covered by the psychotherapist–patient privilege against nondisclosure, created by Evidence Code section 1014.
>
> There can, of course, be no reasonable objection to appellants' election to describe the persons with whom they work as their "clients." But, nevertheless, the term neither connotes nor confirms the special legal relationship suggested by appellants. More appropriately, the handicapped persons are "clients" of the state and its Department of Social Welfare acting through its employees, psychiatric and other social workers. A commonly accepted definition of the term is "a person served by or utilizing the services of a social agency or a public institution."
>
> A frequently repeated truism of our law is that "activities [of public] employees may not be allowed to disrupt or impair the public service.... It is therefore essential to the public service that its employees obey all *lawful orders* given them in the course of their employment. Of course, a public employee may not himself, in "good faith" and without penalty, determine whether such a lawful order shall be obeyed, for nothing would seem better calculated to "disrupt or impair the public service." And when " 'an employee of the state, under civil service, accepts a position, he does so with knowledge of the fact that... his conduct [is] subject to the law....' "
>
> So without further consideration of any assumed special "client" relationship, or statutory privilege, or higher duty of allegiance to a "code of ethics," we enter upon our inquiry. The basic question before us, as it was before the Department, the Board, and then the superior court, is simply whether the Department's order to its psychiatric social workers was a *lawful order*.
>
> In 1965 the Legislature created the "Department of Social Welfare" to be managed by a "Director" who was given broad power, among other things, to formulate and adopt policies, regulations, orders and standards implementing the "public social service" statutes of California. The order here under dispute was promulgated by the Director pursuant to that authority.
>
> Appellants appear to concede that the subject information of this case was properly in the possession of the Department, and could properly be used by "authorized persons" including such persons in the related county and federal welfare agencies.
>
> Instead, they state: "[T]he issue is whether the collection and storage of data by government in a *computerized data bank* is [*on the facts of this case*], an invasion of the privacy of the persons whom the data concerns." (Emphasis added.) They argue that the Department's

order requiring them to participate in such an invasion of privacy contrary to the Fourth Amendment, is unlawful and therefore need not be obeyed.

Principal reliance is placed by appellants on the case of Parrish v. Civil Service Commission, 66 Cal.2d 260, 57 Cal.Rptr. 623, 425 P.2d 223. But there a social worker was held to have been wrongfully penalized for refusing to participate in an *unlawful activity*, an early morning "bed check" of the homes of welfare recipients, in clear violation of the Fourth Amendment. Parrish v. Civil Service Commission is authority for the proposition that a state employee may properly refuse to obey an *unlawful order*, a point which is here wholly undisputed. . . .

It is first asserted that the subject welfare recipients were not asked for permission to use the pertinent information, or told that they need not supply it, or advised that it would be fed into the computer system. It is conceded that no "directly applicable" authority is to be found supporting appellants' claim that obtaining, storing, and using the information under these circumstances is unlawful. The persons with whom appellants work are, as indicated, receiving welfare aid from the state. The data was obviously sought by the Department from its psychiatric social workers pursuant to its duty to administer such aid efficiently and effectively. There could be no reasonable objection to its use by the Department and related county and federal welfare agencies with, or without, the consent or knowledge of the welfare recipients. This proffered evidence would establish neither unlawfulness nor constitutional impropriety in the Department's order.

Appellants also offered to prove that computer storage of the data, or some of it, by the Department was "unnecessary." Such a determination is best left to the agency charged by law with making it. But in any event, we observe no reason why the Department is legally or constitutionally restricted to the use of such information as is *necessary* to its functioning; some *relevancy* to the agency's administrative functions would reasonably be sufficient.

The third area of appellants' offer of proof may be summarized as follows: (1) inadequate steps are taken to ensure privacy of the data; (2) persons with access to the data are not known with "certainty"; (3) some "authorized" persons have "little or no use for such sensitive information," while (4) others "have access to more information than necessary"; (5) more security could be had "with the expenditure of relatively little time, money, and effort"; and (6) "The Department either did not consider or rejected several very practical and relatively inexpensive methods of improving the security" of the data processing system.

Many of these complaints concern administrative decisions, the responsibility for which is placed by statute in the Director of the Department. To the extent that they relate to the right of privacy of the welfare recipients, that right was and is the concern of Welfare and Institutions Code section 10850. . . .

We are of the opinion that Welfare and Institutions Code section 10850 (since 1969 amended in substantially similar form), imposing criminal sanctions for its breach, adequately protected the right of privacy of the welfare recipients served by the state's psychiatric social workers. No constitutional breach by the Department of that right was established by this segment of the offer of proof.

We observe that the sanctions of section 10850 are equally operative with respect to county welfare agencies and also, that a similar statute safeguards the security of such information in the hands of the Department of Health, Education and Welfare. (See 42 U.S.C., § 1306.)

The fourth and remaining assertion of the offer of proof is that: "Once the information concerning appellants' clients has been supplied to the Department's [electronic data processing] system, appellants have no control over its dissemination or distribution."

It does not appear, nor do appellants even contend, that "control" over the Department's records is any part of the duties of psychiatric social workers. The Department is obviously free to place that responsibility elsewhere.

From all of the foregoing it follows that the Department's and the Legislature's purpose to make "maximum use of electronic data processing" in the handling and storage of welfare recipient information, under the facts embraced by appellants' offer of proof, flouted neither the "right of privacy" nor other Fourth Amendment principle.

Appellants having, as a matter of law, willfully refused to obey a lawful order of the Department, the judgment of the superior court will be affirmed.

5.68 CLARK V. GERACI
29 Misc.2d 791; 208 N.Y.S.2d 564 (New York, 1960)

The plaintiff in this case was a civilian who worked for the Air Force as an accountant. He had taken off time from work owing to respiratory difficulties that stemmed from his alcoholism. In response to an official request for information concerning the causes of the plaintiff's absences, the defendant psychiatrist revealed that the plaintiff had a drinking problem (despite the fact that the plaintiff had explicitly objected to the revelation of that information). The plaintiff was subsequently fired from his job, and he brought suit against the doctor for breach of confidentiality.

The court recognized that breach of doctor–patient confidentiality is an actionable offense, but it declined to find in favor of the plaintiff in this case. The court held that the plaintiff had probably lost his job not because of the mere revelation of confidential material, but because of repeated absences from work. Furthermore, the court held the doctor's duty to the United States government to be above the doctor's duty to the patient.

5.69 BERRY V. MOENCH
8 Utah 2d 191; 331 P.2d 814; 73 A.L.R.2d 315 (Utah, 1958)

Berry was a patient seen by Dr. Moench, a psychiatrist, seven years prior to this litigation. Berry was about to remarry, and the father of his bride-to-be asked a Dr. Hellewell to write Dr. Moench to find out information about Berry. Hellewell wrote to Moench, specifically stating that the reasons he was soliciting information about Berry was to advise the father of the prospective bride-to-be. Dr. Moench's letter to Hellewell said that Berry had been diagnosed as "manic depressive depression in a psychopathic personality." Moench went on to offer the following advice in his letter:

> My suggestion to the infatuated girl would be to run as fast and as far as she possibly could in any direction away from him. . . . Of course, if he doesn't marry her, he will marry someone else and make life hell for that person.

Berry brought suit against Moench for breach of confidentiality. The court found in favor of the defendant, holding that the parents of the woman Berry was dating were concerned only with the welfare of their daughter and that that concern was a sufficient interest to legally protect. The court wrote that, according to generally accepted standards of decent conduct, "the privilege exists if the recipient has the type of interest in the matter, and the publisher stands in such a relation to him that it would reasonably be considered the duty of the publisher to give the information."

5.70 (Citation Withheld)

The plaintiff claimed that a psychologist gave damaging information to his employer without his permission. The amount in damages sought was approximately $150,000. The case was eventually dismissed, and no award was made.

5.71 (Citation Withheld)

The plaintiff, a member of a therapy group, spoke during a group session of some illegal manipulations in which he had been involved. Another member of the therapy group talked about the plaintiff's actions to a non–group member at a party. The plaintiff brought suit against the group's psychologist, claiming that there was a breach of confidentiality. The plaintiff agreed to drop the matter if the psychologist would not attempt to collect his bill. The case was closed.

5.72 FURNISS v. FITCHETT
(Case cited in *New Zealand Law Review*, 1958, p. 396)

A psychiatrist treating a husband and wife gave some information about the wife to the husband. One year later, that information was revealed by the husband's attorney in a public proceeding. The revelation of this material caused great distress and shock on the part of the wife, and she brought suit against the psychiatrist for breach of confidentiality. The court found the psychiatrist liable for failing to exercise reasonable care in foreseeing that the revelation of that material might cause harm to the plaintiff.

5.73 SCHAFFER V. SPICER
215 N.W.2d 135 (South Dakota, 1974)

A husband and wife were involved in a family court dispute, each desiring custody of their child. The husband introduced testimony from his wife's psychiatrist which divulged in detail information obtained in psychotherapy sessions. The wife had not given permission to the psychiatrist to divulge such information, and she filed suit against the psychiatrist for violating the doctor–patient privilege. The court found in favor of the plaintiff, but there was a strong dissenting opinion in this case:

> Although there is but limited authority, precedent does exist for the proposition that, without any claim of consent or waiver, the physician–patient privilege must yield in a custody proceeding to the paramount rights of the infant. In People v. Fitzgerald, 40 Misc. 2d 966, 244 N.Y.S.2d 441, the Supreme Court of New York so held, over objection of a husband, in granting a request by his wife in a custody proceeding for an examination by a court of the husband's hospital records containing allegedly confidential records pertaining to the psychological examination of the husband's mental condition. The court stated [that] "[t]he precise question as to whether the court may disregard the patient–physician privilege in a custody proceeding does not appear to have been ruled upon by the courts of this state. There is, of course, ample authority indicative of the court's right to discover the mental condition of a party in a matrimonial matter. . . . The individual rights of infants to invoke the protection of the state in which they reside cannot be ignored." It is thus clear to me that, in the exercise of the court's inherent power to do what is best to protect the welfare of the infant, the right of the petitioner to invoke the patient–physician privilege must yield to the paramount rights of the infant.

5.74 HANNAWAY V. COLE
311 N.E.2d 924 (Massachusetts, 1974)

A patient filed suit against his psychiatrist, claiming breach of confidentiality. The plaintiff did not set forth the circumstances of the alleged disclosure or the identity of the persons to whom the disclosure was made. The court decided that the mere claim of breach of confidentiality would not be sufficient for the plaintiff to recover damages.

DEFAMATION

5.75 IVERSON V. FRANDSEN
      237 F.2d 898 (Idaho, 1956)

In his psychological report, Arden Frandsen, a psychologist at
State Hospital South, Blackfoot, Idaho, described a nine-year-old
Jo Ann Iverson as being feeble-minded and a high-grade moron.
Carmel Iverson, Jo Ann's mother, brought suit against the psychologist alleging that his psychological report contained libelous statements on the mental level and capacity of her daughter. A United
States District Court entered judgment in favor of the defendant
psychologist, and the plaintiff appealed. The facts of the case as well
as the decision of the United States Court of Appeals appear in the
opinion written by Circuit Judge Murrah:

> Since very early childhood, the appellant [Jo Ann] has admittedly
> suffered from claustrophobia—a fear of enclosed places. Early in Sep-
> tember 1951, the guardian ad litem [Jo Ann's mother] took her nine-
> year-old daughter, the appellant, to the State Hospital South,
> Blackfoot, Idaho, a state institution for the mentally ill, for assistance
> in overcoming this fear which prevented her child from attending pub-
> lic school. After a short discussion with Dr. Isabella Ralph, a staff
> psychiatrist, she was advised to return at a later date for a more
> thorough inquiry. At the subsequent meeting Dr. Ralph directed the
> mother and daughter to the appellee, Frandsen, an experienced psy-
> chologist employed part time at the hospital. It was standard institu-
> tional procedure to have all patients examined by psychologist-
> psychiatrist teams—the psychologist doing the testing and evaluating
> and the psychiatrist administering the treatment. As a part of his exam-
> ination Frandsen gave the daughter a Stanford–Benet [sic] test—a
> universally recognized method for determining the intelligence quotient
> and mental capacity of an individual. He then forwarded to psychia-
> trist Ralph his report which stated in part that the intelligence quotient
> of the child classified her as " 'feeble-minded', at the high-grade moron
> level of general mental ability." The report further stated that "at the
> time she is about sixteen, she should have progressed to about the
> fourth grade level in reading, arithmetic, writing, etc." These two
> statements are the basis for this libel action. Subsequently, on request
> of the appellant's school guidance director, and following the practice
> of the hospital, a copy of Frandsen's report was forwarded to the
> school officials. It was from this source that embarrassing rumors ap-
> parently emanated concerning the mental condition of the appellant.
> Upon contacting the local school authorities, the mother was shown
> Frandsen's report and another report made three years later by the
> school's guidance director which gave her daughter about the same
> I.Q. rating.
>   Without taking issue with any of the foregoing facts, the appellant
> rests her case squarely on the proposition that she went to Dr. Ralph

for advice and treatment concerning claustrophobia; that the Stanford–Benet test was beyond the scope of the consultation, wholly unauthorized and therefore not qualifiedly privileged.

There was positive and uncontradicted proof to the effect that the Stanford–Benet test was standard procedure for all patients to ascertain whether such patients had the mental capacity to respond to psycho-therapy and, if so, at what level it must be based; that the report was prepared at the request of Dr. Ralph, in accordance with standard procedures and intended only for hospital officials or professionally interested persons; that Frandsen only saw the appellant on this one accasion; that the report was as accurate as Frandsen could make it; that Frandsen had never seen it since forwarding it to Dr. Ralph; and that he had never been consulted concerning the use of the report by any one other than the hospital officials to whom it was directed. The report was clearly within the duties of Frandsen as a staff psychologist of the state hospital and it contained matter which certainly was of professional interest both to the appellee and Dr. Ralph.

[5] The report is said to be absolutely privileged under the rationale of Glass v. Ickes, supra. But, we have seen no Idaho decisions indicating a disposition to extend the doctrine of absolute privilege to communications of this kind. See Dwyer v. Libert, 30 Idaho 576, 167 P. 651, 652, citing Foster v. Scripps, 39 Mich. 376, 33 Am.Rep. 403, which denied privilege to the communications of an appointed physician in public service " 'except a bona fide representation made without malice to the proper authority' ". In the view we take of this case, however, it is unnecessary for us to delineate the field of absolute privilege in Idaho. For, we are convinced that the assailed report, though qualifiedly privileged, was positively free from any actionable malice whatsoever. In the first place, it was incumbent upon the appellant to offer some evidence of an extrinsic character to show actual malice on the part of the appellee. The appellant admittedly consulted a psychiatrist at a public institution for the purpose of receiving psychiatric therapy. And, it is also true that, as a part of the contemplated treatment, she voluntarily submitted herself to an examination by a duly recognized psychologist, and having done so, she cannot prescribe the diagnostic procedure incident to such treatment. To be sure, she is not libeled by the contents of the report. It was a professional report made by a public servant in good faith, representing his best judgment, and therefore could not be maliciously false.

The judgment is affirmed.

5.76 MODLA V. PARKER
495 P.2d 494 (Arizona, 1972)

Shortly before a hospital patient was to be discharged, a hospital administrator remarked to her, "Do me a favor and see a psychiatrist." The patient brought suit against the administrator for slander. The court found the administrator not liable, on the grounds that no compelling testimony or evidence had been adduced to prove that the patient's personality or professional life had been injured.

5.77 (Citation Withheld)

A psychologist testified at a family court hearing that the plaintiff beat his children, harassed his wife, and was in need of psychiatric care. The plaintiff brought suit against the psychologist in the amount of one million dollars. (In litigation.)

5.78 GASPERINI V. MANGINELLI
196 Misc. 547; 92 N.Y.S.2d 575 (New York, 1949)

In filling out a request for an order for psychiatric hospitalization, a psychiatrist omitted the word "Jr." from the patient's name. The father of the patient brought suit against the psychiatrist, charging libel. The court held that whether or not anyone had in fact read what the psychiatrist wrote and interpreted the name to be that of the patient's father was a matter for a jury to decide.

5.79 (Citation Withheld)

A patient disrupted a therapeutic workshop, and the psychologist allegedly stated in front of the group members that he had treated the patient before and that the patient was suffering from a character disorder. A suit claiming defamation was filed in the amount of $200,000. The claim was settled out of court for approximately $1,000.

5.80 (Citation Withheld)

A psychologist brought suit against another psychologist for allegedly publishing and disseminating a written report that contained false and malicious statements about her. The plaintiff further alleged that her privacy had been violated by the defendant's reading of her mail and monitoring of her private phone calls and telephone service. The suit was brought in the amount of $100,000 in compensatory damages and $60,000 in punitive damages. (In litigation.)

SEXUAL IMPROPRIETIES

5.81 ROY V. HARTOGS
381 N.Y.S.2d 587 (New York, 1975)

Dr. Renatus Hartogs, a psychiatrist, had used sexual intercourse as therapy over a period of thirteen months, according to the plaintiff, Ms. Julie Roy. The defense attorney argued that Roy did not have a valid cause of action as actions for seduction, alienation of affection, and breach of contract to marry had been abolished in New York State. The court ruled that a valid cause of action for malpractice had been brought. Dr. Hartogs was subsequently found to be liable for malpractice. (See pp. 94–95 for a more detailed description of the circumstances of this case). A memorandum filed by one of the justices who concurred that Hartogs should be held liable for malpractice is reprinted below, followed by the opinion of a dissenting justice who did not believe that Hartogs should have been found liable.

Presiding Justice Markowitz (concurring):

The subject matter of this case was highly sensational, forcing the participants to operate in a charged atmosphere rather than the calm, almost cloistered, climate of the routine civil courtroom. However, since this State has not closed the door on all actions merely because sexual relations are part of the core facts, and does permit civil prosecutions where the wrong alleged is grounded on conventional tort (*Tuck v. Tuck*, 14 N.Y.2d 341, 251 N.Y.S.2d 653, 200 N.E.2d 554) there is no question that the facts adduced in this record were properly presented to the jury as a possible basis for malpractice which had a causal connection to plaintiff's subsequent psychotic episodes.

While cultists expound theories of the beneficial effects of sexual psychotherapy, the fact remains that all eminent experts in the psychiatric field including the American Psychiatric Association abjure sexual contact between patient and therapist as harmful to the patient and deviant from accepted standards of treatment of the mentally disturbed.

Dr. Ernest Jones, in his encyclopedic treatment of "The Life and Work of Sigmund Freud" (New York, Basic Books, Inc., 1953) sets forth (Vol. 3, p. 163) a letter written by Freud to a colleague which is relevant to the discussion here.

It reads in pertinent part as follows:

"13. XII. 1931

"Lieber Freund:

". . . You have not made a secret of the fact that you kiss your patients and let them kiss you; . . .

"Now I am assuredly not one of those who from prudishness or from consideration of bourgeois convention would condemn little erotic gratifications of this kind. . . . But that does not alter the facts . . . that with us a kiss signifies a certain erotic intimacy. We have hitherto in our technique held to the conclusion that patients are to be refused erotic gratifications. You know too that where more extensive gratifications are not to be had milder caresses very easily take over their role, in love affairs, on the stage, etc.

"Now picture what will be the result of publishing your technique. There is no revolutionary who is not driven out of the field by a still more radical one. A number of independent thinkers in matters of technique will say to themselves: why stop at a kiss? Certainly one gets further when one adopts 'pawing' as well, which after all doesn't make a baby. And then bolder ones will come along who will go further to peeping and showing—and soon we shall have accepted in the technique of analysis the whole repertoire of demiviergerie and petting parties, resulting in an enormous increase of interest in psychoanalysis among both analysts and patients. The new adherent, however, will easily claim too much of this interest for himself, the younger of our colleagues will find it hard to stop at the point they originally intended, and God the Father Ferenczi gazing at the lively scene he has created will perhaps say to himself: maybe after all I should have halted in my technique of motherly affection *before* the kiss.

"Sentences like 'about the dangers of neocatharsis' don't get very far. One should obviously not let oneself get into the danger. I have purposely not mentioned the increase of calumnious resistances against analysis the kissing technique would bring, although it seems to me a wanton act to provoke them. . . .

With cordial greetings

Your

Freud"

Thus from the font of psychiatric knowledge to the modern practitioner we have common agreement of the harmful effects of sensual intimacies between patient and therapist.

Of interesting note is an annotation entitled Civil Liability of Doctor or Psychologist for Having Sexual Relationship With Patient (33 A.L.R.3d 1393), in which the notewriters state: "Apart from *Nicholson v. Han* [12 Mich.App. 35, 162 N.W.2d 313, 83 A.L.R.3d 1386, a case whose facts are not applicable here], research has failed to disclose any case in which the courts have discussed or passed upon the civil liability of a doctor or a psychologist, as such, who while the doctor–patient relationship subsisted, had established a sexual relationship with a patient." However, where the sexual contacts are themselves the prescribed course of treatment and where such treatment is outside of accepted professional standards, what remains is a simple malpractice action as to which research would be merely cumulative.

On the question of punitive damages, such recovery is allowed in cases where the wrong complained of is morally culpable, or is actuated by evil and reprehensible motives, not only to punish the defendant but to deter him as well as others, from indulging in similar conduct in the future. (*Walker v. Sheldon*, 10 N.Y.2d 401, 404, 223 N.Y.S.2d 488, 490, 179 N.E.2d 497, 498.)

In the instant case all that has been established is professional incompetence. It was established that plaintiff was influenced to participate on a theory that it would solve her problems.

Sex under cloak of treatment is an acceptable and established ground for disciplinary measures taken against physicians either by licensing authorities or professional organizations (see 15 A.L.R.3d 1179). Whether defendant acted in such manner as to seriously affect his performance as a practitioner in the psychiatric field should be left to these more competent fora, rather than by seeking deterrence by way of punitive damages. The only thing that the record herein supports is that his prescribed treatment was in negligent disregard of the consequences. For that, and that alone, he must be held liable.

Justice Riccobono (dissenting):

The plaintiff pursued her action for malpractice by alleging that over a period of some 13 months the defendant made sexual advances towards her with a lewd and lascivious motive and that he did in fact engage in sexual intercourse and other acts of carnal knowledge with her, in a purported furtherance of psychiatric treatment. Plaintiff further asserts that instead of assisting and curing her, the defendant's therapeutic methods caused her permanent mental and emotional harm. This harm, it is alleged, was caused by the defendant's failure to treat the plaintiff by acceptable medical procedures.

The right of action to recover a sum of money for seduction was abolished by virtue of former Article 2–A of the Civil Practice Act, now Civil Rights Law, section 80–a et seq. Article 8 of the Civil Rights Law must be liberally construed to effectuate this purpose (Civil Rights Law, § 84). This legislation was passed as a matter of public policy because of the threat or danger of an action to recover money damages and the embarrassment and humiliation emanating from such scandalous causes of action.

In the case at bar, although the plaintiff was suffering from a number of emotional problems her competency was never placed in issue. Is it not fair to infer, therefore, that she was capable of giving a knowing and meaningful consent? For almost one and a half years while this "meaningful" relationship continued, the plaintiff was not heard to complain. Upon the defendant terminating the relation, this lawsuit evolves.

The defendant obviously did not help his cause by denying what the jury found to be the fact, viz., that the defendant did have sexual relations with the plaintiff. Nevertheless, however ill-advised or ill-conceived was the choice of his defense, in my view this did not constitute malpractice. The plaintiff was still obliged to prove her case by the preponderance of the credible evidence, regardless of the defendant's defense.

I neither condone the defendant's reprehensible conduct, nor maintain that it was not violative of his professional ethics and Hippocratic oath. If, however, the defendant has committed a crime, let him be brought before the criminal halls of justice. For violation of his Hippocratic oath, if there be any, let him suffer the sanctions of the Medical Ethics Board or other appropriate medical authority. But let him not be convicted of his acts of misfeasance and malfeasance by virtue of an action in malpractice. I might parenthetically add, that if the plaintiff is to succeed I am in total agreement with my colleagues that the plaintiff is not entitled to punitive damages and am likewise in full accord that her recovery should not exceed $25,000.

The relief sought by this plaintiff constitutes the closest approach to a conventional action for seduction, and hence must be treated as such. This is barred by section 80–a of the Civil Rights Law (*Fernandez v. Lazar*, N.Y.L.J., September 15, 1971, p. 19, col. 6, N.Y. Supreme Ct., *Leff, J.*; *Nicholson v. Han*, 12 Mich.App. 35, 162

N.W.2d 313 [1968]). As so inextricably intertwined, I would reverse
and dismiss the complaint.

5.82 ZIPKIN V. FREEMAN
436 S.W.2d 753 (Missouri, 1968)

After four months of treatment with psychiatrist Dr. Freeman,
Mrs. Zipkin told her doctor that she loved him and he told her that
he loved her, too. Dr. Freeman began taking Mrs. Zipkin to
functions outside of the consultation room, such as a nude swimming
party which Freeman described as "group therapy." Some of the evidence presented alleged that Dr. Freeman had advised Mrs. Zipkin

- to divorce her husband, as this was necessary to become "completely well";
- to bring a lawsuit against her brother (which she did attempt
  to do);
- to make an investment of $14,000 to help him buy a farm;
- to move in with him (along with her three children); and
- to rid herself of her hostility by breaking into her husband's
  home and stealing a desk, two beds, a television, and some suits
  for Dr. Freeman.

Mrs. Zipkin testified that during her treatment with Dr.
Freeman she had gone on overnight trips with him, had been his
mistress, and had done anything that he asked. She said that
Freeman had advised her that she needed a "stronger" man than
her husband and that he (Freeman) was that man. It was alleged
that at one point in the treatment Freeman had placed a pistol in
Mrs. Zipkin's hand and told her to return to her home, take anything she wanted, and "shoot anyone who got in the way." An
expert witness at the trial testified that the actions described above
were not generally regarded as the proper treatment for neurosis.

Dr. Freeman was found liable for malpractice. The court held
that "the damages sustained by Mrs. Zipkin were directly and proximately connected with the professional services which Dr. Freeman
rendered or failed to render" and that some of the defendant's
actions "probably constituted crimes." The plaintiff was awarded
$5,000 (plus interest) in damages. (Dr. Freeman's insurance com-
pany refused to pay the damages, on the grounds that Freeman's
actions could not have been construed as having been performed
within the context of a doctor–patient relationship. The court compelled the insurer to pay the damages, however, holding that
Freeman's actions were the result of his mishandling of the transference phenomenon.)

5.83 LANDAU V. WERNER
Queens Bench Reports, March 1, 1961; 105 *Solicitor's Journal* 1008 (Great Britain, 1961)

In Great Britain, an intelligent, middle-aged woman told her psychiatrist that she loved him after she had been treated for about five months for anxiety. The psychiatrist explained the phenomenon of transference to the woman. The psychiatrist began dating the patient over the next several months, going out for tea or dinner and talking of taking a vacation together. When the patient's condition worsened formal treatment was resumed, but to no avail. The trial court found evidence of malpractice and awarded the plaintiff £6,000 in damages. The doctor lost an appeal to a higher court, which also found his departure from standard practice unjustified. The doctor had argued that his continuing to see the patient on a social basis was necessary because a sudden withdrawal might have precipitated a relapse. The appellate court disagreed, holding that the trial court judge was "justified in his view that this unwise treatment had led to the grave deterioration in the plaintiff's health."

5.84 (Citation Withheld)

A patient charged her psychologist with forcing himself sexually on her and causing "irreparable emotional injury." The psychologist admitted to having had sexual relations with the patient on a weekly basis for a period of one year. The psychologist also admitted to having recommended extramarital dating. The amount sued for was $1 million. (In litigation.)

5.85 (Citation Withheld)

A suit was brought against a psychologist alleging that the psychologist had committed adultery with the plaintiff's wife and that the psychologist had been instrumental in instigating the subsequent divorce. The psychologist admitted to having had sexual relations with the plaintiff's wife. During litigation the psychologist died. The suit had been in the amount of $400,000 compensatory damages and $600,000 punitive damages, and it is not known whether or not the plaintiff will continue the suit against the psychologist's estate.

5.86 ANCLOTE MANOR FOUNDATION V. WILKINSON
263 So.2d 265 (Florida, 1972)

A psychiatrist at a psychiatric clinic told his patient that he planned to divorce his wife and marry her (the patient). The woman had been under the psychiatrist's care at a clinic for approximately two years and had paid a total of approximately $29,000 for services. Ten days after the psychiatrist informed the woman of his plans, she was discharged from the clinic. About one year later she committed suicide. The woman's husband (who had divorced his wife in the interim) filed suit against the clinic for breach of contract. The plaintiff's argument was that the breach of contract committed by the psychiatrist destroyed the possibility of any benefit that could have been anticipated under skillful treatment. Expert witnesses at the trial testified that the psychiatrist's acting out of counter-transferential feelings fell below accepted medical standards. The court found in favor of the plaintiff, and the jury awarded the amount sued for. The clinic appealed the decision on the grounds that it was not possible to determine exactly what damages were suffered by the plaintiff as a result of the psychiatrist's action. The court of appeals, however, upheld the trial court's decision:

> [Plaintiff] contends that he is entitled to full reimbursement for monies paid under the contract on the theory that where there is a breach of contract on the part of a physician which destroys the possibility of any benefit which could have been anticipated under skillful treatment in the first instance, he is entitled to recover all expenses incurred by him in the entire course of treatment of his wife. We agree that this is the correct measure of damages if supported by the evidence....

5.87 NICHOLSON V. HAN
12 Mich. App. 35; 162 N.W.2d 313 (Michigan, 1968)

Mr. Nicholson, the plaintiff, began treatment with psychiatrist Dr. Han in late December of 1960. Nicholson complained of marital problems, and soon both he and his wife were being seen in treatment by the defendant doctor. Nicholson and his wife were divorced in 1962. In 1964, the plaintiff learned that Dr. Han had been having sexual relations with his wife in 1961. A suit was brought against Dr. Han, claiming that he had committed malpractice, fraud, breach of contract, assault and battery, and trespass on the case. The plaintiff's action was dismissed on procedural technicalities attendant to the action; the court held that the claim had been based on torts which had been abolished by statute.

5.88 (Citation Withheld)

A patient claimed that her psychologist had convinced her that it was necessary for her treatment that she engage in certain sexual behavior with him. The psychologist admitted to having had sexual relations with the patient and that the matter had been discussed in group therapy. The amount sought was approximately $1 million in compensatory damages and $1 million in punitive damages. (In litigation.)

5.89 (Citation Withheld)

A psychologist at a psychotherapy center assigned a therapist to treat the plaintiff. Away from the center and without the psychologist's knowledge, the therapist allegedly engaged in sexual relations with the plaintiff. A lawsuit was brought against the psychologist, claiming that he negligently allowed an unlicensed person to treat the plaintiff. The therapist denied having had sexual relations with the plaintiff. (In litigation.)

5.90 SAVADER v. KARP
(New York, 1978, in litigation)

Mrs. Penny Savader and her husband, Louis, sought help for marital difficulties and consulted with a thirty-six-year-old psychologist, Nita Karp. Court papers filed by Mrs. Savader's attorney alleged that the defendant, Dr. Karp, "advised the husband to remove himself from the plaintiff's home, prevented them improperly from resuming their marital relationship, commenced a meretricious relationship with the husband and during the period continued to treat the plaintiff wife in an unprofessional and damaging manner, causing her injury." It was also alleged that the plaintiff suffered "mental and emotional discomfort and retarded psychological progress" when the defendant Dr. Karp terminated treatment. Approximately four months after treatment was terminated, the couple were divorced. One month after that Mr. Savader married Dr. Karp.

In a hearing to determine whether the case should go to trial, the attorney for the defendant argued that there were no grounds for a charge of malpractice but only for "alienation of affection"—an invalid cause of action in New York State since 1935. State Supreme Court Justice Martin Stecher denied the motion to dismiss the lawsuit, holding that "this action is not, on its face, an action for alienation of affection, criminal conversation, seduction or breach of contract to marry; it is an action of malpractice by a licensed psychologist."

5.91 PEOPLE v. BERNSTEIN
171 Cal. App.2d 279; 340 P.2d (California, 1959)

This was a criminal case in which a psychiatrist was convicted of statutory rape. The patient, a minor, had been referred to the defendant psychiatrist because her mother had heard that the girl had had sexual relations with a number of boys at a party. The psychiatrist was found guilty of having had sex with the patient.

VIOLATION OF CIVIL RIGHTS

5.92 WYATT V. STICKNEY
344 F. Supp. 373 (Alabama, 1972); (See also *Wyatt v. Aderholt*, 503 F.2d 1305 [1974])

When ninety-nine employees in Alabama's state mental institutions were fired owing to a lack of funds, suit was brought claiming inadequate care in the affected hospitals. The court agreed that mental patients confined to institutions are entitled to a number of rights, some of which are

- the right to treatment by adequate staff;
- the right to treatment that represents the "least restrictive" alternative;
- the right to privacy, a comfortable bed, adequate diet, and recreational facilities;
- the right not to be subjected to experimental treatments or to electroshock therapy or to psychosurgery or to related treatments without fully informed consent and consultation with an attorney; and
- the right to receive monetary compensation for any work done in the institution, with the exception of activities of daily living and therapeutic activities that do not involve the institution's maintenance.

5.93 MORALES V. TURMAN
383 F. Supp. 53 (Texas, 1974)

A suit brought on behalf of incarcerated adolescents against a rehabilitation facility claimed that the youths' right to be rehabilitated was being violated by inadequate staffing and nonexistent treatment. The court agreed that the incarcerated individuals did have a right to treatment. In writing its decision, the federal district court rejected the defendant's argument that merely providing a structured environment for these offenders was therapeutic. The court held that

> [I]t is not sufficient for defendants to contend that merely removing a child from his environment and placing him in a "structured" situation constitutes constitutionally adequate treatment.... Nor do the Texas Youth Centers' sporadic attempts at... "behavior modification"

through the use of point systems rise to the dignity of professional treatment programs geared to individual juveniles.

Furthermore, the court suggested that treatment or supervision by unqualified persons might represent cruel and unusual punishment and that some of the treatment programs in effect at the institution may have infringed on individual liberty to the point that due process should have been required before they were attempted.

5.94 IN RE GAULT
387 U.S. 1 (U.S. Supreme Court, 1967)

Gault was an adolescent who had been sent to a reformatory for making obscene telephone calls. A suit brought on his behalf alleged that the state had denied him due process in sending him to the reformatory. The state's defense was that due process was not required, since the proceedings were not of a criminal nature. The Supreme Court ruled against the state, holding that any proceeding which might deprive an individual of liberty—whether or not that proceeding was undertaken in the name of "treatment" for the individual—required due process. Accordingly, Gault should have had the right to be notified of the charges that were being lodged against him, the right to retain an attorney who might confront and cross-examine his accusers, the Fifth-Amendment right to avoid self-incrimination, and the right to appeal.

5.95 ROUSE v. CAMERON
373 F.2d 451 (Washington, D.C., 1966)

The plaintiff was a man who had pleaded insanity as a defense to a criminal charge. The criminal court had acquitted him of the crime and remanded him to a mental institution for treatment. The plaintiff then brought a suit which sought his release from the mental institution on the grounds that he was not receiving any treatment there. The court ruled that the plaintiff, by statute, had to either be treated or be released from the institution.

5.96 McNEIL v. DIRECTOR, PAXTUXENT INSTITUTION
407 U.S. 245 (U.S. Supreme Court, 1972)

McNeil had been convicted of criminal assault and sentenced to five years imprisonment. In order to determine if he needed psychiatric treatment, he was sent to Paxtuxent Institution for evaluation. McNeil refused to cooperate with the authorities at the institution, however, and he was held there indefinitely pending his cooperation with a psychiatrist. After five years had elapsed,

McNeil brought suit to gain his freedom. The Supreme Court agreed with McNeil that he had a constitutional right to refuse to cooperate under the Fifth Amendment: it held that no person need participate in a process that might result in his loss of liberty. It further held that Paxtuxent Institution could neither force a psychiatric examination nor hold him there for more than five years.

5.97 O'CONNOR V. DONALDSON
422 U.S. 563; 95 Supreme Court 2486 (U.S. Supreme Court, 1975)

An institutionalized individual with a diagnosis of paranoid schizophrenia brought suit against a psychiatrist and other physicians employed at the state hospital, claiming that his right to liberty as guaranteed by the Fourteenth Amendment had been violated. The plaintiff had been hospitalized for fifteen years after his father had initiated a civil commitment proceeding. The trial court heard evidence that the defendants had, on numerous occasions, refused to let the patient leave the facility, although they believed him not to be harmful to himself or others. The plaintiff was awarded $28,000 in compensatory damages and $10,000 in punitive damages, a finding upheld by the Court of Appeals.

This case was subsequently heard by the United States Supreme Court, which ruled in favor of the plaintiff. The majority opinion held that

> [a] finding of "mental illness" alone cannot justify a State's locking a person up against his will and keeping him indefinitely in simple custodial confinement. Assuming that the term can be given a reasonably precise content and that the "mentally ill" can be identified with reasonable accuracy, there is still no constitutional basis for confining such persons involuntarily if they are dangerous to no one and can live safely in freedom.[4]

5.98 IN THE MATTER OF CLEMENT
340 N.E.2d 217 (Illinois, 1976)

A patient voluntarily admitted himself to an Illinois mental health center. Soon after his admission, the patient's condition worsened to the point where he was attacking other patients and staff. Six weeks after his admission, a committee met to consider the transfer of the patient to a more structured facility. A psychologist who had attended the committee meeting filed a petition for commitment, which was accompanied by a statement from two psychia-

---

[4]Opposing views on the question of the significance of *O'Connor* for mental health professionals, particularly psychologists, appear in Bernard (1977) and Siegel (1978).

trists claiming that the patient was mentally ill and unable to care for himself. At a hearing on the matter of the commitment petition, the state of Illinois called nine witnesses (all health center staff) who testified to the patient's violent proclivities. The judge interviewed the patient himself during a recess and observed that the patient did not appear to know what was going on and did not appear to be able to make a rational decision concerning his treatment. Nevertheless, the court found that the voluntary patient had been denied due process. He was entitled to object to the transfer because he had been admitted on a voluntary basis and Illinois law stipulates that

> [e]ach voluntary admittee shall be allowed to leave the hospital within 5 days, excluding Saturdays, Sundays, and holidays, after he gives any professional staff person written notice of his desire to leave, unless prior to leaving the patient withdraws such notice by written withdrawal, or unless within said 5 days a petition and the certificates of 2 examining physicians, at least one of whom shall be a psychiatrist, are filed with the court, and the court shall order a hearing pursuant to Section 8.8. The patient may continue to be hospitalized pending a final order of the court in the court proceedings.

5.99 WINTERS v. MILLER
306 F. Supp. 1158 (New York, 1969)

A patient at a state hospital claimed that her rights under the Fourth, Fifth, and Fourteenth amendments (rights of privacy, due process, and equal protection of the law, respectively) had been violated by the taking of her photograph and fingerprints. The court ruled that fingerprints and photographing were reasonable and necessary in identifying the patient and dismissed the suit.

5.100 PEOPLE v. SANSONE
309 N.E.2d 733 (Illinois, 1974)

On initial examination at an Illinois mental health center, a psychiatrist diagnosed a patient as paranoid schizophrenic, noting, among other things, that the patient claimed to be a United States Senator. At a civil commitment proceeding, the psychiatrist testified that the patient was "fairly" but "not completely" oriented and that he had "quite unrealistic thinking." The psychiatrist further testified that the patient was able to care for himself and that he did not appear to be dangerous to himself, but that he could potentially be harmful to others. In the psychiatrist's words, the patient might "start a fight with someone telling them to clear off his property." In granting the petition to commit this patient, the court cited the state's duty to "protect society from dangerous conduct of the mentally ill" and noted that the patient being deprived of his liberty would be receiving treatment. The patient's lawyer argued that his commitment would be unconstitutional because no proof of prior dangerous conduct had been made. The court rejected the lawyer's argument, stating that

> [i]n the area of mental health law, the State must balance the curtail-ment of liberty against the danger of harm to the individual or others. The paramount factor is the interest of society which naturally includes the interest of the patient in not being subjected to unjustified confine-ment. We agree with [the patient] that the "science" of predicting future dangerous behavior is inexact, and certainly is not infallible. We also agree that the mere establishment of a mental problem is not an adequate basis upon which to confine a person who has never harmed or attempted to harm either himself or another. However, we are of the opinion that a decision to commit based upon a medical opinion which clearly states that a person is reasonably expected to engage in danger-ous conduct, and which is based upon the experience and studies of qualified psychiatrists, is a determination which properly can be made by the State.

GENERAL DIAGNOSIS AND TREATMENT

5.101 CHATMAN V. MILLIS
        517 S.W.2d 504 (Arkansas, 1975)

A woman sought the assistance of a psychologist to put an end to her divorced husband's visitation rights with their child. The woman maintained that her ex-husband had engaged their two-and-a-half-year-old son in homosexual acts. A psychologist was con-sulted to determine whether or not the son had been sexually molested by the father and to comment on the child's future psychosexual development if he had been molested. The psycholo-gist interviewed the mother and son but not the father. Drawing on this interview material, the psychologist concluded that

> [w]hile it will be the court's decision, and not mine, I feel that it would not be a good idea to allow the child to continue to visit his father at all. If it is necessary that visitation rights be continued, I would strongly urge that the presence of a third person, preferably a relative, be in their presence at all times.

The woman's husband sought to bring suit against the psycholo-gist. The court, however, ruled that suit could not be brought be-cause a doctor–patient relationship had never existed between the husband and the psychologist; hence the latter could not be sued for negligence. One of the judges wrote a dissenting opinion:

Defendant was negligent and careless in making such diagnosis by failing to exercise the degree of skill and care, or to possess the degree of
knowledge, ordinarily exercised or possessed by other psychological
examiners or psychologists engaged in this type of practice . . . in that
he failed and neglected to ever interview the plaintiff and in fact did not
even know him, failed to administer any diagnostic tests which would
reveal any homosexuality tendencies or to use any of the proper
methods that psychologists use in exercising ordinary care to protect
others from injury or damage; the defendant acted in a manner
willfully and wantonly in disregard to the rights of plaintiff. . . .

Our statutes make the practice of psychology a profession of the
healing arts. . . . They provide for licensing of psychological examiners
and psychologists and for suspension and revocation of licenses, for
privileged communication between such a licensee and his client, and
for a code of ethics governing practice and behavior. It seems so clear
such a malpractice action can lie against such a practitioner as to be
beyond argument.

5.102 OLINDE V. SEGHERS
280 So. 657 (Louisiana, 1973)

The plaintiff alleged that a psychiatrist's treatment of his wife
was worthless and that the fee charged was excessive. The court
rejected the claim that the treatment was worthless, because no
expert-witness testimony was offered to substantiate that claim. The
claim that the fee was excessive was also rejected, since the patient
had paid two previous bills at the agreed-upon rate. The testimony
in this case suggested that the real reason the suit was being brought
was that the husband had been sued for divorce by his wife and did
not want to pay her psychiatrist's bill. Since no professional services
had been rendered subsequent to the divorce action, the husband
was found to be legally obliged for the entire bill.

5.103 HESS V. FRANK
367 N.Y.S.2d 30 (New York, 1975)

A patient sued his psychiatrist for using abusive language which
allegedly caused anguish and grave injury to the patient's health.
The patient alleged negligence on the part of the psychiatrist, claiming that the doctor knew or should have known that such words and
phrases would have a deleterious effect. The suit sought to recover
$100,000 in damages and $20,000 previously paid to the psychiatrist. The court did not find that a valid claim of malpractice had
been presented. The court further did not find that, as the plaintiff
claimed, the abusive language constituted a breach of an agreement
to render service:

> . . . the complaint failed to set forth the traditional elements of a claim
> for malpractice. As stated. . . . "Negligence is the basis of a malpractice

action which is tortious in nature and predicated upon a failure to use requisite skill.'' The conduct complained of, however, was not part of the course of treatment and there is no claim or indication that defendant failed to provide medical services in accordance with accepted standards or that he did not exercise requisite skills in the treatment of the patient. The argument which ensued between the parties and the abusive language allegedly employed by the defendant, if it may in some manner be considered a tortious act, may not be considered an act of professional misconduct, and indeed, was unrelated to the medical treatment which was being rendered.

... papers demonstrated that plaintiff paid defendant a fee for each visit that plaintiff made to defendant's office for the purpose of receiving psychiatric treatment. There is nothing in the papers to indicate that such treatment was not in fact rendered during plaintiff's visit, or that defendant had agreed to refrain from uttering the allegedly abusive words in consideration for plaintiff's payments.

5.104 (Case Cited in Slawson, 1970) ·

A twenty-four-year-old woman sued her thirty-two-year-old psychiatrist after more than two years of treatment, alleging "improper medical care, treatment, acts, and conduct resulting in permanent mental injuries." The patient further alleged that the psychiatrist's treatment made her more upset and nervous. The psychiatrist described the patient as "lonely and frightened" and said that he "helped her, brought her various gifts, let her do routine work in the office and helped her find an apartment." The psychiatrist denied that he dated the patient or had ever engaged in sexual acts with her. Because the psychiatrist reported difficulty in locating his records, he asked his insurance company to settle quickly at any cost. The suit was settled for $3,500 plus legal fees.

5.105 (Citation Withheld)

The plaintiffs claimed that their son had been labeled in such a manner that the child's entire future had been jeopardized. Investigation disclosed that the psychologist had examined the plaintiffs' child to determine whether the child was eligible to attend a school for physically disabled children and obtain state assistance. The psychologist had diagnosed the child as having an emotional disturbance rather than a brain dysfunction, thus leading to a nonreimbursable situation for the parents. Subsequent findings supported the psychologist's diagnosis, and the claim went no further.

5.106 (Citation Withheld)

A psychologist recorded therapy sessions with a woman and then let her take home the tapes for review. The woman's husband listened to the tapes and discovered that his wife had been unfaithful. The husband brought suit against the psychologist for $1 million, claiming that the psychologist was incompetent. When the psychologist received notice of the suit he threatened a countersuit on the grounds of slander. No action was taken by either party.

5.107 (Citation Withheld)

A patient alleged that a psychologist breached a contract to render adequate counseling, breached the doctor–patient confidential relationship, and harassed him over nonpayment of the bill. Investigation revealed that the suit seemed to have originated when the psychologist attempted to collect his bill through a lawsuit. Eventually the patient decided to pay the psychologist's fee, and the suit was dropped.

5.108 PARRISH V. CIVIL SERVICE COMMISSION OF COUNTY OF ALAMEDA 425 P.2d 223 (California, 1967)

Benny Max Parrish, a social worker, was discharged for "insubordination" after he refused to participate in the county's "Operation Bedcheck." "Operation Bedcheck" was the code-name for a series of unannounced searches of the homes of welfare recipients for the purpose of discovering "unauthorized males." Social workers were instructed to work in pairs, presenting themselves at the clients' homes on a Sunday morning at 6:30 A.M. One social worker would position himself at the rear door, the other would seek entry from the front door and once inside "would proceed to the rear door and admit his companion. Together the two would conduct a thorough search of the entire dwelling, giving particular attention to beds, closets, bathrooms, and other possible places of concealment."

Parrish sought reinstatement on the grounds that the operation was unconstitutional. The county counsel "did not seek to establish the constitutionality of the searches but urged that, whatever the legal status of the operation, the county could still discharge plaintiff because, at the time he refused to participate in it, he had not yet learned of the unconstitutional nature of the contemplated searches." The Supreme Court of California held the searches to be unconstitutional and found in favor of the plaintiff citing uncontradicted evidence that the plaintiff's refusal to participate had been based on his suspicions concerning the illegality of the operation. One of the justices dissented for the reasons expressed by Mr. Justice Taylor in a lower court ruling (see *Parrish v. Civil Service Commission*, 51 Cal. Rptr. 589).

5.109 IN RE STERILIZATION OF MOORE
   221 S.E.2d 307 (North Carolina, 1976)

A director of a county's Department of Social Services requested the court to order authorization for the sterilization of a
minor who, according to a psychological report, had a full scale IQ
of under 40. The constitutionality of the order was challenged. Citing the opinion of the United States Supreme Court in *Buck v. Bell*
(47 S.Ct. 584), the Supreme Court of North Carolina held that: A
state does have the right to sterilize a retarded or insane person
provided that the sterilization is not prescribed as punishment, the
policy is applied equally to all persons, and notice and hearing are
provided; according to mental health laws, the interest of the un-
born child is sufficient to warrant the sterilization of a retarded
individual; and, further, the People also have the right to prevent
the procreation of children who will become a burden on the State.

5.110 (Citation Withheld)

A patient had been treated for several years by several defendants who had failed to diagnose the existence of a brain tumor. One
of the defendants, a psychologist, had administered a Wechsler
Adult Intelligence Scale test. (In litigation.)

5.111 (Citation Withheld)

A psychologist treated a patient, a minor, with play therapy, for
his difficulty in sleeping. In the course of the therapy the psychologist played a game which the child invented, involving turning off
the lights. On the occasion in question, the patient became excited
when the lights were turned off and grabbed for the psychologist,
knocking him over. In the process, the patient struck his face on
something and chipped a tooth. This case was settled out of court for
approximately $1,500.

5.112 (Citation Withheld)

A patient who attempted suicide by slashing her wrists then sued
her psychologist, claiming that his negligent diagnosis and treatment
had resulted in the wrist-slashing episode. The amount sued for was
approximately $200,000. (In litigation.)

5.113 (Citation Withheld)

A psychologist received a letter advising him of a patient's intention to sue on the grounds that the treatment provided to the plain-

tiff and to the plaintiff's wife had resulted in a divorce proceeding initiated by the plaintiff's wife. Investigation revealed that the threat of legal action seemed to have arisen from a dispute regarding the psychologist's rates. No further action was taken by the plaintiff. It is a reasonable inference that the psychologist did not attempt to collect his fee for professional services.

5.114 (Citation Withheld)

The plaintiff, a minor, fell, injuring a hand, while playing dodge ball during a school gym period. Suit was brought against a school psychologist who happened to be supervising the play at that time. The psychologist was not found to be legally liable.

5.115 ESTATE OF FINKLE
385 N.Y.S.2d 343 (New York, 1977)

Before psychiatrist Theodore H. Finkle died, he had left instructions to his executor, "Smith," to "sell" his practice. He had also entrusted the keys to his office to a fellow psychiatrist, "Jones." After Dr. Finkle's death, Dr. Jones began attending to those patients requiring prompt medical attention. When Smith obtained the keys to the office from Jones he found that all of the medical records were missing. Smith demanded that Jones return the records so that the estate could collect debts. Further, every day that the records were not returned would make it more difficult to sell the practice. When Jones refused to return the records legal action was taken by Smith.

In a discovery proceeding it was ruled that Jones was not entitled to possession of the records. Whether the estate had sustained any loss as a result of the retention of the records was a matter of fact to be determined at a trial: "If [Jones's] alleged actions went beyond proper authorization and interfered with the estate's right to notify the patients . . . he may be liable to compensate the estate for any proven loss caused by his actions."

5.116 (Citation Withheld)

Plaintiff claimed that in violation of ethical and legal principles, a psychologist sought to terminate therapy at a time of crisis. After the patient agreed to try another psychologist the suit was dismissed "without prejudice," meaning that it could be refiled within the Statute of Limitations.

5.117 (Citation Withheld)

In preparation for group therapy, the plaintiff was doing

warm-up exercises at a psychologist's direction, which consisted of running up and down a flight of stairs. In the process the plaintiff slipped and fell on the carpeting, resulting in a torn tendon. (In litigation.)

5.118 WELLS V. CREIGHTON MEMORIAL HOSPITAL
321 N.W.2d 570 (Nebraska, 1975)

A fifty-year-old woman who had a history of ten psychiatric hospitalizations in the past thirty years was admitted to a hospital under the care of the physician who had been treating her since her first hospitalization. The physician ordered that his patient, a diagnosed catatonic schizophrenic, be given freedom to move about the ward and the hospital sun porch. Approximately three weeks after her admission to the defendant hospital, the patient complained of pain in her arm. The arm was red and swollen, and it was later diagnosed to be broken. The patient brought suit against the hospital, claiming that it was negligent in not providing sufficient supervision to prevent her from falling.

At the trial no evidence concerning how the patient fell was presented by anyone except the plaintiff, and so the details of how the broken arm occurred were not known. The physician did testify that because of the patient's episodic withdrawals from reality it was possible for her to have sustained the injury and not told anyone about it immediately. The court found no evidence indicating negligence on the part of the hospital and observed that the plaintiff's having sustained a broken arm did not automatically imply negligence on the part of the staff. Since no evidence that the hospital failed to provide "reasonable care" was present, the court found in favor of the defendant hospital.

5.119 RODRIGUEZ V. STATE
355 N.Y.S.2d 912 (New York, 1974)

A profoundly retarded five-year-old girl who could not sit, crawl or move her legs because of medical complications was a resident of a state mental hospital. A hospital attendant observed a swelling on the child's leg while routinely checking her temperature and noted this finding on the child's chart. The next day the child's mother visited her and also noticed the swelling. The child was x-rayed, and a fracture was discovered. The mother brought suit against the hospital, claiming that since the child could not in any way move when placed on a flat surface, the state should be held liable for damages under the doctrine of *res ipsa loquitur*. Exactly what caused the fracture could not be determined from the child or from any agent of the hospital. The court found in favor of the plaintiff, invoking the doctrine of *res ipsa loquitur*.[5]

5.120 (Case Cited in Ledakowich, 1976e; 1977)

A physician in a hospital treated an eleven-month-old infant for a fractured leg. At that time the infant also had bruises and lacerations on her back and a skull fracture which was in the process of healing. No explanation for the injuries was provided by the patient's mother. Within three months after the treatment, the infant was taken to a second hospital for treatment of traumatic blows to the eye, puncture wounds on the leg and back, burns on the hand, and bites on the face. Battered child syndrome was diagnosed, and the child was taken into protective custody (and subsequently placed with foster parents).

A court-appointed guardian brought suit against the physician and the hospital who had treated the child three months before, charging a failure to diagnose battered child syndrome at that time. The doctor's negligence was allegedly responsible for the permanent physical injuries and mental distress suffered by the infant.

The plaintiff's complaint was dismissed by the trial court, and an appeal was taken. The court of appeals (123 Cal. Rptr. 713, 1975) held that because battered child syndrome was so rarely seen by physicians and because its diagnosis was by no means clear-cut, "there is no basis for imposing a legal duty upon the members of the medical profession for the failure to recognize the syndrome." The appellate court pointed out, however, that California (like all of the states) has a statute mandating that all suspected cases of child abuse seen by physicians be reported to the proper authorities. It therefore remanded the case back to a trial court to determine whether or not the doctor and the hospital had violated their statutory duty to report suspected child abuse cases.

In 1976, the Supreme Court of California heard and ruled on the case. As reported by Ledakowich (1977), the court

> ... reversed and vacated the decision of the Court of Appeals. Citing such leading medical authorities in the field as Doctors Kempe, Fontana and Helfer, the Court noted the abundant medical literature available for the instruction of the medical practitioner. Nevertheless, the Court pointed out that whether or not a reasonably careful physician examining the infant plaintiff in 1971 should have suspected an

---

[5]The legal doctrine of *res ipsa loquitur* ("the act speaks for itself") is invoked when the mere fact that an injury occurred suggests that there probably was negligence on the part of the defendant. For example, in a malpractice action claiming damage as a result of a surgeon's negligently leaving a sponge inside of a patient, the doctrine of *res ipsa loquitur* might be invoked.

intentional abuse of the child from the particular injuries and circumstances presented to him is a question which "remains one of fact, to be decided (by the jury) on the basis of expert testimony." (p. 112)

5.121 ESTATE OF BURKS V. ROSS
438 F.2d 230 (Michigan, 1971)

A psychiatric patient escaped from a locked Veterans Administration hospital ward and was killed in a train accident. Suit was brought against the attending doctors and nurses for negligence in allowing the patient to escape. The court dismissed the suit against the doctors on the grounds that they were federal employees with "executive privilege." Thus, even if the doctors were negligent, they could not be held liable. The nurses, on the other hand, who were not covered by the doctrine of "executive privilege," were held liable. It should be noted that since this case, "executive privilege" has been extended by Congress to all federal employees. However, whether or not the immunity offered by such privilege will be enforced may vary with the specific fact situation of the case.

5.122 (Case cited in Slawson, 1970)

A forty-two-year-old pharmacist was advised by his lawyer to see a psychiatrist because he had been taking various tranquilizers for extreme anxiety. The psychiatrist the patient saw was a prominent Beverly Hills psychoanalyst who, after a course of treatment, recommended hospitalization. The psychiatrist saw the patient at a Los Angeles teaching hospital for one hour a day, during which time the patient complained about the food, his roommate, and the confined atmosphere. Still, the patient remained there for approximately three weeks. He was described as somewhat improved when he left, but he never saw the doctor again. One year later he became depressed and was treated at another hospital. Two years later the Beverly Hills psychoanalyst and the teaching hospital were named as co-defendants in a malpractice action.

The plaintiff's suit alleged "negligent care and treatment and having claimant hospitalized in a psychopathic ward with sexual perverts." The case was eventually settled for $2,000.

5.123 SCHWARTZ V. THIELE
242 Cal. App. 2d 799; 51 Cal. Rptr. 767 (California, 1966)

Judith Schwartz's suit against psychiatrist David A. Thiele alleged that they were strangers when they met in a restaurant parking lot about 9:30 in the morning. As stated in the court record, Judith and her sister "after having had breakfast at a restaurant in the city of Los Angeles, were walking to her automobile (when) the defendant, a total stranger to the plaintiff, and without her consent, purported to make an examination of plaintiff as to her mental illness." Exactly why Thiele had occasion to "examine" Schwartz or what, in fact, transpired in the parking lot is not clear from the court record:

> In the case at the bench, so far as it may be determined from the pleading, the defendant had some contact with the plaintiff, the exact nature of which is not disclosed.

After that contact, Thiele wrote a letter to the psychiatric department of the Superior Court of Los Angeles County stating that Schwartz was mentally ill and that she was likely to injure herself or others if not immediately hospitalized. After receiving the letter, a judge of the superior court signed an order appointing a physician to examine Schwartz. The court-appointed physician tried, through Schwartz's lawyer, to arrange an appointment for an examination. However, Schwartz was examined by her own physician, who did not find her to be mentally ill.

Schwartz's suit against Thiele claimed $100,000 in damages. She alleged that her right of privacy had been invaded and as a consequence of that invasion she had suffered "great mental pain and physical suffering, humiliation, annoyance, and mortification" and she had been exposed to "public ridicule and disgrace."

The court found in favor of the defendant, holding him immune from liability and noting that there was no publication of the letter. The court further stated:

> The restraint and treatment of persons who are mentally ill is a matter of public concern. If a person in good faith and for probable cause makes a written statement to an agency charged with the duty of enforcement of the law, designed to give such agency information upon which it can conduct an investigation, such a communication is not an invasion of the right of privacy of the person who is the subject of the communication.

6

Other Illustrative Cases

- Who qualifies as an expert and when is expert testimony needed?
- Are you, as a supervisor, responsible for the negligence of your trainees?
- Is one member of a "team" of health professionals liable for the negligence of another member of the team?
- Can health professionals be sued for breach of contract if they do not effect cures?

These are some of the questions that will be touched on in the sampling of cases presented in this chapter. A detailed discussion of the legal and professional ramifications of these and other questions as they may apply to mental health professionals will appear in Part IV. The areas to be treated here have been arbitrarily grouped in the following order:

- Expert Testimony (6.1–6.9)
- Supervisory Liability (6.10–6.18)
- Referrals (6.19–6.23)
- Teams (6.24)
- Pain, Suffering, and Emotional Distress (6.25–6.28)
- Standard of Care (6.29–6.33)
- The Statute of Limitations (6.34)
- Contributory Negligence (6.35–6.37)
- Informed Consent (6.38–6.39)
- Breach of Contract (6.40–6.42)
- Invasion of Privacy (6.43)
- Undue Influence (6.44)

- Insurance (6.45–6.46)
- Medical Practice and Religion (6.47–6.48)
- Physical Ministrations (6.49)

EXPERT TESTIMONY

6.1   RAGAN V. STEEN
Supreme Court of Pennsylvania, September 23, 1974 (cited in Cases
Unlimited, Inc., 1975a).

A patient was advised by a radiologist to use radiation therapy
to remove a colony of planter warts on his foot. Following the treatment and corrective surgery, the patient was left permanently disabled and brought suit. One of the expert witnesses that the patient
brought to testify at the trial was a surgeon. The plaintiff won the
case but the defendants appealed, arguing that a surgeon was not a
radiologist and that his testimony amounted to tracing the poor
course of treatment, which was not in itself a proof of negligence.
The Supreme Court said they would allow the surgeon's testimony to
stand as that of an expert if he as a witness had "any reasonable
pretention to specialized knowledge on the subject under investigation." The court did allow the testimony and the trial court's decision was upheld, but one of the judges was unconvinced that the
surgeon could qualify as an expert. In his dissenting opinion, the
judge wrote, "It is time that Pennsylvania joined the states which
have recognized the absurdity of permitting witnesses to testify as
experts simply by virtue of their license or degrees."

6.2   KRONKE V. DANIELSON
499 P.2d 156 (Arizona, 1972)

A plaintiff bringing suit in the State of Arizona was unable to
obtain a board-certified expert witness to testify against a board-
certified specialist in a malpractice action. The plaintiff asked the
court to accept testimony from a board-certified specialist from
another state who had never practiced in Arizona. The court consented, writing in part that

> it is well known that the various specialties of medicine have set up
> uniform requirements for certification of specialists. The length of
> residency training, subjects to be covered, and even examinations are
> established by the national boards. Since medicine recognizes a stan-
> dard for specialists not based on geography, the law should join in
> upholding such standards.

6.3   MITZ V. STERN
183 N.W.2d 608 (Michigan, 1970)

The defendant had trouble urinating and consulted a urologist. The urologist performed a surgical procedure during which the sphincter muscle was damaged, and the plaintiff thereafter suffered incontinence. The urologist was sued for malpractice. At the trial, the urologist testified that it was not usual that the sphincter muscle be damaged during the surgical procedure. The court ruled that this expert testimony by the defendant himself was enough to hold the defendant liable.

6.4   ROBERTSON V. LaCROIX, M.D.
534 P.2d 17 (Oklahoma, 1975)

Less than a week after a surgeon removed the plaintiff's uterus, Fallopian tube and appendix, the plaintiff noticed a leakage of urine, which she reported to the surgeon. In diagnosing the problem as an injury to the plaintiff's bladder, the surgeon casually commented that he had "racked his brain trying to figure out what he had done differently or he had done wrong, but the only thing he knew was that he just made a mistake and got over too far." At the trial, the defendant surgeon was called as an expert witness on behalf of the plaintiff. He testified that the complication may have been caused by a puncture of the bladder or by a blood circulation problem in the area, but leaned toward the latter explanation. The trial court found in favor of the defendant, noting that insufficient evidence of negligence had been presented. The plaintiff appealed, arguing that the surgeon had, in essence, admitted his guilt to her, thus resolving any doubt regarding the question of negligence. The appeals court reversed the decision of the trial court and found in favor of the plaintiff, stating that "the defendant's statment that he 'just made a mistake and got over too far' is more than a mere statement of mistaken judgment; it constituted an admission of negligence during the performance of the surgery."

6.5   PHELPS V. VANDERBILT UNIVERSITY
Court of Appeals of Tennessee, July 26, 1974; review denied by Supreme Court, February 3, 1975 (Cited in Cases Unlimited, Inc., 1975b)

A man was taken to a hospital emergency room after he had been struck by a truck while walking. After examining the patient and his x-rays, the doctor (a resident from Vanderbilt Medical School) sent the patient home with some drugs to relieve the pain and instructions for home care. As was customary, the x-rays were read the next morning by the radiologist, who noted fractures of the pelvic bone which the resident had failed to diagnose. The resident called the family, asking that the man be returned to the hospital at once. The man returned to the hospital, was given additional medication, and was confined to bed, but he died the next morning. An autopsy suggested that the possible cause of death was bone fragments that had become lodged in the deceased's lungs. The deceased's wife brought suit, arguing that negligence in failing to diagnose the fracture resulted in the deceased's movement away from and then back to the hospital and that this movement may have been instrumental in dislodging the fracture fragments, resulting in her husband's death. The court ruled against the plaintiff because she did not present an expert witness to offer any affirmative evidence. The jury was not qualified to determine the standard of care without expert testimony.

6.6   SANDERS V. FROST
251 N.E.2d 106 (Illinois, 1970)

The plaintiff was advised by the court that his case could not be tried without expert testimony. In the past, the plaintiff had not expressed the intention of getting expert testimony, and he did not express the intention of seeking expert testimony in the future. The trial court made a summary judgment in favor of the defendant. The opinion of the trial court was upheld on appeal:

> Since plaintiff failed to indicate that he had expert medical opinion to sustain the charges in his complaint, or that he would be able to obtain such opinion in the future, the trial court correctly entered a summary judgment in favor of the defendants.
> The proving of negligence in medical malpractice cases usually depends upon the ability of the plaintiff to secure the services of a member of the medical profession to give expert testimony as to the proper method of treatment in the particular case. The reluctance of the members of the medical profession to testify against a fellow disciple of Aesculapius makes the search for a medical expert very difficult in most cases and well nigh impossible in some cases. For this reason, the trial court should be extremely cautious in entering summary judgment in this type of case.
> Here, however, plaintiff did not urge in the trial court, nor does he urge in this court, that he has, intends to, or may be able to prove his case by expert testimony. Therefore, there is no triable issue of fact for us to consider.

6.7   (Case cited in Ledakowich, 1972a)

A woman suing for medical malpractice arranged to obtain the services of another doctor to testify on her behalf as an expert witness. She had paid the doctor his fee in advance, but when the case went to court, he did not show up. The following morning the doctor was present in court, but it was ruled that he would not be allowed to testify, since the defendant's expert witness was not present and would not be able to counter any testimony. Without the benefit of medical evidence, the court awarded $2,500 to the plaintiff. The plaintiff thought that she could have gotten more had her expert witness been present to testify. She brought suit against her expert witness for breach of contract. The amount she sued for was the difference between what she was awarded and what she thought she would have gotten had he been there to testify. The defendant moved for dismissal of the case, arguing that any award that a jury might make in such a case could be based only on conjecture and speculation. The defense maintained that the correct legal procedure would be for the plaintiff to simply appeal the judgment, but the trial court disagreed and allowed the woman to bring an action against her expert witness. An appeals court upheld the trial court's decision, stating that

> it may very likely be difficult to prove damages, but this is no reason for denying plaintiff the chance to try. "Difficulty of proof" should not bar the plaintiff from the opportunity of attempting to convince the trier of fact of the truth of her claim. Many difficulties of proof seemingly as intractable as that before us have given way before the imaginative ingenuity and resourcefulness of counsel.

6.8   SANZARI V. ROSENFELD
167 A.2d 625 (New Jersey, 1961)

Violet Sanzari visited the office of Rosenfeld and Shepard (two partners in the practice of dentistry) in order to have a filling replaced. In preparation for replacing the filling, defendant Dr. Rosenfeld injected an anesthetic solution (a mixture of Xylocaine and epinephrine) into the patient's gums. After the injection, the patient asked the defendant dentist to wait a few minutes before beginning work. The dentist waited about three to five minutes and then proceeded to fill the tooth, a process that took about twenty minutes. Upon completion of the filling, the patient rose from the chair and prepared to leave. However, as she did she fell, having suffered a cerebral hemorrhage or stroke from which she subsequently died.

As administrator of the deceased's estate Angelo Sanzari brought suit against Rosenfeld and Shepard charging that a careful history was not taken and that this negligence resulted in wrongful death. The deceased had suffered from high blood pressure (hypertension). Epinephrine is a drug that has the effect of constricting blood vessels. Raising the patient's already high blood pressure even higher had the effect of bursting blood vessels causing the cerebral hemorrhage. In his deposition, Rosenfeld stated that he routinely asked all of his patients on their first visit how their general health was. Rosenfeld had stated that, to the best of his recollection, the patient had not told him anything about hypertension. It was for this reason that no mention of the patient's hypertension appeared in the dental records.

After the plaintiff's case was presented, the trial court granted the defendant's motion to dismiss on the grounds that (1) there was no expert testimony as to the method of treatment approved by dentists for administering anesthesia, and (2) there was no evidence that the defendant dentist failed to obtain a history from the patient.

On appeal to the Supreme Court of New Jersey the plaintiff argued that the decision of the lower court should be reversed on the grounds that (1) if the applicable standard of care was not established it was because the trial court erroneously ruled that the plaintiff's expert witness was incompetent, (2) in fact, the applicable standard of care was established, and (3) it was unnecessary to establish a standard of care in this case.

In regard to the issue of the qualifications of an expert witness, the New Jersey Supreme Court Justice who delivered the opinion of the court noted, "It is generally held that the witness must be a licensed member of the profession whose standards he professes to know." The plaintiff's expert witness was not a dentist but a medical doctor who specialized in dental anesthesiology. The Supreme Court ruled that the trial court erred in not admitting into evidence the anesthesiologist's testimony. It said, "The facts that he is not a licensed dentist, did not attend dental school, and is unfamiliar with the curriculum pertaining to anesthesiology in the ordinary dental school, go to the weight to be accorded his opinion and not to his competency to testify."

The plaintiff's argument that the brochure accompanying each container of Xylocaine was proof of the applicable standard of care among dentists was rejected by the court:

> In the present case, the standard from which defendant is alleged to have departed is the taking of a medical history or adequate medical history before administering anesthesia. The brochure accompanying Xylocaine says nothing about taking a history from the patient. It merely states that Epinephrine constricts the blood vessels and that where such constriction is contraindicated Xylocaine without Epinephrine may be administered. The jury could not find *from these statements in the brochure alone* that proper practice among dentists required the taking of a history before injecting Xylocaine with Epinephrine into a patient. The brochure was therefore not evidential of the standard of care demanded of the defendant.

However, the court did hold that the pharmaceutical company's brochure was admissable for a purpose other than proving a standard of care:

> Defendant argues that if a medical treatise does not constitute substantive evidence of statements contained therein, *a fortiori*, a drug manufacturer's brochure does not. But the defendant's argument is irrelevant to the admissibility of the brochure in the present case. The defendant stated that he had read the brochure at least when he first started using Xylocaine. And even if he had not read it, the jury could reasonably conclude that under the circumstances he should have read it. It is therefore admissible as indicating that he was or should have been alerted to the possible dangers in the use of Xylocaine with Epinephrine. In other words, the brochure is evidence of the fact that Dr. Rosenfeld was on notice Epinephrine might be harmful to hypertensive patients.

The plaintiff argued that it was not necessary to establish a standard of care in that the doctrine of *res ipsa loquitur* was applicable: "In the absence of negligence the routine filling of a tooth does not result in death." The court rejected this argument holding that were such a rationale to become law it would make every untoward result in medicine or dentistry a *res ipsa* case:

> There are a variety of reasons why a patient may die while being operated on by a dentist—none of which may be related to the dentist's failure to exercise proper skill and care. While there is proof in the present case that Mrs. Sanzari died from the injection, the fact does not of itself evidence negligence. In other words, the probabilities are such that one cannot reasonably say that in the absence of negligence a patient would not die in the dentist's chair. Since the fundamental postulate of the *res ipsa* doctrine cannot be assumed upon the facts in the present case, application of the doctrine is inappropriate.

Invoking the doctrine of common knowledge,[1] the Supreme Court of New Jersey reversed the lower court's decision and remanded the case for retrial:

> We believe that the doctrine of common knowledge combined with the manufacturer's brochure admitted in evidence was sufficient to avoid a dismissal, especially in the light of defendant's testimony that he was unaware that the drug was contraindicated for patients suffering from hypertension. The brochure stated that Epinephrine is administered with Xylocaine to prolong the anesthetic effect of the latter drug; that to achieve greater constriction of the blood vessels (haemostasis) the concentration of Epinephrine should be increased; and that in cases where vasopressor drugs (Epinephrine) are contraindicated (dangerous) Xylocaine can be used alone. From this evidence the jury could

---

[1]This doctrine is explained on p. 235.

reasonably conclude that defendant knew or should have known that it was dangerous to administer Epinephrine to a hypertensive patient. We believe that it is within the common knowledge of laymen that a reasonable man, including a dentist, who knows a drug is potentially harmful to a certain type of patient should take adequate precaution before administering the drug or deciding whether to administer it. The jury could reasonably conclude from the evidence that defendant took no precautions or inadequate precautions before injecting Xylocaine with Epinephrine into Mrs. Sanzari. Defendant said it was his "guess" that he asked her how her general health was. But his chart contained no notations at all about her condition. His lack of assurance about what he did, plus the absence of any record would support a legitimate inference that he did nothing. See Ferdinand v. Agricultural Ins. Co. of Watertown, New York, 22 N.J. 482, 494, 126 A.2d 323, 62 A.L.R.2d 1179 (1956).

The judgment below is reversed and the case is remanded because (1) the trial court erroneously refused to allow the plaintiffs expert to testify to the standard of care accepted by dentists administering anesthesia, and (2) even in the absence of expert testimony as to standard of care, the plaintiff submitted sufficient proof to avoid a dismissal at the end of his case.

6.9   STEINKE V. BELL
107 A.2d 825 (New Jersey, 1954)

A dentist who extracted the wrong tooth was sued by his patient. At the trial, the defense argued that the plaintiff could not recover unless she could offer expert testimony to establish what the applicable standard of care was. The appellate court ruled that a jury was competent to determine what the applicable standard was:

> We think laymen, looking at this case in the light of their common knowledge and experience, can say that a dentist engaged to remove a lower left second molar is not acting with the care and skill normal to the average member of the profession if, in so doing, he extracts or causes to come out an upper right lateral incisor. Expert testimony was therefore not necessary under the circumstances of this case.

SUPERVISORY LIABILITY

6.10   YORSTON V. PENNELL
153 A.2d 255 (Pennsylvania, 1959)

A resident who was technically under the supervision of a surgeon removed a nail embedded in a workman's leg and ordered postoperative penicillin. The penicillin was administered three times by nurses. A fourth-year medical student had previously taken the patient's history and noted that the patient was allergic to penicillin. The patient developed a severe allergic reaction to the penicillin.

The plaintiff did not bring suit against the hospital, because of a Pennsylvania law that made the hospital immune from liability, and he declined to bring suit against the impecunious resident in favor of suing the supervising surgeon (under the doctrine of *respondeat superior*).[2] Since the defendant surgeon had use of the hospital for private-practice purposes and the patient was admitted as a private patient, the court ruled that the surgeon (who had assigned the resident to treat the patient) was liable for damages under *respondeat superior*.

6.11 MINOGUE V. RUTLAND HOSPITAL
125 A.2d 796 (Vermont, 1956)

A nurse pressed on the rib of a woman during childbirth, causing a fracture, and a lawsuit followed. The court found the hospital to be free of liability but held that the nurse was a "borrowed servant" of the obstetrician and held the obstetrician liable for the nurse's action.

6.12 RULE V. CHESSMAN
317 P.2d 472 (Kansas, 1957)

A surgeon who taught residents at a hospital was sued when a resident he had supervised and advised during surgery left a sponge in the patient's abdomen. The trial court directed a verdict against the surgeon. The state supreme court, however, ruled that the resident and his advisor were *jointly* liable for negligence.

6.13 NORTON V. ARGONAUT INSURANCE COMPANY
144 So.2d 249 (Louisiana, 1962)

A physician prescribed some medication for a patient, but in writing the prescription in the hospital chart, he neglected to note that it was to be administered orally. The nurse administered the prescribed amount by injection (which was equivalent to about five times the prescribed dosage), and the patient died. In the subsequent lawsuit, the physician was found liable for the nurse's negligence.

6.14 MARVULLI V. ELSHIRE
103 Cal. Rptr. 461 (California, 1973)

The plaintiff sought to hold a surgeon liable for the alleged

---

[2] *Respondeat superior* ("let the master respond") is a legal doctrine that provides that a "master" can be held liable for the negligence of his "servants." More detail on this doctrine is provided in the following chapter, pages 237–238.

negligence of an anesthesiologist. The court did not find the surgeon liable, since the anesthesiologist had been selected in the normal course of events from among available, qualified, reputable, and competent anesthesiologists, and the surgeon therefore had no control over his performance.

6.15 SESSELMAN V. MUHLENBERG HOSPITAL
306 A.2d 474 (New Jersey, 1973)

During childbirth the plaintiff suffered injuries as the result of an anesthetist's negligence. In a suit to recover damages, the plaintiff named several defendants, including the obstetrician who was supervising in the operating room. The court did not find the obstetrician liable. The nurse, it noted,

> did not become a legal servant or agent of the defendant [obstetrician] merely because she received instructions from him as to the work to be performed. During the administration of the anesthesia and the dynamics of the childbirth, we find nothing in the record whereby we can fairly say that the defendant undertook to exercise control over [the nurse's] activities to warrant removing him from the general rule of not being liable for the negligence of a third party.

6.16 (Case cited in Ledakowich, 1976a: Court of Civil Appeals of Texas, Amarillo, Texas, October 31, 1975)

A sponge was left in a patient's abdomen as the result of an incorrect sponge count by hospital nurses. The patient brought suit against the surgeon for failing to observe the sponge in his abdomen before he was stitched up. Suit was also brought against the employer of the nurses (the hospital) for negligence. The court found the hospital liable for $21,000 but did not find the surgeon liable. The hospital appealed the decision and tried to shift liability back to the surgeon. The surgeon argued that, though he was in charge of auxiliary personnel in the operating room, there were certain duties that did not usually entail his supervision. The surgeon's argument was that the nurses' negligence with regard to such duties as counting sponges or instruments was the hospital's liability, under the doctrine of *respondeat superior*.

The appeals court reversed the trial court's judgment with regard to the surgeon and found him equally liable, noting that "as a matter of law, the surgeon had such control of the nurses in the operating room as to render him liable for their negligence in making an incorrect sponge count." Because the nurses were serving not only the surgeon but the hospital as well, the hospital was again found to be liable for negligence. The suit was successful against the surgeon and the hospital "jointly and severally" for $21,000.

6.17 MARCUS V. FRANKFORD HOSPITAL
283 A.2d 69 (Pennsylvania, 1971)

In answer to an advertisement placed in a newspaper by the American Red Cross, a fourteen-year-old girl became a hospital volunteer (a Candy Striper). She told the hospital interviewers that her preference was either to work with children or to do office work. She was told that hospital policy prohibited volunteers from working in pediatrics. The girl obtained written permission from her parents and health clearance from her family physician and subsequently took a two-day training program in which Candy Stripers were taken on a tour of the hospital and given demonstrations of the kinds of functions that they would be involved in (e.g., serving meals, arranging flowers, making beds). After performing comparable functions on her first two days of work, the girl was asked to assist two nurses in bathing an elderly man ridden with bed sores. The man was unconscious, and there was excrement covering the lower portion of his nude body. The girl, who had been assigned the task of supporting the patient's shoulders, told the nurses after a few minutes that she didn't feel well. She subsequently fainted, hitting her face on an oxygen tank. The girl was not an employee of the hospital and therefore was not entitled to workmen's compensation for the fractured nose she sustained. In the subsequent lawsuit, the court awarded the girl $11,000 in damages, stating that

> given the nature and purpose of the services to be performed by the plaintiff, the circumscribed extent of the training she received, the limited experience she had during her two—to three—day period of work at the hospital, and combined with her extreme youth, it cannot be said as a matter of law that the hospital owed no duty to its nurse's aid not to subject her, without warning or preparation of any kind, into a situation as unpleasant and emotionally disturbing as that to which this child was subjected. That in such circumstances the minor might become so upset as to faint, with injurious consequences to herself, was not beyond the bounds of foreseeability to a reasonably prudent master.

It is noteworthy that a strong dissenting opinion was filed at this trial:

> Hospitals are not pleasant institutions by definition. The struggle between life and death occurs daily within their walls. People with horrible diseases and unpleasant appearances are likely to be encountered.

We cannot agree that the hospital, with its carefully regulated volunteer program, was negligent in any way towards the plaintiff.

6.18 SEARS v. CITY OF CINCINNATI
285 N.E.2d 735 (Ohio, 1972)

A charge of negligence that allegedly led to amputation of part of the plaintiff's right foot was brought against the University of Cincinnati Hospital. The City of Cincinnati (which was the owner and operator of the hospital) claimed governmental immunity as a defense from liability. The court ruled that a city-owned hospital was not providing a service essential to municipal government and therefore could not be granted governmental immunity.

REFERRALS

6.19 STOVALL v. HARMS
522 P.2d 353 (Kansas, 1974)

A general practitioner referred a patient to a psychiatrist for psychiatric care. The patient was subsequently involved in a car accident, allegedly caused by his psychiatrist prescribing an excess of medication. Suit was brought against the general practitioner for injuries incurred in the auto accident. The general practitioner was not found to be liable, since it had not been proved that he had been negligent in selecting a psychiatrist. The psychiatrist was fully qualified, and the general practitioner had had no control over the treatment administered.

6.20 STATE v. STUBBS
485 S.W.2d 152 (Missouri, 1972)

A physician was admittedly negligent in the treatment of the plaintiff. Subsequent treatment by other doctors had aggravated the plaintiff's injuries, and the plaintiff sought to hold the treating physician liable for the subsequent injuries. The court found in favor of the plaintiff, stating that

> a person who has received an injury due to the negligence of another is entitled to recover all damages proximately traceable to the primary negligence, including subsequent aggravation which the law regards as a sequence and natural result likely to flow from the original injury, even though there may have been some intervening agency contributing to the result. Thus, it has been held that the original wrongdoer who negligently causes injury to another may be held liable to the latter for the negligence of the physician who treats such person where such negligent treatment results in the aggravation of such injuries.

6.21 McCoy v. Mitchell
463 S.W.2d 710 (Tennessee, 1970)

A child's parents called an orthopedic surgeon and were told
that it was his day off but that they could call another number for
another physician. The patient consulted the other physician, and
subsequently the child's arm had to be amputated. The parents
brought suit against both physicians. The court ruled that the orthopedic surgeon could not be held liable for the acts of the substitute physician unless the substitute physician was either his partner
or acting as his agent. As long as the physician had taken reasonable
care in deciding who should substitute for him, it would then be up
to a jury to decide whether the substitute had acted as his agent or
not.

6.22 Modica v. Battista
339 N.Y.S.2d 599 (New York, 1973)

A consultant physician was not paid by a patient, and he sued
the patient for his fee. At the trial the referring doctor was not
considered a disinterested party, since he would be held responsible
for the consultant's fee if a judgment was made in favor of the
defendant patient. In this case, the patient was not found to be liable
for the fee of the consultant physician. The court noted that in order
for the suit to be successful the consultant must prove by the preponderance of the evidence that the patient expressly, impliedly, or
through ratification approved of the rendering of professional services.

6.23 Brandt v. Grubin
329 A.2d 82 (New Jersey, 1974)

An adult patient consulted the defendant physician, a general
practitioner (GP), for problems related to anxiety, loneliness, and
insomnia. The GP diagnosed the patient as "anxiety syndrome" and
prescribed chlorpromazine "to take the edge off his anxiety." The
GP recommended psychiatric care, both directly to the patient and
in a note that the patient brought home with him to his family. The
note specifically referred the patient to the county's psychiatric
clinic. About one month later, the patient showed up at a hospital
emergency room and was again advised to go to the county's
psychiatric clinic. Two days later the patient again came to the
hospital emergency room, and this time he was admitted for two
days to a medical and then a psychiatric service. The following day
the patient committed suicide. The suit brought against the GP by
the deceased's next of kin alleged that the doctor had been negligent

in assessing the seriousness of the situation, that he had offered inadequate treatment, and that he had abandoned the patient. The physician did admit to knowing that chlorpromazine was contraindicated in the case of depression.

In its decision in favor of the defendant doctor, the court observed that the doctor's treatment of the patient had ended when he referred the patient to the psychiatric clinic. The physician had further notified the patient's family of the seriousness of the problem and had, in essence, placed the responsibility for obtaining the appropriate care in their hands. The court also noted that:

> in malpractice actions, unlike most other negligence cases, the trial itself may have an adverse effect upon defendant's professional life. Courts should be aware that even allegations of malpractice against physicians and other professionals may have such effect. As noted in this opinion, the application of the principles of negligence law to the facts alleged by plaintiff should be terminated at this stage insofar as [the defendant] is concerned. A physician who upon an initial examination determines that he is incapable of helping his patient, and who refers the patient to a source of competent medical assistance, should be held liable neither for the actions of subsequent treating professionals nor for his refusal to become further involved with the case.

TEAMS

6.24 (Case cited by Ledakowich, 1976b)

An orthopedist recommending surgery for a patient consulted with a neurosurgeon and an internist. The internist had been consulted because the patient had had a heart attack some years before and the feasibility of surgery for him had to be evaluated. The internist's data showed some cardiac irregularities and an abnormal enzyme count, but the internist assessed the man as a "fair" risk for surgery. The orthopedist and the neurosurgeon performed the surgery. The attending anesthesiologist ordered an electrocardiogram (EKG) just after the surgery and another one on the following morning. The morning EKG report had indices of heart abnormalities, including atrial fibrillation. The following day fluid in the lungs appeared, and the neurosurgeon ordered that the patient try to walk around, assisted by hospital personnel. Subsequently, the patient's temperature rose and his pulse increased. Sometime between midnight and 2 A.M. the next day the patient developed difficulty breathing, and he subsequently died.

The patient's widow sued the orthopedist, the neurosurgeon, and the internist, claiming that each of them had had a part in the allegedly substandard medical care that led to her husband's death.

At the trial, all three of the doctors denied having knowledge of the EKG ordered by the anesthesiologist. The trial court granted judgment in favor of the orthopedist and the neurosurgeon but denied judgment for the internist. The plaintiff appealed the trial court's decision, arguing that when doctors act as a "team" in treating a patient, one should be liable for the negligence of the other. The decision of the trial court was affirmed by the Court of Appeals of Arizona, which ruled:

> It is generally held that physicians who are engaged to treat the patient concurrently and who serve together by mutual consent necessarily have the right, in the absence of instructions to the contrary, to make such a division of services as in their honest judgment the circumstances may require.
>
> The responsibility of such independent treating physicians has been held to be that one is not liable for the malpractice of the other, in the absence of evidence that he observed the wrongful act or omission, or in the exercise of ordinary care, should have observed it.

PAIN, SUFFERING, AND EMOTIONAL DISTRESS

6.25 FERRELL v. CHESAPEAKE & OHIO RAILWAY EMPLOYEES HOSPITAL ASSOCIATION
336 F. Supp. 833 (Virginia, 1971)

While eating dinner with his family, Thomas Cecil Ferrell swallowed a chicken bone. Complaining of discomfort in his throat, Ferrell was taken by his wife, Mary, to Greenbriar Valley Hospital, where he was examined by a board-certified general and thoracic surgeon. The surgeon was not able to locate the chicken bone, and he noted that the patient was uncooperative, irrational, and at times seemed to be hallucinating. The surgeon did not think it was an emergency, so he sent the patient home with instructions to come back the following morning. Later that night Mr. Ferrell was in severe pain and discomfort and his wife brought him to the Chesapeake & Ohio Railway Employees Hospital (C&O Hospital). The patient was examined in the C&O Hospital emergency room by Dr. Melvin Antonio, who could not find the chicken bone and whose opinion it was that there was no immediate danger. At the request of Mary Ferrell, Mr. Ferrell was given an injection and some pills to help calm him down. Antonio advised the patient to return the next morning.

The following morning the Ferrells did not go to Greenbriar Valley or C&O Hospital but instead to their family physician. This physician instructed the Ferrells to return to C&O Hospital, where he would arrange for Mr. Ferrell to be seen by Dr. Stuart Harris, a thoracic surgeon. The Ferrells arrived at the C&O Hospital at approximately 11:15 A.M. and were told to go to the waiting room and wait for Dr. Harris. Dr. Harris was performing surgery at the time and was not able to see Mr. Ferrell until approximately 3 P.M. The three-and-a-half-hour wait caused Mr. Ferrell to become extremely upset and angry. When Dr. Harris did examine him and attempted a bronchoscopy he found the patient to be uncooperative and confused. Dr. Harris told Mrs. Ferrell that he had another appointment and had to leave, but he was going to admit her husband to the hospital and contact an ear, nose, and throat specialist, Dr. Murdo M. MacKay, about handling the case.

Mr. Ferrell was admitted to the hospital with the diagnosis, "chicken bone in throat, bilateral bronchopneumonia." He was wheeled into his hospital room at 3:15 P.M. and was seen by Dr. MacKay at 3:30. At that time, Ferrell was confused and disoriented, and he was given Probanthine (a relaxant) for a muscle spasm in the throat. At about 4:45 Sparine was administered for restlessness and confusion. Approximately one hour later Mr. Ferrell was placed in a restraining sheet. Ferrell was also seen by Dr. Charles F. Ballou, III, who had been asked by Dr. MacKay to investigate the possibility that the patient was suffering from delirium tremens. An x-ray taken on the day of admission did indicate that a foreign object was lodged in the esophagus.

In the week that followed Dr. MacKay informed Mrs. Ferrell that her husband appeared to be suffering from delirium tremens, a diagnosis that Mrs. Ferrell insisted was incorrect. Also in the subsequent week, Dr. MacKay received medical records from two other hospitals on the patient. The records indicated that Mr. Ferrell had a history of alcohol abuse and schizophrenia. One week after the admission to C&O hospital another x-ray of Mr. Ferrell's esophagus was taken. Dr. MacKay informed Mrs. Ferrell that the x-ray indicated that the chicken bone had passed. Mr. Ferrell died the following week. A postmortem pathological report indicated that there was a chicken bone in the throat at the time of death. Listed on the death certificate were the following three causes of death: (a) bilateral bronchopneumonia, (b) cerebral edema, and (c) acute schizophrenia.

Mrs. Ferrell brought suit against C&O Hospital and Doctors Antonio, Harris, MacKay, and Ballou. As stated in the opinion of the federal district court that heard the case, Mrs. Ferrell's suit alleged two causes of action against the defendants:

The first cause of action charged that the defendants negligently and carelessly failed and refused to remove a chicken bone from the throat of her husband, Thomas Cecil Ferrell, and that they negligently and carelessly diagnosed her husband as suffering from delirium tremens. She further alleged that as a direct and proximate cause of the defendants' negligence and carelessness, she was subjected to unnecessary humiliation and embarrassment by having her husband diagnosed as an alcoholic; and she suffered unspeakable mental anguish witnessing the painful and agonizing demise of her husband for lack of proper medical treatment and attention. The second cause of action in the plaintiff's original complaint alleged that the defendants breached their duty to render proper medical care to her husband and that they fraudulently and deceitfully represented to her that her husband had passed the chicken bone from his throat when in fact the chicken bone remained lodged in his esophagus.

Following the defendants' motion to dismiss, the court ruled the plaintiff's first cause of action should be dismissed on the grounds that her alleged mental anguish was not accompanied by any actionable injury on her part and that the court could find no basis in Virginia law for awarding damages for humiliation suffered as a result of a negligent diagnosis of delirium tremens. The plaintiff subsequently amended her first complaint and alleged that the defendants' conduct had been "wilfull and wanton" instead of "negligent and careless." The second cause of action was dismissed as against Doctors Antonio, Harris, and Ballou but allowed to stand as against the C&O Hospital and Dr. Murdo M. MacKay. In determining that the two complaints stated causes of action upon which relief could be granted, the trial proceded.

The court found in favor of the defendants, stating,

> . . . upon examination of the evidence in this case, this court is unable to find any acts on the part of any of the defendants which constituted willful, wanton, intentional, or vindictive conduct.
>
> As to the plaintiff's second cause of action alleging breach of contract to perform proper medical treatment by the C&O Hospital and Dr. MacKay, this court fails to find that the treatment administered to Mr. Ferrell was improper, but under the circumstances discussed herein that treatment is deemed to have been proper.

6.26 CAPELOUTO V. KAISER
500 P.2d 880 (California, 1972)

The parents of an infant patient brought suit against the patient's physician to recover for damages for pain and suffering. Testimony at the trial indicated that the patient had begun to dehydrate at the age of two months and had required at least five hospitalizations before reaching one year of age. The court found in favor of the plaintiff, stating in essence that a one-year-old infant could recover damages for pain and suffering on the same basis as an adult.

6.27 ROCKHILL V. POLLARD
485 P.2d 28 (Oregon, 1971)

Two victims of an automobile accident, a woman and her unconscious baby daughter, came to a doctor's office seeking treatment. The doctor allegedly stated that there was nothing wrong with
either of them, and he made them wait outside his office in freezing
temperature until someone came to pick them up. The woman
charged that the doctor's rudeness caused her severe emotional
distress. The question of whether or not the case should go before a
jury was decided affirmatively:

> Under these circumstances we think that a jury could find the defen-
> dant's conduct was outrageous in the extreme. Defendant contends
> that the evidence discloses at most rudeness and a mistaken diagnosis.
> The plaintiff, however, is not attempting to recover for her hurt feel-
> ings at defendant's rudeness or for any harm she or the baby suffered
> as a direct result of the defendant's failure to diagnose their injuries
> properly. Her complaint charges him with abandoning her and her
> child, when he knew or should have known that they were in need of
> medical treatment. She charges that the defendant, by his behavior,
> intentionally or recklessly caused her severe emotional distress. The
> defendant's rudeness is simply evidence of his intention or reckless-
> ness; we think the jury could find that his statement that there was
> nothing wrong with the child was more than simply a mistaken diag-
> nosis. It could infer that he refused to give or suggest any treatment
> even though he must have known that there was a possibility the child
> had been seriously injured.

6.28 (Case cited by Ledakowich, 1976c)

While being inserted into the patient's shoulder during surgery,
a catheter broke and two pieces of it could not be found. The patient
was, in fact, stitched up with the two pieces lodged inside her body.
The patient brought suit against the doctor, claiming pain, suffering, and disability. Additionally, she claimed that she had developed
a phobia that she would develop cancer as a result of the two pieces
of catheter. The trial court awarded the plaintiff $45,000, as well as
an additional $3,350 for medical and hospital expenses. The defen-
dants appealed, conceding that negligence had taken place but arguing that the patient's fear of cancer was not compensable. The Supreme Court of Wisconsin noted that such damages were not recov-
erable, and a new trial to consider damages alone was ordered. In
coming to this conclusion, the court stated that

> although there is no question about there being in fact a fear of future
> cancer, the claim of damages is so remote and is so out of proportion to
> the culpability of the tortfeasor that, as a matter of public policy, we

conclude that the defendants are not to be held liable for this element of damages.

STANDARD OF CARE

6.29 HICKS v. UNITED STATES
368 F.2d 626 (Virginia, 1966)

Carol Greitens, the twenty-five-year-old wife of a Navy enlisted man, was brought by her husband to the dispensary at a Navy base about 4 A.M. Mrs. Greitens complained of vomiting and severe abdominal pain, which had come on suddenly approximately one hour before she sought treatment. The events that followed are set forth in the court record:

The corpsman on duty in the examining room procured her medical records, obtained a brief history, took her blood pressure, pulse, temperature, and respiration and summoned the doctor on duty, then asleep in his room at the dispensary. The doctor arrived 15 or 20 minutes later and after questioning the patient concerning her symptoms, felt her abdomen and listened to her bowel sounds with the aid of a stethoscope. Recording his diagnosis on the chart as gastroenteritis, he told Mrs. Greitens that she had a "bug" in her stomach, prescribed some drugs for the relief of pain, and released her with instructions to return in eight hours. The examination took approximately ten minutes.

The patient returned to her home, and after another episode of vomiting, took the prescribed medicine and lay down. At about noon, she arose and drank a glass of water, vomited immediately thereafter and fell to the floor unconscious. She was rushed to the dispensary, but efforts to revive her were unsuccessful. She was pronounced dead at 12:48 p.m. and an autopsy revealed that she had a high obstruction, diagnosed formally as an abnormal congenital peritoneal hiatus with internal herniation into this malformation of some of the loops of the small intestine. Death was due to a massive hemorrhagic infarction of the intestine resulting from its strangulation.

Harry J. Hicks, as administrator of Mrs. Greitens's estate, brought suit against the United States charging that the dispensary doctor negligently failed to thoroughly examine the patient or order immediate hospitalization. Expert witnesses for the plaintiff testified that, according to prevailing practice in the community, the dispensary doctor should have inquired whether the patient had had diarrhea. Additionally, the dispensary physician should have done a rectal examination to rule out an obstruction before diagnosing gastroenteritis. An expert witness for the government said that the dispensary physician had exercised "average judgment." The trial court ruled in favor of the defendant, holding that the evidence was insufficient to establish (1) that the physician was negligent, and (2) that the physician's admittedly erroneous diagnosis and treatment was the proximate cause of death.

The United Sates Court of Appeals rejected the testimony of the government's expert witness, observing that analysis of his testimony pointed to contrary conclusions. The court also questioned that witness's assumption that the dispensary physician's diagnosis was a "working" or "tentative" diagnosis. In fact, it was not:

> By releasing the patient, the dispensary physician made his diagnosis final, allowing no further opportunity for revision, and this prematurely determined final diagnosis was based on an investigation not even minimally adequate.

The Court of Appeals next dealt with the question of proximate cause:

> The government further contends that even if negligence is established, there was no proof that the erroneous diagnosis and treatment was the proximate cause of the death, asserting that even if surgery had been performed immediately, it is mere speculation to say that it would have been successful. The government's contention, however, is unsupported by the record. Both of plaintiff's experts testified categorically that if operated on promptly, Mrs. Greitens would have survived, and this is nowhere contradicted by the government expert....
>
> When a defendant's negligent action or inaction has effectively terminated a person's chance of survival, it does not lie in the defendant's mouth to raise conjectures as to the measure of the chances that he has put beyond the possibility of realization. If there was any substantial possibility of survival and the defendant has destroyed it, he is answerable. Rarely is it possible to demonstrate to an absolute certainty what would have happened in circumstances that the wrongdoer did not allow to come to pass. The law does not in the existing circumstances require the plaintiff to show to a *certainty* that the patient would have lived had she been hospitalized and operated on promptly.

The Court of Appeals reversed the lower court's decision and remanded the case for the determination of damages.

6.30 HELLING V. CAREY
519 P.2d 981 (Washington, 1974)

The plaintiff, Barbara Helling, first consulted the defendant physician, Dr. Thomas F. Carey, in 1959 for myopia (nearsightedness). Dr. Carey, an ophthalmologist, fitted the patient with contact lenses. The defendant was subsequently consulted at various times in 1963, 1967, and 1968 for various problems which, the defendant believed, were associated with the wearing of contact lenses. On one such consultation in 1968, Carey tested the plaintiff's eye pressure and her field of vision and diagnosed primary open angle glaucoma. This is a condition that results in an abnormally high pressure leading to optic nerve damage with consequential impairment of vision. Glaucoma can usually be detected by a pressure test, but in the absence of such a test the disease may progress, causing extensive, permanent damage before it becomes detectable.

In 1969, after consulting with other physicians, Helling brought suit against Carey claiming that her loss of vision and the permanent damage to her eyes was a proximate result of his negligence. It was alleged that if the doctor had performed a pressure test on the eye the injury could have been prevented. Expert witnesses at the trial testified as to what the applicable standard of care was. Witnesses for both the plaintiff and the defense agreed that the standards of the profession of ophthalmology would not require a routine pressure test for glaucoma in the same or similar circumstances. This is so because the incidence of glaucoma in patients under forty years of age is approximately 1 in every 25,000 persons, and the patient was thirty-two years old at the time of the consultation. Incidence over age forty is about 2 to 3 percent in the general population.

The trial court found in favor of the defendant doctors, a finding that was upheld by the court of appeals. The plaintiff then petitioned the Supreme Court of Washington to review the case. The Washington Supreme Court reversed the decision of the lower courts and remanded the case back for a trial on the issue of damages only. Associate Justice Hunter wrote in his opinion as follows:

> We find this to be a unique case. The testimony of the medical experts is undisputed concerning the standards of the profession for the specialty of ophthalmology. It is not a question in this case of the defendants having any greater special ability, knowledge and information than other ophthalmologists which would require the defendants to comply with a higher duty of care than that "degree of care and skill which is expected of the average practitioner in the class to which he belongs, acting in the same or similar circumstances." Pederson v. Dumouchel, 72 Wash.2d 73, 79, 431 P.2d 973 (1967). The issue is whether the defendants' compliance with the standard of the profession of ophthalmology, which does not require the giving of a routine pressure test to persons under 40 years of age, should insulate them from liability under the facts in this case where the plaintiff has lost a substantial amount of her vision due to the failure of the defendants to timely give the pressure test to the plaintiff.
>
> The defendants argue that the standard of the profession, which does not require the giving of a routine pressure test to persons under the age of 40, is adequate to insulate the defendants from liability for negligence because the risk of glaucoma is so rare in this age group. The testimony of the defendant, Dr. Carey, however, is revealing as follows:

"Q. Now, when was it, actually, the first time any complaint was made to you by her of any field or visual field problem? A. Really, the first time that she really complained of a visual field problem was the August 30th date. [1968] Q. And how soon before the diagnosis was that? A. That was 30 days. We made it on October 1st. Q. And in your opinion, how long, as you nor have the whole history and analysis and the diagnosis, how long had she had this glaucoma? A. I would think she probably had it ten years or longer. Q. Now, Doctor, there's been some reference to the matter of taking pressure checks of persons over 40. What is the incidence of glaucoma, the statistics, with persons under 40? A. In the instance of glaucoma under the age of 40, is less than 100 to one per cent. The younger you get, the less the incidence. It is thought to be in the neighborhood of one in 25,000 people or less. Q. How about the incidence of glaucoma in people over 40? A. Incidence of glaucoma over 40 gets into the two to three percent category, and hence, that's where there is this great big difference and that's why the standards around the world has been to check pressures from 40 on."

The incidence of glaucoma in one out of 25,000 persons under the age of 40 may appear quite minimal. However, that one person, the plaintiff in this instance, is entitled to the same protection, as afforded persons over 40, essential for timely detection of the evidence of glaucoma where it can be arrested to avoid the grave and devastating result of this disease. The test is a simple pressure test, relatively inexpensive. There is no judgment factor involved, and there is no doubt that by giving the test the evidence of glaucoma can be detected. The giving of the test is harmless if the physical condition of the eye permits. The testimony indicates that although the condition of the plaintiff's eyes might have at times prevented the defendants from administering the pressure test, there is an absence of evidence in the record that the test could not have been timely given.

Justice Holmes stated in Texas & Pac. Ry. v. Behymer, 189 U.S. 468, 470, 23 S.Ct. 622, 623, 47 L.Ed. 905 (1903):

"What usually is done may be evidence of what ought to be done, but what ought to be done is fixed by a standard of reasonable prudence, whether it usually is complied with or not."

In The T. J. Hooper, 60 F.2d 737, on page 740 (2d Cir. 1932), Justice Hand stated:

"[I]n most cases reasonable prudence is in fact common prudence; but strictly it is never its measure; a whole calling may have unduly lagged in the adoption of new and available devices. It never may set its own tests, however persuasive be its usages. *Courts must in the end say what is required; there are precautions so imperative that even their universal disregard will not excuse their omission.*" (Italics ours.)

Under the facts of this case reasonable prudence required the timely giving of the pressure test to this plaintiff. The precaution of giving this test to detect the incidence of glaucoma to patients under 40 years of age is so imperative that irrespective of its disregard by the standards of the opthalmology profession, it is the duty of the courts to say what is required to protect patients under 40 from the damaging results of glaucoma.

We therefore hold, as a matter of law, that the reasonable standard that should have been followed under the undisputed facts of this case was the timely giving of this simple, harmless pressure test to this plaintiff and that, in failing to do so, the defendants were negligent, which proximately resulted in the blindness sustained by the plaintiff for which the defendants are liable.

There are no disputed facts to submit to the jury on the issue of the defendants' liability. Hence, a discussion of the plaintiff's proposed instructions would be inconsequential in view of our disposition of the case.

The judgment of the trial court and the decision of the Court of Appeals is reversed, and the case is remanded for a new trial on the issue of damages only.

Associate Justice Utter concurred and filed an opinion which, in part, suggested that liability in such a fact situation might better be based on strict liability rather than upon negligence:

I concur in the result reached by the majority. I believe a greater duty of care could be imposed on the defendants than was established by their profession. The duty could be imposed when a disease, such as glaucoma, can be detected by a simple, well-known harmless test whose results are definitive and the disease can be successfully arrested by early detection, but where the effects of the disease are irreversible if undetected over a substantial period of time.

The difficulty with this approach is that we as judges, by using a negligence analysis, seem to be imposing a stigma of moral blame upon the doctors who, in this case, used all the precautions commonly prescribed by their profession in diagnosis and treatment. Lacking their training in this highly sophisticated profession, it seems illogical for this court to say they failed to exercise a reasonable standard of care. It seems to me we are, in reality, imposing liability, because, in choosing between an innocent plaintiff and a doctor, who acted reasonably according to his specialty but who could have prevented the full effects of this disease by administering a simple, harmless test and treatment, the plaintiff should not have to bear the risk of loss. As such, imposition of liability approaches that of strict liability.

Strict liability or liability without fault is not new to the law. Historically, it predates our concepts of fault or moral responsibility as a basis of the remedy. Wigmore, Responsibility for Tortious Acts: Its History, 7 Har.L.Rev. 315, 383, 441 (1894). As noted in W. Prosser, The Law of Torts § 74 (3d ed. 1964) at pages 507, 508:

"There are many situations in which a careful person is held liable for an entirely reasonable mistake. . . . in some cases the defendant may be held liable, although he is not only charged with no moral wrongdoing, but has not even departed in any way from a reasonable standard of intent or care. . . . There is 'a strong and growing tendency, where there is blame on neither side, to ask, in view of the exigencies of social justice, who can best bear the loss and hence to shift the loss by creating liability where there has been no fault.' " (Footnote omitted).

Tort law has continually been in a state of flux. It is "not always neat and orderly. But this is not to say it is illogical. Its central logic is the logic that moves from premises—its objectives—that are only partly consistent, to conclusions—its rules—that serve each objective as well as may be while serving others too. It is the logic of maximizing service and minimizing disservice to multiple objectives." Keeton, Is There a Place for Negligence in Modern Tort Law?, 53 Va.L.Rev.886, 897 (1967).

When types of problems rather than numbers of cases are examined, strict liability is applied more often than negligence as a principle which determines liability. Peck, Negligence and Liability Without Fault in Tort Law, 46 Wash.L.Rev. 225, 239 (1971). There are many similarities in this case to other cases of strict liability. Problems of proof have been a common feature in situations where strict liability is applied. Where events are not matters of common experience, a juror's ability to comprehend whether reasonable care has been followed diminishes. There are few areas as difficult for jurors to intelligently comprehend as the intricate questions of proof and standards in medical malpractice cases.

In applying strict liability there are many situations where it is imposed for conduct which can be defined with sufficient precision to insure that application of a strict liability principle will not produce miscarriages of justice in a substantial number of cases. If the activity involved is one which can be defined with sufficient precision, that definition can serve as an accounting unit to which the costs of the activity may be allocated with some certainty and precision. With this possible, strict liability serves a compensatory function in situations where the defendant is, through the use of insurance, the financially more responsible person. Peck, Negligence and Liability Without Fault in Tort Law, *supra* at 240, 241.

If the standard of a reasonably prudent specialist is, in fact, inadequate to offer reasonable protection to the plaintiff, then liability can be imposed without fault. To do so under the narrow facts of this case does not offend my sense of justice. The pressure test to measure intraocular pressure with the Schiotz tonometer and the Goldman applanometer takes a short time, involves no damage to the patient, and consists of placing the instrument against the eyeball. An abnormally high pressure requires other tests which would either confirm or deny the existence of glaucoma. It is generally believed that from 5 to 10 years of detectable increased pressure must exist before there is permanent damage to the optic nerves.

Although the incidence of glaucoma in the age range of the plaintiff is approximately one in 25,000, this alone should not be enough to deny her a claim. Where its presence can be detected by a simple, well-known harmless test, where the results of the test are definitive, where the disease can be successfully arrested by early detection and where its effects are irreversible if undetected over a substantial period of time, liability should be imposed upon defendants even though they did not violate the standard existing within the profession of ophthalmology.

The failure of plaintiff to raise this theory at the trial and to propose instructions consistent with it should not deprive her of the right to resolve the case on this theory on appeal. Where this court has authoritatively stated the law, the parties are bound by those principles until they have been overruled. Acceptance of those principles at trial does not constitute a waiver or estop appellants from adapting their cause on appeal to such a rule as might be declared if the earlier precedent is overruled. Samuelson v. Freeman, 75 Wash.2d 894, 900, 454 P.2d 406 (1969).

6.31 (Case cited in Ledakowich, 1974)

A child who complained of pain in the lower right abdomen had a temperature of 101 degrees and was vomiting. The child was taken to the hospital, and after laboratory tests and x-rays, the defendant doctor's diagnosis was tonsilitis. Medication was prescribed and ordered to be given at home. Five days later the parents complained that their child still was in pain, and the child was rehospitalized. Subsequently two operations were necessary to remedy the child's condition (ruptured appendix and peritonitis). The first operation involved the placement of tubes to drain the infection; the second was for removal of the appendix. The patient's parents brought suit against the doctor for negligence. Medical testimony offered at the trial led the trial judge to direct a verdict in favor of the defendant doctor. The plaintiffs appealed, arguing that sufficient evidence of negligence had been presented to warrant sending the case to the jury. The plaintiffs contended that even without expert testimony the doctor's negligence was so obvious as to be apparent even to laymen. The state supreme court reaffirmed the trial court's decision, stating that

> the symptoms of appendicitis are so well known and recognized . . . that the illness on the surface appeared to be appendicitis. But the experts pointed out that the symptoms and x-ray findings are consistent with other diseases including tonsilitis. The high white blood cell count generally associated with appendicitis was not present. No findings of the examination have been shown to be inconsistent with tonsilitis, but a low white cell blood count is not consistent with appendicitis.
>
> The layman would have no conception of the complex nature of the problem. In this case the obvious was correct and the doctor's diagnosis was wrong. But, recovery is not permitted merely because a doctor makes a wrong diagnosis. If the examination was thorough and competent, and no negligence is shown, the patient cannot recover. The record here discloses an honest mistake in the doctor's judgment, but does not show he was negligent in arriving at his opinion.

6.32 EBAUGH V. RABKIN
99 Cal.Rptr. 706 (California, 1972)

Ms. A was scheduled for a breast biopsy by Dr. X in the same hospital, on the same day, and in the same hour that Ms. B was scheduled to undergo gall bladder surgery by Dr. Y. A mix-up led to each patient's being operated on by the other's doctor. Dr. Y opened up Ms. A, saw a normal gallbladder, and realized his error when he looked at her wristband and chart. Meanwhile, Dr. X had made an incision in Ms. B's breast, but he soon realized his error and terminated the procedure. Ms. A's suit against both doctors and the hospital was successful, and she was awarded $7,500 in compensatory damages and punitive damages in the amount of $10,000 against Dr. X, $5,000 against Dr. Y (who had technically committed a battery), and $30,000 against the hospital.

6.33 ANDERSON V. JOHNS HOPKINS HOSPITAL
272 A.2d 372 (Maryland, 1971)

A surgeon performed two operations on a woman: the first was to elevate her breast, and the second involved silicone implantation. The woman and her husband were dissatisfied with the results and brought suit against the surgeon, even though the surgeon had made no guarantees about the outcome. The court ruled in favor of the defendant surgeon, noting that in order for the surgeon to be held liable it would have to be demonstrated that the standard of care associated with this type of treatment had been violated.

THE STATUTE OF LIMITATIONS

6.34 (Case cited in "Six court decisions," 1974)

After undergoing a radical mastectomy, the patient received radiation treatment from a radiologist that led to several severe complications. She was then treated by an osteopath, who hospitalized her fifteen times subsequent to the treatments. She then sought treatment elsewhere, and while in the hospital overheard her doctor saying to his colleagues: "And there you see, gentlemen, what happens when a radiologist puts a patient on the table and goes out and has a cup of coffee." The woman brought suit against the radiologist and the osteopath for malpractice and for conspiracy in concealing the negligent cause of her injuries. The defendants moved for a summary dismissal of the case on the grounds that the legal period of time within which the defendant was entitled to bring suit had expired. The attorney for the plaintiff, however, sought to invoke the discovery rule—the rule that says that the Statute of Limitations can be exceeded if the plaintiff had no way of knowing, within the legal time limit, that negligence had occurred. The plaintiff argued that the first occasion she had to suspect negligence was when she overheard her doctor discussing the case. The defense argued that the discovery rule was not applicable since it applied only to "hidden" negligence, and if any negligence was involved in the treatment of the plaintiff it had been "blatant" enough to warrant bringing suit earlier. The New Jersey trial court awarded a summary judgment to the defendant, but the Appellate Division returned the case for trial. The defendants then appealed to the New Jersey Supreme Court, and the Appellate Division's decision that the case be remanded for trial was upheld by the supreme court. The supreme court ruled, however, that whether or not the statute of limitations can be applied must be decided by a judge rather than a jury:

> It is not every belated discovery that will justify an application of the rule lifting the bar of the limitations statute. The interplay of the conflicting interests of the competing parties must be considered. The decision requires more than the simple factual determination; it should be made by a judge and by a judge conscious of the equitable nature of the issue before him.

CONTRIBUTORY NEGLIGENCE

6.35 RAY V. WAGNER
176 N.W. 101 (Minnesota, 1971)

A patient being examined for a contraceptive device underwent a Pap smear, which came back from the lab with a note that it was suspicious for malignancy. The patient did not try to contact the physician to find out what the result of the test was. The physician tried to contact the patient but was unable to do so, because she could not be reached by phone and had given him only vague information about her living arrangements. The woman subsequently became sterile as a result of cobalt and radium therapy and sought to recover damages from the doctor for negligence. The court found the woman to be contributorily negligent—to have contributed to her condition by her own negligence—and ruled in favor of the defendant doctor.

6.36 BYRD V. PRITCHARD
291 N.E.2d 769 (Ohio, 1973)

After cutting her hand, a woman was treated by an osteopathic surgeon. Though instructed by the surgeon to visit his office again in three days, the woman failed to keep the appointment. She later brought suit against the surgeon, claiming that permanent damage had been done to her hand. The surgeon's defense was that of contributory negligence. The court found against the doctor, holding that nerve damage which was not treated by the doctor during the first visit could not have been repaired even if the woman had kept her second appointment.

6.37 ROCHESTER V. KATALAN
320 A.2d 704 (Delaware, 1974)

"John" and "Bill" were brought by the police to a hospital emergency room for treatment, since both claimed to be heroin addicts suffering from withdrawal symptoms. Both men were observed by the emergency room doctor to be exhibiting symptoms consistent with the claim that they were suffering from heroin withdrawal; John had referred to himself as a "junkie" requiring four to five bags of heroin daily. When asked if they had ever attended a methadone clinic, both men answered affirmatively. John stated that he had attended for four months but had then dropped out. On the basis of this history and clinical observation, the physician ordered that John and Bill each be medicated with 40 milligrams of methadone. Approximately thirty to forty minutes after the administration of the methadone, Bill had calmed down but John had become more violent, banging his head against the wall and shouting at the physician that he needed more medication. The doctor ordered the administration of another 40 milligrams of methadone and ordered a nurse to watch John for thirty minutes thereafter. John quieted down after the administration of the second dose, and both men were brought to cells to spend the night. The following morning the turnkey was unable to arouse John, who was subsequently pronounced dead.

It was later learned that although Bill was indeed a heroin addict, John was not. It was discovered that shortly before being taken into custody by the police, John had consumed an unknown quantity of beer and tranquilizers. The plaintiff sought to hold the defendant emergency room doctor liable for John's death, claiming that the doctor was negligent in not doing enough to ascertain that John was not (and had never been) a heroin addict or a participant in a methadone program. The court found in favor of the defendant doctor, stating that

> the undisputed facts show that the decedent put on an act, tragic in its consequences but effective in the emergency room under the circumstances in which it was performed. For reasons of his own, he demonstrated the clinical symptoms associated with heroin withdrawal and confirmed them by insisting that he was an addict. It is no answer to this to say, as the plaintiff argues, that the doctor and staff could have done more to determine the truth of his assertions. We have already assumed negligence in that respect. The critical issue involves the decedent's conduct, not that of the defendants. Whatever the decedent's purpose, his conduct was a true tragedy for all who were involved. And he continued the contribution to his own destruction by failing to tell the medical people present the facts (he was not an addict, he had been drinking and taking tranquilizers) and by asking for more.... Our

analysis of the record persuades us that, beyond doubt, the decedent causally contributed to his death up to the time when it occurred. Had he informed the defendants or hospital personnel that he neither was currently nor had ever been a heroin addict (even after the original deliberately misleading statements and actions), proper measures might have been taken to avoid potential ill effects from administration of the methadone. It is the failure to exercise the power to correct the situation which rendered the decedent's actions continuing negligence on his part. What is significant is that aside from being at least partially responsible for causing use of the methadone, the decedent possessed the power to thereafter set in motion procedures which might have prevented the result.

INFORMED CONSENT

6.38 FUNKE V. FIELDMAN
512 P.2d 539 (Kansas, 1973)

A spinal anesthetic was administered by an anesthesiologist who told the patient that the only possible complications of the procedure might be headaches. The patient suffered nerve damage as a result of the procedure and brought suit against the doctor, claiming that informed consent for the procedure had not been obtained. The court ruled in favor of the plaintiff, finding that the defendant knew or should have known that spinal anesthesia carried with it more risks than simple headaches and that, in the absence of an emergency situation, the doctor did have the legal obligation to disclose inherent risks and possible consequences of the treatment.

6.39 MEIDMAN V. REHABILITATION CENTER
444 S.W.2d 78 (Kentucky, 1970)

A patient was asked by a rehabilitation center to sign a written release of liability before receiving treatment. The release said:

> I further agree, that I will assume all risks which have been explained to me in detail that can result from my attending the Center and at prescribed activities outside the Center, and from diagnosis and treatment. I will not assert any claim against the center, its employees, or its volunteers that results from unintentional acts or conduct on their part.

The legal question of whether or not the patient could then sue the rehabilitation center was raised. The court ruled that the plaintiff could sue the center, since such a release was contrary to public policy and therefore void.

BREACH OF CONTRACT

6.40 HERRERA V. ROESSING
Colorado Court of Appeals, Division II, February 19, 1975 (cited in Cases Unlimited, Inc., 1976)

A woman underwent a tubal ligation for contraceptive purposes. Before undergoing the surgery, she signed a form stating that no guarantee of any kind was made to her as a result of her treatment or examination in the hospital. After the procedure, the physician had told her informally "not to worry about the tubes coming undone," that he was sure she wouldn't become pregnant and that she need not take any other precautions against becoming pregnant. The woman brought suit against the physician when she did become pregnant. The court found that since the patient had not paid any money to the physician for a "warranty" after surgery, she could not recover for a breach of the alleged warranty. The court found the statements made by the physician to be mere opinions and reassurances and held that they did not constitute a guarantee.

6.41 GUILMET V. CAMPBELL
385 Mich. 57; 188 N.W.2d 601; 43 A.L.R.3d 1194 (Michigan, 1971)

The plaintiff, a peptic ulcer patient who had twice suffered near-fatal bleeding, alleged that prior to his gastric resection the surgeon made some of the following remarks in the course of recommending the surgery:

- "Once you have an operation it takes care of all your troubles. You can eat as you want to, you can drink as you want to, you can go as you please."
- "There's nothing to it at all. It's a very simple operation. There's no danger at all in this operation."
- "You will be out of work three to four weeks at the most."
- "After the operation, you can throw away your pill box. If you figure out what you would spend for antacids and doctor calls over, say twenty years, you could buy an awful lot. Weigh it against an operation."

Following the operation, in which 80 percent of the patient's stomach was removed, the patient suffered a ruptured esophagus due to surgical trauma. The patient then needed three additional operations to draw fluid from his body and developed hepatitis as a result of the many transfusions. Persistent vomiting and coughing caused his weight to drop from 170 to 88 pounds. The plaintiff sought damages on the grounds that he had relied upon the surgeon's representations in consenting to the surgery and that subsequent events amounted to a breach of contract. The trial court found in favor of the plaintiff. The surgeon lost an appeal to the state appeals court and subsequently lost an appeal to the state supreme court, which stated that

> we do not say that everytime a doctor says, "I recommend an immediate appendectomy. It will fix you up fine. You will be back to work in no time. Do not worry about it—I have done hundreds of these operations . . ." that he contracted to "cure" his patient.
>
> What we are saying is that under some circumstances the trier of fact might conclude that a doctor so speaking did contract to "cure" his patient. . . .
>
> What was said, and the circumstances under which it was said always determines whether there was a contract at all and if so what it was. These matters are always for the determination of the fact finder.
>
> The jury must have found from the evidence that the doctor made a specific, clear and express promise to cure or effect a specific result which was in the reasonable contemplation of the parties and which was relied upon by the plaintiff.

6.42 STEWART V. RUDNER
349 Mich. 459; 84 N.W.2d 816 (Michigan, 1957)

A physician told his patient that her baby would be delivered by a Cesarean section. The baby was not delivered by a Cesarean section but by other, usual procedures. The suit brought against the defendant physician charged breach of contract. The court found in favor of the plaintiff.

INVASION OF PRIVACY

6.43 (Case cited in Ledakowich, 1977: Supreme Judicial Court of Maine, 1976)

An otolaryngologist/surgeon defendant had taken photographs of a patient suffering from cancer of the larynx at various stages of the patient's treatment. The last series of photos was taken two weeks after the defendant had completed his treatment and only hours before the patient died. According to the patient's widow, the patient had objected to the picture taking and had tried to move himself from camera range, raising a clenched fist to make his objection known. The patient's widow sued the surgeon, charging invasion of privacy. The trial court directed a verdict in favor of the defendant, noting that "the mere taking of pictures is not an invasion of privacy" and that "medical science must have some information in its effort to track down and search for a cure."

The plaintiff appealed to the Supreme Judicial Court of Maine, which struck down the lower court's ruling. The court rejected the surgeon's arguments that it was in the interest of medical science to take such photographs and that such picture taking should be legally permissible over a patient's objections. In ordering a new trial, the court ruled that the patient's "right to be let alone" had been violated and that the violation had constituted a tort for which liability could be assessed.

UNDUE INFLUENCE

6.44 MITCHELL V. HARRIS
246 So.2d 648 (Alabama, 1971)

A physician treating a patient for approximately seven months bought some land from the patient about one month before the patient died. A suit was subsequently brought against the doctor, alleging that he had taken unfair advantage of the doctor–patient relationship in purchasing the land. The court found no evidence of undue influence and noted that the doctor had paid the full fair-market value for the land.

INSURANCE

6.45 (Case cited in Ledakowich, 1972a)

As a result of a doctor's treatment of a cheek tumor, the tumor's size swelled instead of reducing. Neither the doctor nor any of his colleagues could determine why the treatment had failed. The doctor continued to treat the patient for over twelve years, and ultimately the patient lost a portion of her jawbone and suffered other facial scarring. The doctor was notified of a suit against him for malpractice, and he immediately notified his insurance company. The insurance company agreed to defend the doctor, but reserved the right to deny him coverage in the event that he was found liable. After a settlement of the plaintiff's claim was reached the doctor sued the insurance company for payment under the policy, but the insurance company argued that he had not complied with the terms of his policy, which specifically stated that

[u]pon the Insured becoming aware of any alleged injury covered hereby, written notice shall be given by or on behalf of the Insured to

the company or any of its authorized agents as soon as practicable together with the fullest information obtainable.

In other words, the insurance company argued that the terms of the insured's policy made it incumbent upon him to notify them as soon as he was "aware of any alleged injury," not after he was formally charged with negligence. The trial court denied the doctor's right to try the case, and the doctor appealed the decision. On appeal, the lower court's decision was reversed. The court affirmed the doctor's right to proceed with a jury trial, stating that

> [i]t must be understood that the practice of medicine is not an exact science. It frequently happens that anticipated or hoped-for results do not follow treatment in connection with the healing arts. If a doctor had to report every such occasion to his insurer, the insurer would be endlessly annoyed, for in the great majority of cases the patient recovers. That which will benefit one patient may not be helpful to the next one, and so a doctor must of necessity watch the progress of his patient and change the treatment from time to time in an effort to obtain favorable results. If he had to report to his insurer every adverse reaction of his patients, he would scarcely have time to practice his profession, and the constant efforts of the insurer to make a defense would greatly hamper the doctor in his attempt to heal the patient.
>
> We hold that a doctor should notify his insurer of a claim of malpractice when it is alleged to have been committed or when it is or should be obvious to him that he has caused harm to his patient through neglect of duty or ignorance of the standards of practice amongst his fellow doctors and that a claim is likely to be made against him.
>
> Whether this plaintiff knew or should have known that the condition of his patient was due to his own lack of due care in treating her at any time prior to the time of giving notice, would be a question of fact for a jury to determine.

6.46   (Case cited in "Six court decisions," 1974)

The patient, a pregnant woman, came to a hospital emergency room complaining of pain and high fever. The emergency room doctor, an obstetrician, diagnosed the cause as a kidney infection and anemia and admitted the woman to the hospital under his sole care. After release from the hospital the woman and her husband decided to obtain a family health insurance policy. The insurance salesman told the couple that the policy would be retroactive to a certain point once the requirements needed to put the policy in force were met. One of the requirements was that the obstetrician who had treated the woman fill out a one-page form with five questions on it. The form was sent to the obstetrician, who promised to fill it out but neglected to do so. Even after the obstetrician delivered the woman's babies (she had twins), the forms had still not been sent in.

Subsequent to the delivery, the insurance company notified the family that because the doctor had not sent in the forms their application for insurance was being turned down. The family was told that their application would be reconsidered when they received the form. All efforts on the part of the family to get the doctor to fill out the forms were in vain, and this was particularly unfortunate because they were incurring numerous medical problems in the meantime. (The twins had been born with congenital illnesses, necessitating a prolonged hospital stay; the mother had to be hospitalized for a ruptured appendix; and the husband apparently suffered a seizure which resulted in a fall that required hospitalization.)

The insurance company refused to extend the family's retroactive coverage after it finally received the form, and the family brought suit against the doctor for negligence. The defendant doctor argued for a dismissal of the charges against him on the grounds that the plaintiff was not his patient. The court denied the defendant's motion, however, holding that,

> [u]nder the particular circumstances here, if a doctor–patient relationship is shown to exist, it must have given rise to a duty of reasonable care in the disposition of the form. . . .
>
> In the absence of special circumstances it was the doctor's duty to recognize his unique position as the treating physician who alone could comply with the insurance requirement without the expense and delay of a further examination. Upon actual receipt of the form, he was under a duty to exercise reasonable care in the disposition of the form. He might discharge that duty by completing and returning the form within a reasonable period of time to the insurance company, or by promptly notifying the applicants and the insurance company that he would not complete the form and perhaps referring them to another source for the vital information.
>
> Whether under the circumstances the doctor acted within a reasonable time is a question of fact to be decided by the trier of fact upon familiar negligence principles. There are issues of material fact as to the relationship of the parties, the details of their communications and the reasonableness of defendant's delay.

MEDICAL PRACTICE AND RELIGION

6.47 (Case cited in "Six court decisions," 1974)

A pregnant woman in her late thirties was brought to the hospital after accidentally fracturing her thigh. The woman was placed in traction, and it was decided that the infants (she was expecting a multiple birth) would be delivered by Caesarean section. The woman was unwed, epileptic, and supported by welfare and had consulted a physician early in her pregnancy about obtaining a tubal ligation for contraceptive purposes at the time of delivery. Because the hospital she was brought to was owned and operated by the Roman Catholic Church, however, the hospital administrators refused on religious grounds to allow the sterilization to take place. The woman was in no condition to be moved to another hospital, and she brought suit to allow the procedure to take place at that hospital. A United States district court found in the hospital's favor, stating that

> [t]he Court does not find that there is such emergency existing or overriding interest of the plaintiff that would justify this Court's intervention in the hospital's operating policies and regulations. The interest that the public has in the establishment and operation of hospitals by religious organizations is paramount to any inconvenience that would result to the plaintiff in requiring her to either be moved or await a later date for her sterilization.

6.48 (Case cited in "Six court decisions," 1974)

A twenty-two-year-old victim of an automobile accident was brought to a hospital emergency room unconscious and in critical condition, in serious need of a blood transfusion. The patient's mother told the doctor that both she and her daughter were Jehovah's Witnesses and as such could not receive blood. The mother signed a document releasing the hospital of liability for any contingency that might arise from respecting her wishes. As the girl's condition worsened, the hospital obtained court-ordered permission to give blood and perform the necessary surgery. Though the girl was saved, the mother brought suit against the hospital for violating her wishes. Specifically, the plaintiff alleged that her constitutional liberty of religious freedom had been violated. The hospital argued that once a person came under its care it was its duty to treat that person with the best possible medical care and not let the patient dictate what the treatment should be. The court found in favor of the hospital, stating that

> [t]here is no constitutional right to choose to die. Nor is constitutional right established by adding that one's religious faith ordains his death. Religious beliefs are absolute, but conduct in pursuance of religious beliefs is not wholly immune from governmental restraint.
>
> The relevant question is whether there is a "compelling state interest" justifying the state's refusal to permit the patient to refuse vital aid. Indeed, the issue is not solely between the state and the patient, for the controversy is also between the patient and a hospital and staff who did not seek her out and upon whom the dictates of her fate will fall as a burden.
>
> Hospitals exist to aid the sick and injured. The medical and nursing professions are consecrated to preserving life. That is their professional creed. To them, a failure to use a simple, established procedure

in the circumstances of this case would be malpractice, however the law may characterize that failure because of the patient's private convictions. A surgeon should not be asked to operate under the strain of knowing that a transfusion may not be administered even though medically required to save his patient. The hospital and its staff should not be required to decide whether the patient is or continues to be competent to make a judgment upon the subject, or whether the release tendered by the patient or a member of his family will protect them from civil responsibility. The hospital could hardly avoid the problem by compelling the removal of a dying patient, and the patient's family made no effort to take her elsewhere.

When the hospital and staff are thus involuntary hosts and their interests are pitted against the belief of the patient, we think it reasonable to resolve the problem by permitting the hospital and its staff to pursue their functions according to their professional standards. The solution sides with life, the conservation of which is, we think, a matter of state interest.

PHYSICAL MINISTRATIONS

6.49 COREY V. DALLAS
352 F.Supp. 977 (Texas, 1973)

A Dallas law that made it illegal to administer a massage to someone of the opposite sex was challenged. The court found the law to be unreasonable and arbitrary, since it denied the right of all persons (including physicians and nurses) to administer a massage, simply because there was a potential for misuse. (The court did allow that the city could lawfully regulate the licensing and dress of massage parlor personnel, the dress of the clientele, and the hours of operation.)

IV

AVOIDING LEGAL JEOPARDY

Laws in the area of negligence and the interpretation of those laws have been undergoing rapid change. Still, health professionals interested in avoiding such litigation have much to learn from previous court decisions. In Chapter 7, we shall review some of the cases presented in Part III and attempt to provide some guidelines for avoiding legal jeopardy. In the final chapter, some more global recommendations for protecting your practice will be made. Nothing in the present or preceding material is intended to imply a standard of care or a definitive statement of the law.

7

Principles of Malpractice Law: A Review of the Cases

The great complexity of negligence law precludes an in-depth discussion of the numerous and multifaceted issues underlying each of the cases presented in Part III. It is hoped, however, that the brief discussion of these cases presented in this chapter will be useful in acquainting mental health professionals with a sampling of the legal principles that have been invoked by various jurisdictions in such litigation.

SUICIDE OR ATTEMPTED SUICIDE

All of the states now have what are called "wrongful death" statutes, which provide for a civil cause of action if the death of an individual is brought about wrongfully (such as by the negligence of another). The wrongful death action must have a basis in tort. That is, all of the elements of the alleged tort (e.g., negligence or battery) must be proven before damages for wrongful death will be awarded. Courts have held that mental health professionals have an affirmative duty to prevent the suicide of their patients. If professionals negligently breach that duty of due care, they may be sued by the decedent's next of kin or estate for wrongful death.[1] In *Meier* (5.2),[2] for example, a patient committed suicide by jumping out of an open window in a hospital where the psychiatric facility maintained an "open door" policy. In its decision, the court held that "the 'open door' policy does not necessarily call for an

---

[1] In some states, such as New York, it is only the next of kin who may bring a wrongful death action, *not* the decedent's estate. The estate can, however, still sue for whatever claim the decedent had up to the time of his death.
[2] Numbers in parentheses refer to case numbers in Part III.

openable window; the objectives of the policy can be achieved without leaving an openable window for the patient."

As early as 1941 the courts were beginning to recognize the value of freedom of movement in the treatment of psychiatric patients. The 1941 case of *James v. Turner* (201 S.W.2d 691) involved a voluntary patient at a private sanitarium who had threatened to commit suicide. In his treatment, the physicians had allowed this patient some freedom of movement such as excursions to the town barber shop. One day while walking with an attendant the patient suddenly darted to a reservoir, climbed the water tank tower ladder, threw himself in and drowned. Rejecting the plaintiff's argument that the defendant physicians were negligent in that they failed to properly supervise and restrain this patient, the court held that "the use of ropes or handcuffs or other restraining forces would have retarded his natural progress in regaining his health, both mental and physical."

More recently, opinions expressed in *Baker* (5.1), *Gregory* (5.3), and elsewhere are reflective of judicial acknowledgement of the value of "open" wards. However, in all cases, the therapeutic value of an open ward must be balanced against the probability of the patient's doing harm to himself (or others). In this context, even the most casual survey of the cases presented in Chapter 5 should impress mental health professionals with the importance of taking a very careful history of their patients. In case after case, the questions that inevitably get raised by the court are, "Had this person previously attempted suicide or expressed suicidal ideation? What evidence was there that this individual was suicidal?" These questions are also of primary importance at the institutional level, since the answers will often be instrumental in a court's assignment of liability as regards the extent of supervision provided by the institution. Compare for example, the liability assigned to hospitals and individuals in cases where the patient did (5.4–5.10) and did not (5.11) have a suicidal history.

The legal literature is replete with cases concerning individuals who have committed or attempted to commit suicide regardless of the closeness of the supervision they were under at the time. In *Fernandez v. Baruch* (52 N.J. 127; 244 A.2d 109) it was alleged that the defendant psychiatrist was negligent in failing to take proper precautions in transferring a patient from a general hospital to the county jail; after four days in jail the patient hanged himself with his socks. In *Mills v. Society of New York Hospital* (1 N.E.2d 346) an institutionalized patient who was out on a walk with nine other patients and two aides suddenly ran from the group and committed suicide by jumping in front of an oncoming bus. Another instance of a patient jumping in front of a bus while out on a supervised walk is cited in *Noel v. Menninger Foundation* (180 Kan. 23; 299 P.2d 38). In *Benjamin v. Havens, Inc.* (60 Wash.2d 196; 373 P.2d 109), suit was brought against a psychiatrist and Havens, Inc. (a mental hospital) for alleged negligence in failing to provide proper supervision for a patient. The patient had been diagnosed as "agitated depression, probably involutional in character" and admitted to the defendant hospital with a note that read, "Watch patient—depressed." On the eighth day after her admission, the patient fled through an unlocked door and leaped or fell down a hill, landing on a concrete patio. An excerpt from the opinion in *Benjamin* provides more detail about the circumstances under which the injury occurred:

> The hospital... was operating upon the psychiatric concept whereby mental patients, in its custodial care, were allowed as much freedom as possible in an effort to resocialize them. Such type of therapy, within the framework of the evidence presented, would appear to involve a reasonably foreseeable risk that patients, such as plaintiff wife, may impetuously flee. The exercise of ordinary care could well compel the maintenance of reasonable safeguards against such risk, consistent with the type of treatment, the patients' mental condition, and the physical surroundings. The defendant hospital staff recognized this in their practice or policy of either having a nurse present in the main corridor leading to the unlocked outer door, or in maintaining vigilant observation thereof. At the time in question, one of the nurses on duty was downstairs, another in plaintiff wife's room, and the third purportedly in the office telephoning or otherwise out of visual contact with the main corridor. Whether the defendant hospital was, under these conditions, providing to plaintiff wife such custodial care or attention as a reasonable man would provide, under the circumstances, we conclude presented a question for the jury.

How "reasonable" must the "reasonable care" accorded to suicidal patients be for a professional or an institution to avoid liability for suicide? The general rule of thumb here is "as reasonable as that level of care provided by the ordinary, reasonable, and prudent professional or institution acting under the same or similar circumstances in the same or similar community." The caution that "the therapist who does not have facilities for emergency hospitalization at his disposal... should not treat severely depressed patients, let alone suicidal patients" (Lesse, 1965, p. 105) must be given due consideration by psychologists and other mental health professionals who may not have hospital admitting privileges. However, there are few hard-and-fast rules in the assignment of liability for suicide. Readers interested in pursuing additional sources on this subject are urged to consult Perr (1965), Schwartz (1971), Slawson, Flinn, and Schwartz (1974), Tarshis (1972), Morse (1967), *Vistica v. Presbyterian Hospital and Medical Center* (67 Cal.2d 465; 62 Cal. Rptr. 577), *Cauverien v. De Metz* (188 N.Y.S.2d 617), *Hebel v. Hinsdale Sanatorium and Hospital* (119 N.E.2d 506), *White v. United States* (317 F.2d 13), *Dimitrijevic v. Chicago Wesley Memorial Hospital* (236 N.E.2d 309), and *Deitz v. Bumstead* (168 N.Y.S.2d 669; 5 App. Div.2d 739).

In some instances, courts have held institutions and individuals liable neither for the death of an individual "bent on" taking his own life (5.15) nor for the death of a patient who committed suicide when the guard assigned to watch her left for five minutes to go to the bathroom. In some cases, immunity for government institutions and employees has served as a shield from liability (5.17). As in other areas of professional practice, honest errors in judgment are not sufficient grounds to prove negligence (5.18; 5.21; see also *Dillman v. Hellman*, 283 So.2d 388). Theoretically, another possible defense to a wrongful death action is the defense of contributory negligence, according to which the victim's own negligence contributed to the consequences (see p. 248 below). If a victim had signed some release of liability prior to his suicide attempt or commission, a court might consider that certificate to be a valid defense against a wrongful death action. Finally, some courts have held professionals to be free of liability because their actions (negligent or otherwise) could not reasonably be seen as causally related to the consequences (5.23).

Physician/attorney Irwin Perr (1965) has addressed himself to the feeling of helplessness mental health professionals may feel when working with suicidal patients. Perr observed that a professional may feel anxious or helpless

> in that there are limits to control and to predictability as to what will happen—where, how or by whom. The law demands reasonable care in foreseeable situations. This is a sound and logical principle. We can ask only that it be applied in an intelligent and rational manner. (p. 637)

ASSAULT AND/OR BATTERY BY PATIENT

Much of our previous discussion concerning wrongful death statutes, honest errors in professional judgment, the importance of careful history taking, and the concept of "reasonable care" is applicable to a discussion of the potential liability that mental health professionals may incur for the assaults upon others by their patients. The major difference in the latter situation is, of course, that the welfare of a third party must now be considered. The decision in *Tarasoff* (5.24) clearly holds that therapists are under a legal obligation to warn endangered third parties of patients' threats. The rationale of *Tarasoff* would appear to be an extension of the long-standing obligation doctors have had to warn endangered third parties of their patients' contagious physical diseases (Harris, 1973; also see *Hofman v. Blackmon*, 241 So.2d 752) and violent proclivities (5.25; 5.43).

As in suicide cases, mental health professionals have been held liable for negligence with respect to restraining and supervising assaultive patients. In this context, Rothblatt and Leroy (1973) cited the case of a patient who had recently been released from a hospital. At a meeting with his attorney the patient became enraged, and he leaped across the desk, biting off the lower half of his attorney's nose. The attorney brought suit against the patient's doctor and the hospital that had released him, claiming that they were negligent in not confining a dangerous person. The court found in favor of the attorney and awarded him $200,000 in damages. Other examples of what evidence has and has not been sufficient to prevail in a cause of action in related cases are presented in cases 5.24 through 5.43.

Like professionals who work in institutions with suicidal or potentially suicidal patients, professionals who work with potentially assaultive patients are frequently called upon to balance what may be therapeutic against what may be catastrophic. Specifically, the potential benefits of the "open ward," with its free movement and potential for gains in terms of the patient's self-respect, must be weighed against the need for adequate supervision and restraints. The courts have recognized the value of open wards (e.g., 5.28; 5.29; 5.33; 5.35) and have acknowledged that the purpose of hospitalizing the suicidal or assaultive individual is treatment, not merely incarceration:

> Treatment requires the restoration of confidence in the patient. This in turn requires that restrictions be kept at a minimum. Risks must be taken or the case left as hopeless. . . . The standard of care which stresses close observation, restriction and restraint has fallen in disrepute in modern hospitals and this policy is being reversed with excellent results. (*Baker v. United States* [5.1])

In one case, however, the meaning of the words "confined" and "treated" used in combination by a lower court were deemed to be "at the most contradictory and at the least confusing" by a higher court. The case involved Arthur Harold Robinson, an individual who, within the meaning of a Florida statute, had been adjudged to be a "mentally disordered sex offender." In connection with an incident of child molestation, the Palm Beach County Circuit Court had ordered as follows:

> ORDERED AND ADJUDGED that the defendant will be transported to the appropriate Florida State Hospital and committed, confined, detained and treated by the Division of Mental Health until the further Order of the Court and, in the event that the defendant shall cease to be manifestly dangerous to others, said fact shall be reported to the Court for further Order.

While being treated at South Florida State Hospital, Robinson was given furloughs to visit his wife in West Palm Beach for short periods. The Palm Beach County Circuit Court held the hospital and related defendants in criminal contempt of court for violating the terms of the court order. In the appeal that followed, it was argued that the hospital and the

other defendants should not be held in criminal contempt for releasing
Robinson on furloughs to visit his wife. The District Court of Appeal
reversed the contempt judgment, holding that the language of the circuit
court order had been unclear:

> We hold that the order, in using the terms "confined" and "treated" in
> combination was at the most contradictory and at the least confusing.
> (*Department of Health and Rehabilitative Services, Division of Mental
> Health, South Florida State Hospital v. State*, Fla. App., 338 So.2d
> 220.)

In *Semler v. Psychiatric Institute of Washington, D.C.* (5.27) a probationer being treated at the institute was put on outpatient status (without the approval of the court) and subsequently committed murder. The
defendants argued that under the terms of the state court order their only
duty was to rehabilitate the probationer. However, the court rejected this
argument, holding that the defendants had a duty to treat the probationer
and a duty to protect the public. The probation officer who approved the
probationer's change of status to outpatient without consulting the court
claimed immunity from liability as a government employee. However, the
court denied him immunity, and a $12,500 judgment was levied against
him. The institute's breach of its duty to the public was adjudged to be
proximately related to the murder.

Generally, in order for a mental health professional to be held liable
for a patient's assault or battery on a third party, it must be shown by the
preponderance of the evidence that

1. the professional owed a duty to the third party who was injured;
2. the professional knew or should have known of the patient's potential
   for such violent acts;
3. the professional's actions were the proximate cause of the third party's
   injury.

ASSAULT AND/OR BATTERY BY THERAPIST

Unlike negligence, the torts of assault and battery are *intentional*
torts, which require volition on the part of the defendant as an element of
proof. The difference between intentional and unintentional torts is frequently a crucial one for insurance purposes; some policies might only
cover claims of malpractice (i.e., negligence) and not intentional torts.
Definitions of "assault" and "battery" will vary from jurisdiction to
jurisdiction, but there are some rules of thumb which are generally applicable. For a plaintiff to prove assault, he has to prove that without his

authorization, the defendant engaged in some action that caused the plaintiff to be placed in apprehension of a harmful or offensive touching of his person. Additionally, the plaintiff has to prove that the defendant intended the act to be harmful or offensive. To prove battery, the plaintiff has to prove that without his authorization, the defendant acted with an intent to inflict some harmful or offensive touching and that some harmful or offensive touching was legally caused by the defendant's act.[3] A "harmful" touching is typically defined as one that causes pain, injury, or any bodily impairment. An "offensive" touching is typically defined as one that would be offensive to "a reasonable person's" sense of dignity.

To clarify the distinction between what constitutes an assault and what constitutes battery, consider the example of Jones and Smith, who are standing around watching some construction. For the purpose of getting a rise out of Smith, Jones suddenly shouts, "Watch out, Smith! That steel ball's headed right toward you!" Jones might very well incur liability for *assault* for his false statement to Smith—a statement that placed Smith in a state of apprehension. In *battery*, the plaintiff would have to have actually been touched by the defendant or in some way physically hurt by a process set in motion by the defendant. Suppose Green, while firing at White's head with a sawed-off shotgun, misses White but hits a chandelier which falls, causing injuries to White. In addition to the criminal action that the state would probably initiate against Green, White (or his estate) could sue for battery.

From our sampling of cases in Chapter 5, it can be seen that suits have been brought against mental health professionals for physically stimulating a patient's rib cage (tickling?) in the name of "Rage Reduction Therapy" (5.44), for beating a patient as a means of treatment (5.45), and for ordering injections and medication administered to an involuntary patient in a private hospital (5.46). We note in passing that the judgment against Dr. Zaslow, the psychologist who administered the Rage Reduction Therapy, was the highest judgment awarded to date against a psychologist ($170,000). Presumably, this was because of the evidence of physical injury (i.e., black-and-blue marks) that was presented to the jury. Professionals' defenses to charges of assault and/or battery have typically been grounded on the claim that there existed patient consent (actual, apparent, or implied) to treatment. An additional defense for state or federal employees is that they were working in an official capacity. In *Beaumont* (5.47) for example, a hospital superintendant was adjudged to be free of liability for the assault and battery committed by his "agents and servants" because he was a public official.

---

[3]It should also be mentioned here that, when surgery, injections, and similar procedures are administered to patients without their permission, a battery may be said to have occurred.

FALSE IMPRISONMENT

Intentionally causing the unauthorized confinement of another individual constitutes false imprisonment. In the past, private practitioners and court-appointed psychiatrists have been held to be immune from charges of false imprisonment on the grounds that such physicians are acting in an official or quasi-official capacity rather than as physicians per se (e.g., 5.47 through 5.52). The court in *Dunbar v. Greenlaw* (152 Me. 270, 128 A.2d 218) stated flatly: "The role and function of the examining and certifying physician in insanity detention and commitment cases are those of a witness.... His relation to the alleged insane person is not, *pro hac vice* [for this one occasion], that of a physician with patient." Thus, doctors have traditionally been given "witness" status and immunity even when there appeared to be evidence that their actions were undertaken with malicious intent and in bad faith (e.g., 5.50), although this policy has not prevailed in all cases (5.53).

Interestingly, one California court ruled that, if a patient in some way profits from the false imprisonment, that is a matter to be considered when assessing damages. The false imprisonment referred to in that decision involved an involuntary hospitalization of a patient that did not comply with California statutes (*Maben v. Rankin*, 55 Cal.2d 139; 10 Cal. Rptr. 353). The court in *Maben* ruled that "in determining the damages suffered as a result of a tortious act, consideration may be given, where equitable, to the value of any special benefit conferred by that act to the interest which was harmed."

The amount of communication that a patient is or is not allowed to have with the outside world can be an aggravating circumstance in false imprisonment. In *Stowers v. Wolodzko* (5.46), Mrs. Stowers, the patient, was held incommunicado. When she finally succeeded in contacting her family, she was taken into a room by the defendant physician who had committed her (Dr. Wolodzko) and told: "Mrs. Stowers, don't try that again. If you do, you will never see your children again." The fact that the plaintiff was prohibited from calling her family or an attorney, combined with the fact that when she did contact her family she was set free, was a primary factor in the court's finding for the plaintiff. The court rejected the argument of the plaintiff's expert witness (Dr. Bolter) who argued that it was usual and proper not to let Mrs. Stowers consult with an attorney:

> Dr. Bolter was unable to give any valid reason why a person should not be allowed to consult with an attorney. We do not believe there is such a reason. While problems may be caused in a few cases because of this requirement, the facts in the instant case provide cogent reasons as to why such a rule is necessary. Mrs. Stowers was able to obtain her release after she made the telephone call to her relatives and they, in turn,

obtained an attorney for her. Prior to this, because of the order of no communications, she was virtually held a prisoner with no chance of redress. We, therefore, agree with the Court of Appeals that there was sufficient evidence from which a jury could find that Dr. Wolodzko had committed false imprisonment.

Increasing judicial concern with the rights of mental patients is likely to make judgments like the one that prevailed in the *Whitree* (5.54) case more common than ever before. It is incumbent upon psychologists, psychiatrists and others involved in commitment hearings, therefore, not only to exercise due caution in executing papers for commitment but also to faithfully, comprehensively, and regularly reevaluate the condition of committed patients. (A recent review of commitment statutes in twenty-four states appears in Drude [1978].)

TREATMENT WITH MEDICATION

As physicians, psychiatrists are the only mental health professionals licensed to prescribe and dispense medications. Clinical psychologists, as well trained as they are in the areas of psychopathology, psychodiagnosis, psychotherapy, and related areas, typically have little or no training in biochemistry—and no license to practice medicine—and should therefore steer clear of recommending, prescribing, or dispensing any medication at any time. In one complaint (currently in the claim stage), the defendant psychologist offered the opinion that his patient (who had seen a psychiatrist for medication) didn't need the medication any more. Relying on the psychologist's advice, the patient stopped taking the medication—with allegedly disastrous consequences including the loss of employment.

Psychiatrists who do use medications should be aware of all the side effects and contraindications associated with various drugs and should also have a working knowledge of how to handle toxic reactions and complications. Reading the package insert of medications is a must, for as an attorney for Smith Kline and French Laboratories has noted, "It has been held in some states (California for one) that a drug manufacturer's prescribing brochure is evidence in support of a malpractice claim where a physician deviates from the instructions contained therein" (cited in Appleton, 1968, p. 879). Doctors who dispense experimental drugs may similarly find themselves in court defending their treatment (5.56). It would be wise for doctors who prescribe medication classified by the FDA as "investigational" to obtain their patient's written permission and informed consent for such use.

One of the issues in *Meier* (5.2) concerned the ordering of medication for the severely depressed patient who subsequently committed suicide. The plaintiffs attempted to introduce as evidence a brochure from the drug's manufacturer which stated in part that the medication was contraindicated in the treatment of severe depression. The trial court refused to admit the brochure as evidence (although the defendant physician did admit to knowledge of the contraindication on cross-examination). In remanding the case for retrial the California Supreme Court found that the plaintiffs had not properly introduced the brochure as evidence but that the brochure could be used as evidence at the new trial:

> ... plaintiffs contend that the trial judge erred in refusing to admit a brochure from the manufacturer of a drug (Mallaril) [sic] administered to decedent, which showed the drug to be contraindicated for severely depressed patients. This assignment of error would not, standing alone, require a reversal because plaintiffs' counsel obtained an admission of the contraindication from defendant Stubblebine on cross-examination. Furthermore, the plaintiffs do not present an adequate record for challenging this ruling since they laid no foundation for admission of the brochure and presented no properly informative offer of proof. (*Douillard v. Woodd* (1959) 20 Cal.2d 655, 670, 128 P.2d 6; *Carey v. Lima, Salmon & Tulley Mortuary* (1959) 168 Cal. App.2d 42, 46, 335 P.2d 181; *Blackburn v. Union Oil Co.* (1949) 90 Cal. App.2d 775, 778, 204 P.2d 69.) For the purposes of retrial, however, we believe that the court should permit the introduction into evidence of such a brochure, not to establish the standard of care, but to show that the physician administering the drug had *notice* of the contraindication. (*Sanzari v. Rosenfeld* (1961) 34 N.J. 128, 139, 140, 167 A.2d 625, 631.)

In *Sanzari* (6.8), a dentist, in the course of filling a tooth, injected a solution of Xylocaine and epinephrine into the patient's gums. Because the patient was hypertensive she suffered a cerebral hemorrhage as a result of the injection, from which she subsequently died. The pharmaceutical company's package insert that was supplied with the drug was deemed by the court to have put the defendant dentist "on notice" that the drug might be harmful to hypertensive patients. The court ruled: "We believe that it is within the common knowledge of laymen that a reasonable man, including a dentist, who knows a drug is potentially harmful to a certain type of patient, should take adequate precaution before administering the drug or deciding whether to administer it."

Dawidoff (1973b) has stated that "when a psychiatrist does not, in every particular, follow the precautions laid down in the literature, the door to malpractice litigation may be open" (p. 699). Dawidoff recommended that

> the patient be kept on his drug regimen, and, without endangering the patient's trust in the physician and in himself, it may be helpful to enlist the aid of a family member or roommate in assuring that drugs are taken in their regular and proper dosage and that with the depressed patient,

for example, no pills are hoarded. One must try to assure himself in such instances that more than one physician is not being consulted at the same time for the purpose of building up a supply of drugs which are harmful in large doses. (pp. 699–700)

Doctors who treat their patients with medication must be prepared to justify their treatment on sound medical grounds. Psychiatric treatment of drug abusers may necessitate consultations with an expert in internal medicine if catastrophic consequences are to be avoided (5.55). The use of drugs to restrain a patient (either alone or in combination with other restraints) may be viewed by a court as improper (e.g., 5.57). Similarly, the use of drugs as a punishment or the threat of the use of drugs as punishment has not been endorsed by either legislators or judges. In *Knecht v. Gilman* (488 F.2d 1136), a court described as "cruel and unusual punishment" the involuntary administration of an emetic agent to mental patients who were selected for an aversive-control behavior change program. The court did allow that such treatments could be administered, but only with the patients' informed consent and only if that consent could be withdrawn at any time.

Physician/attorney Don Mills (1974) has noted that "issues raised in malpractice claims have included the decision to use the drug, the manner of administration, the dosage and duration of use, the performance of laboratory tests during prolonged use, [and] the timeliness of diagnosis of reactions and of other untoward results and their management" (p. 35). Mills cautioned against errors involving inadequately trained office personnel and warned that

> permitting office personnel to authorize prescription refills by telephone without direct orders from the doctor have [sic] resulted in embarrassing collateral issues in a number of cases. Prescribing and authorizing refills are legally identical acts, and can be accomplished only by licensed physicians. An office assistant may act as a conduit, but this is the limit of her authority. Whenever a refill is granted by telephone, a note must be entered in the patient's record to this effect, and this note ultimately should be countersigned by the physician for proof that it was his, not his aide's decision. (p. 36)

Patients should be warned of all the possible side effects of a medication and told not to drive or operate certain kinds of machinery if necessary. They should also be given instructions on what to do if side effects occur, and, of course, they sould be told that they can and should contact their physician immediately if serious complications arise. In advertising for its new tranquilizer–antidepressant, Limbitrol (a formula of chlordiazepoxide and amitriptyline), Roche Laboratories included the following advice on "How to make each patient an informed patient":

1. Discuss with your patients the probability that they will experience drowsiness especially during the first week.
2. Reassure your patients that drowsiness is an indication that the medication is working and beginning to help them; indicate that it may help alleviate their insomnia.
3. Encourage your patients to report to you if drowsiness becomes troublesome, so that you can, if necessary, adjust the dosage schedule.
4. Caution your patients about the combined effects with alcohol or other CNS depressants. Let them know that the additive effects may produce a harmful level of sedation and CNS depression.
5. Caution your patients about activities requiring complete mental alertness, such as operating machinery or driving a car.

Psychiatrists or other physicians in hospital settings who joke about their poor penmanship may find it no laughing matter when illegible handwriting leads to a patient's receiving the wrong medication or the right medication in the wrong dosage or mode of administration. If you force the nurse administering the medication to guess what you meant to write in your order, you may be found to have breached a duty of due care. Any requests for laboratory studies should also be written legibly, and the lab reports, once returned, should be read carefully.

ELECTROSHOCK THERAPY

Variously called electroshock therapy, electroconvulsive therapy (ECT), shock therapy, electrotherapy, and "buzzing,"[4] electroshock therapy (EST) is the passing of an electrical current through the brain sufficient to induce a convulsion and a loss of consciousness. EST is a widely practiced treatment (Kalinowsky and Hippius, 1969; Asnis, Fink, and Saferstein, 1978) that is thought to be particularly useful in the treatment of severely depressed, suicidal patients and those suffering from involutional melancholia (Freedman and Kaplan, 1967). Professional opinion concerning the efficacy of EST is divided. There are some psychiatrists who laud this technique (e.g., Andren, 1976; Arnot, 1975) and others who "for sometimes unstated reasons never use this modality" (Bernstein, Bernstein, and Adzick, 1978, p. 252).

A pioneer of the coma therapies, Meduna (1936), held the belief that epilepsy and psychosis were somehow antagonistic to one another. He noted that after a coma was induced, psychotic symptoms would remit—a finding based on an assumption that has since been proved invalid in numerous clinical investigations (e.g., Hoch, 1943; Kalinowsky and Hip-

---

[4]A slang term sometimes used by hospital personnel.

pius, 1969). In his later years, Meduna himself "recognized with admirable candor that the coma therapies were crudely empirical and compared them to kicking a Swiss watch" (Redlich and Freedman, 1966, p. 336). One psychiatrist reviewing proposed explanations for how and why shock therapy works delineated fifty such theories (Gordon, 1948).

But no matter what they are called and no matter how they work, legal obstacles to the administration of shock therapies have grown in recent years, and their use has increasingly been legally restricted (Bernstein, Bernstein, and Adzick, 1977, 1978; L. H. Blackman, cited in "Public Opinion," 1978; Moore, 1973). The sampling of cases presented in Chapter 5 reflects the fact that most of the litigation concerning EST has stemmed either from failure to obtain proper consent for such treatment or from failure to live up to some prescribed standard of care in administration. Although evidence of physical injuries has been the cornerstone of such claims in the past, it seems reasonable to predict that emotional distress will increasingly be claimed by plaintiffs in the future.

Psychiatrists wishing to protect themselves from litigation arising out of their EST treatments should adhere closely to their professional organization's published guidelines for administering such therapy. They should make certain that consents to treatment are informed, and they should be wary of post-treatment complications. In some jurisdictions, there exists a legal duty on the part of psychiatrists using EST to use muscle relaxants as a prerequisite to treatment, and failure to do so may constitute negligence. Therefore, psychiatrists would do well to call their county medical society for additional and up-to-date advice concerning the specific pre-, peri-, and post-EST procedures needed to meet the prescribed standard of care.

BREACH OF CONFIDENTIALITY

Therapists are under a legal duty to safeguard the confidentiality of their patients' communications.[5] If a therapist fails to exercise reasonable care in this matter, he may, according to Shah (1970a), be subject to any of the following consequences: disciplinary action by his professional organization; disciplinary action by the state certifying or licensing authority; a civil suit charging breach of confidentiality and/or defamation. Unauthorized disclosure of confidential information has been held to be justified under certain conditions. In *Clark* (5.68) a physician who re-

---

[5]As explained in Chapter 3, the concept of "confidentiality" is considerably broader than the concept of "privileged communication." As such, the cases in Chapter 5 in which non-authorized disclosure of privileged information was at issue either as a complaint (e.g., 5.73) or as a defense (e.g., 5.67) will be discussed under the more general heading, "breach of confidentiality."

vealed that his patient, an Air Force accountant, was an alcoholic was not held to be liable, because in the opinion of the court the physician was serving a greater interest (the interest of the United States). In *Berry* (5.69) a psychiatrist was not held liable for conveying confidential information about the prospective groom to the father of the bride-to-be (nor was the psychiatrist held liable for defamation; see the discussion of *qualified privilege* (pp. 227–228). A dissenting opinion in *Schaffer* (5.73) questioned the validity of doctor–patient privilege in child custody proceedings. The liability of a group therapist for the breaching of confidentiality by one of his patients to someone outside the group has not, to this author's knowledge, been legally tested, though at least one such claim has been made (5.71). Similarly, whether or not a member of a therapy group could incur liability for a breach of confidentiality will be a matter for a court to decide when and if such a complaint is lodged.

As a matter of course, therapists safeguard the confidentiality of their patients' communications by keeping charts locked in a sturdy file cabinet, by refraining from discussing patients with unauthorized persons, and by not consulting with other professionals in public places (such as restaurants, public transportation, etc.). The question we will focus on here is "Are there any situations that can warrant a breach of confidentiality?"

The answer to this question depends upon whether it is being considered from a legal or ethical perspective. From a legal standpoint there is a clear precedent for breach of confidentiality; although therapists may not be legally compelled to reveal information about crimes their patients have already committed, they may be compelled to report a *prospective* crime, on the grounds that "all citizens have a duty to prevent commission of a crime" (S. Nye, cited in "Duty," 1978, p. 2).

From the standpoint of professional ethics the answer is not as straightforward. Some professionals have argued that *no* conditions justify revelation of patient–therapist communications without the patient's consent. The more moderate position—the one we well argue here—holds that there do exist extreme circumstances under which the breach of confidentiality is ethically conscionable.

At issue here is a delicate balancing of societal versus individual needs and the consequences thereof. My own bias is that there are emergency situations that demand the breach of confidentiality for the sake of the welfare of others as well as the welfare of the patient. One such situation occurred with a fourteen-year-old male who had been seen by me in ongoing therapy at an outpatient clinic of Bellevue Hospital in Manhattan. The youth was struggling to free himself from a gang he had been involved with for two years. In confidence, he told me of the date and place of an upcoming gang battle that had been precipitated by the shooting death of an adolescent member of a rival community. My patient did not really want to fight, but being his gang's leader, he felt that he would lose the respect of all of his peers if he did not. He also expressed concern that this would be a particularly fierce battle, because both sides were arming themselves with firearms instead of the more customary knives, brass knuckles, etc. I discussed the matter with a psychiatrist whose opinions on ethical matters I respected, and we agreed that the patient's act of telling me exactly where and when the fight would take place amounted to a call for help. Accordingly, I contacted the police and informed them of the location and time of the battle. Subsequently, I learned that my patient had contacted the leader of the rival gang and made peace shortly before the fight was to occur.

Not only are there occasions when it would appear to be morally and ethically proper to disclose therapist–patient communications to third parties, there are occasions in which psychotherapists have been or would be legally compelled to make such disclosures (e.g., 5.24–5.26, 5.67).

Mental health professionals should be aware that the privilege in doctor–patient privileged communication belongs to the patient and not the doctor. Barring any extenuating or complicating circumstance (such as the patient's being irrational) or the use of techniques to overcome the patient's will and his ability to resist, it is the patient's right to relinquish that privilege at any time; it is the patient's right to compel a doctor to reveal previously confidential matter to a third party. Therapists may also be legally compelled to breach confidentiality when ordered to do so by a government agency or a court.

Psychotherapists who refuse to divulge confidential communications on the grounds that their doctor–patient communications are absolutely privileged must stand prepared to pay the consequences of their civil disobedience if a court requests such information. In *In Re Lifschutz* (Sup., 85 Cal. Rptr. 829), psychiatrist Joseph Lifschutz was imprisoned after he was adjudged to be in contempt of court for refusing to obey a court order instructing him to divulge information relating to communication with a former patient. Lifschutz's defense was that the court order was unconstitutional in that it infringed on his personal right of privacy, his patients' right of privacy, and his right to practice his profession. He also argued that, since clergymen could not be compelled to reveal certain confidential communications under these circumstances he, as a psychiatrist, should not be compelled either.

The Supreme Court of California held that no constitutional right enables psychotherapists to assert absolute privilege concerning all psychotherapeutic communications. Some excerpts from the opinion of Justice Tobriner follow:

> Although [Lifschutz], in pressing for judicial acceptance of a genuine and deeply held principle, seeks to cast the issue involved in this case in the broadest terms, we must properly address, in reality, a question of more modest dimensions. We do not face the alternatives of enshrouding

the patient's communications to the psychotherapist in the black veil of absolute privilege or of exposing it to the white glare of publicity. Our choice lies, rather, in the grey area. . . .

Although psychotherapists should, of course, be entitled to the constitutional protections requisite to the practice of their profession . . . we doubt that the disclosure involved here goes so far as to constitute the claimed unconstitutional deprivation of that right. . . .

We do not know, of course, to what extent patients are deterred from seeking psychotherapeutic treatment by the knowledge that if, at some future date, they choose to place some aspect of their mental condition in issue in litigation, communications relevant to that issue may be revealed. We can only surmise that an understanding of the limits of section 1016, and the realization that the patient retains control over subsequent disclosure, may provide a measure of reassurance to the prospective patient. . . .

[Lifschutz] maintains, however, that, given the purpose of the clergyman–penitent privilege, the distinction between clergymen and psychotherapists cannot stand. . . . Recognizing that the toleration of religious beliefs and practices forms the basis for this privilege, we cannot say that the Legislature acted irrationally in granting the privilege to clergymen and not to psychotherapists. Although in some circumstances clergymen and psychotherapists perform similar functions and serve similar needs, fundamental and significant differences remain.

The opinion also noted that in the past other organized occupational groups, such as journalists, have argued that required divulgence of information received in confidence would mean the destruction of their calling. However, none of these groups have enjoyed absolute privilege to withhold information gained as a result of confidential communications.

It is incumbent upon mental health professionals to know what the specific extent of their privilege is; they should know which information they can be compelled to reveal, to whom, and under what conditions. In some jurisdictions it is the psychologist who has the broadest privilege. That is, *anything* said to a psychologist or his employee is considered to be privileged communication. What is said in confidence to a social worker may be subject to publication to the entity that employs the social worker (see, for example, 5.67). The privilege of the psychiatrist, like the privilege of any physician, may be limited to only that information which is considered to be "relevant and necessary to treat the illness."

"I have just been subpoenaed to testify and reveal privileged information. What should I do?" Attorneys with a large clientele of mental health professionals frequently receive "emergency" phone calls asking the question above. The situation in which an insurance company, an employer, or some other third party has subpoenaed a professional's records is common enough to be a potential source of difficulty to practitioners in the mental health field. Although clear guidelines on this matter are lacking, the mental health professional would be well advised to refuse to testify immediately. Under the advice of counsel, the steps the practitioner might take are as follows:

1. Wait for (or request) a court order compelling you to testify. In other words, you needn't respond immediately to the third party's subpoena by giving that party all the information requested; wait for or ask the *court* to put on the record an order directing you to testify.

2. Once a court order directing you to divulge information about a patient is put on the record, request the court to notify the patient that you are being called upon to disclose confidential communications. In this context, request the court to provide the patient with a reasonable period of time within which to appeal the order.

3. If you believe that the disclosure of the material in question will be harmful to the patient, your views on this matter should be argued and made clear to the court before the information is revealed. If after your argument and the patient's notification and appeal the court still orders you to testify, failure to do so will be at your own peril. The consequence of refusal to testify at this stage of the proceedings may be a contempt of court citation and a penalty of a fine and/or a prison sentence.

   The state of affairs today as regards the area of privileged communication is that each therapist is ultimately on his own when it comes to making delicate value judgments regarding the disclosure of nondisclosure of information given in confidence. Professional guidelines to help therapists balance individual patient needs with the general public's interest are urgently needed. In this context, Frederick Redlich (cited in Powledge, 1977, p. 46) has said, "We psychiatrists want to save the patient, but also we want to save the world."

DEFAMATION

   The elements necessary for proof of defamation were listed in Chapter 2 (p. 46). The defamation is said to be "published" to a third party when it is communicated either orally (slander) or in writing (libel). A valid defense against charges of defamation is *qualified privilege*. Addressing their article to psychologists, Krauskopf and Krauskopf (1965) offered the following advice:

> The essential elements of a qualifiedly privileged communication are 1) good faith by the defendant, 2) a legitimate interest or duty to be furthered by the statement, 3) a statement limited in its scope to that purpose, 4) a proper occasion, and communication in a proper manner and to proper parties only (*Judge v. Rockford*, 1958). Since psychologists are often requested to comment upon their clients, each psychologist

should insure that his usual procedures render whatever communications he makes privileged ones. (p. 228)

In *Berry* (5.69), a psychiatrist disclosed what might be considered to be defamatory (not to mention confidential) information about his patient to the father of the woman the patient wished to marry. The psychiatrist was protected from liability under the doctrine of qualified privilege, the court holding that a father's concern about his daughter's welfare was a sufficient interest to protect. Thus, it did not really matter that Berry may have been defamed by published statements like "My suggestion to the infatuated girl would be to run as fast and as far as she possibly could in any direction away from him. . . . Of course, if he doesn't marry her, he will marry someone else and make life hell for that person." Legally, all that mattered was that the psychiatrist was doing his duty, and as such was protected by qualified privilege. According to *Berry*, this privilege "must be exercised with certain cautions: (a) it must be done in good fatih and reasonable care must be exercised as to its truth, (b) likewise, the information must be reported fairly, (c) only such information should be conveyed, and (d) only to such persons as are necessary to the purpose." (See also 5.68.) Another defense to a charge of defamation is truth. Even if the defamatory statement was made out of the most malicious of motives, most courts will not find defamation if the statement can be proven to be true.[6]

SEXUAL IMPROPRIETIES

Therapist–patient sexual involvement has been held to be unethical by the American Psychological Association (1977) and the American Psychiatric Association (1973) and held to be actionable under both civil (e.g., 5.81; 5.82) and criminal (e.g., 5.91) law. Although there have been some scattered claims concerning the therapeutic value of therapist–patient sex, the available literature suggests that such claims might best be viewed as self-serving rationalizations for activities initiated by disturbed therapists. (See the review of the literature presented in Chapter 4.) Expert witnesses at trials involving therapist–patient sexual involvement can reliably be expected to testify that such involvement constitutes a mishandling of the transference and as such amounts to negligence on the part of the therapist. Insurance companies have always been reluctant to pay for damages incurred as a result of therapist–patient sex (e.g., 5.82)

---

[6]It should be noted that there is a minority view on this point that holds that the defamatory statement must have been made justifiably. See *Hutchins v. Page*, 72 A. 689.

and have recently begun to write policies that specifically preclude payment for such activities.[7] Hypothetically, a therapist who admitted to having intercourse with his patient might defend himself or herself by arguing that the special circumstances of the case required a deviation from more traditional procedures and that any "reasonable" mental health professional would have acted similarly under the same or similar circumstances. Needless to say, such a defense would be difficult if not impossible to prove.

What about the therapist who has never abused his patients sexually and has never had any intention of doing so—how can he best protect himself against *allegations* of sexual involvement? This dilemma is probably as old as the psychotherapeutic enterprise itself. The well-known hypnotist or "magnetizer" Anton Mesmer reportedly separated from his wife during the course of his treatment of a woman with whom a mutual attraction existed (cf. Ellenberger, 1970, pp. 891–893). Freud's colleague Josef Breuer eventually had to terminate therapy with his famous patient Anna O. after Mrs. Breuer became intensely jealous and depressed over the effect that the attractive Anna seemed to be having on her husband; at one point in the treatment, Anna had charged that Breuer had made her pregnant. Sympathetic to Mrs. Breuer's plight, Mrs. Sigmund Freud asked her husband for reassurances that they would not be subject to a fate similar to the Breuers' (cf. Jones, 1953, pp. 224–225).

No one denies that a working relationship between therapist and patient must exist before therapy can proceed, but exactly how "working" that relationship has to be, so to speak, for treatment to progress is very much an open question. Many behaviorally oriented and community-oriented therapists advise observation of the patient in as many diverse settings away from the consulting room as possible. But at what point, for example, will the meeting at a discotheque between a young male therapist and an attractive female patient with social interaction problems be considered a "date"? How could the behavior therapist in the preceding example—dedicated as he may be—defend himself from an (unfounded) charge that he was "dating" the patient?

Although there are no easy answers to the questions posed above, and the unique needs and resources of different patients may demand different solutions, the therapist who engages in such commendable but out-of-the-ordinary diagnostic and/or therapeutic exercises would be well advised to ask the patient to bring along a "significant other," if possible, as an observer on each and every one of the "dates." The idea of an observer also seems like a good one in less out-of-the-ordinary but equally

---

[7]For example, the new professional liability insurance policy offered to psychologists by American Home Insurance specifically excludes that carrier's liability for payment of damages resulting from the psychologist's sexual involvement with patients.

vulnerable situations, such as the one in which the therapist hypnotizes the patient and the patient is such a good hypnotic subject that there is no recollection of what happened for the last fifty minutes. Of course, observers can be used only with the full knowledge and consent of the patient and with the therapist's understanding that the very presence of the observer will probably change the patient's responses to a greater or lesser degree. The patient will also have to understand that the observer will be privy to otherwise confidential information.

In regular day-to-day office consultations, the therapist will be doing his best to avoid allegations of social or sexual entanglements if he behaves in a thoroughly professional manner with all of his patients, all of the time. I fully appreciate that given the large number of varied approaches to therapy, the term "thoroughly professional" defies any facile explanation. However, what "thoroughly professional" does *not* mean is routinely hugging patients when they come in or depart, asking them out for a drink or a look at the etchings in your apartment, or engaging in related activities.

VIOLATION OF CIVIL RIGHTS

Litigation involving the standard of care provided at mental hospitals and the process by which persons are committed to and detained at such institutions has led to a recent spate of court decisions (e.g., 5.54; 5.92–5.100; see also *Downs v. The Department of Public Welfare*, 368 F. Supp. 454) that have reaffirmed patients' rights to treatment, due process, privacy, etc. Issues regarding the clinical and non-clinical use of psychological tests have long been discussed in the context of civil rights. The potential for misuse of psychological test data has been the subject of numerous sensational (e.g., Gross, 1962; Hoffman, 1962) and scholarly (e.g., Carter, Brim, Stalnaker, and Messick, 1965; "Testing," 1965) reports. Issues related to the use of psychological tests in personnel selection and alleged violations of the equal employment opportunity provisions of the Civil Rights Act of 1964 were touched on in four decisions handed down by the Supreme Court in recent years. Interested readers are referred to *United States v. State of South Carolina*, 98 S.Ct. 756 (1978); *Washington v. Davis*, 96 S.Ct. 2040 (1976); *Albemarle Paper Company v. Moody*, 95 S.Ct. 2362 (1975); and *Griggs v. Duke Power Company*, 91 S.Ct. 849 (1971). (It should be understood that only *state* actions will constitute a deprivation of civil rights in the legal sense. Actions of private individuals are not, legally speaking, deprivation of civil rights regardless of how tortious they may be.)

Mental health professionals interested in keeping up with the judicial decisions and the hundreds of bills introduced in the Senate and House of

Representatives that touch on the area of patients' rights can perhaps most effectively do so by carefully reading the local and national newsletters of their professional organizations. The Washington-based Association for the Advancement of Psychology publishes a regular bulletin designed to keep its membership abreast of mental health legislation and litigation. Other specialized newsletters and journals, such as *Law and Behavior* (published by Research Press) and the *Journal of Legal Medicine*, review judicial decisions, legislation, and administrative regulations. Articles focusing on specialized aspects of patients' rights appear from time to time in various journals (e.g., Bersoff and Prasse, 1978; Bersoff, 1976–77; Miller and Burt, 1977; Bernstein, 1977; Krouner, 1975; Atthowe, 1975; Waterman, 1974), and they can be located via the subject index in *Psychological Abstracts* or *Index Medicus, Psychiatry*.

GENERAL DIAGNOSIS AND TREATMENT

A physician who wrongfully institutionalized an individual in a Pennsylvania mental hospital in 1891 was not held to be liable for his actions. The court held insanity to be such a mysterious phenomenon that even the most prudent and skillful doctor could err by misdiagnosing a sane individual as insane (*Williams v. LeBar*, 141 Pa. 149; 21 A. 525). Modern-day courts have similarly recognized the problems attendant to psychiatric diagnoses. A decision in one recent, important case contained the view that psychiatric diagnosis "is not an exact science" and that "diagnosis with absolute precision and certainty is impossible" (*Baker v. United States* [5.1]).[8]

In addition to complex issues regarding the diagnosis of psychiatric patients, the courts have tackled equally complex issues regarding treatment. At issue are various questions concerning treatment goals and strategies (individual versus group treatment, experimental versus traditional treatment) and the assessment of damages arising from treatment. A recent article in *Roche Report Frontiers of Psychiatry* ("Malpsychotherapy," Note 4) quoted the views on these matters of Dr. Ralph Slovenko, Professor of Law and Psychiatry at Wayne State University School of Law:

---

[8]Mental health professionals themselves have expressed considerable concern over the reliability of psychiatric diagnoses and the validity of the process by which psychodiagnoses are made. Some representative studies in this voluminous literature include Arnhoff (1954), Chapman and Chapman (1967), Gauron and Dickinson (1966), Goldfarb (1959), Hollingshead and Redlich (1958), Kreitman et al. (1961), Masling (1960), Mischel (1968), Sarbin, Taft, and Bailey (1960), Schmidt and Fonda (1956), and Zigler and Phillips (1961a, 1961b).

Negligence, he says, "is the absence of such care, skill and diligence as it was the duty of the person to bring to the performance of the task." But, in psychotherapy, he feels, there is no consensus on what constitutes skill, or technique or standards of care.

"Given the same diagnosis, a person may be involved in individual or group psychotherapy, or in a primal scream or behavior therapy, hypnotherapy, drug therapy, or electroshock, or hospitalized," he notes, and the courts have refused to consider which of two reputable treatment forms is likely to be more effective in a particular case. But even assuming that negligence is established, it would be difficult in psychiatry to establish that it caused damage or injury, the basis for any legal action.

"What can be said to constitute damage?" Professor Slovenko asks. "Some say that breakdown or disintegration of personality is essential to a redevelopment of personality, so 'breakdown' ironically is a 'breakthrough.' Some say divorce is 'a step forward when married life is arid.' Suicide at times might even be a good idea. And so on." (p. 2)

In *Legal Challenges to Behavior Modification*, attorney Reed Martin (1975) pointed out that "the law does not prefer the substance of one strategy over another, but one should be familiar with advantages and disadvantages of a range of alternatives" (p. 33). For institutions, staffing and related considerations might dictate that patients be given group and not individual treatment. That is all right, according to Martin, provided that two important points are kept in mind:

The grouping must come after an individual determination of goal and treatment plan, not before: An individual should not be placed in a program simply because that is the one available. Second, the progress should not be lock step. As an individual progresses, his program must change; he must not be held back until everyone in the group is ready. Individualized programs are more difficult to create and run, but they are worth it. And the law is beginning to require it. (p. 64)

With regard to institutional treatment, Martin also pointed out that "the main legal test to be applied to any strategy is whether a balance between effectiveness and restrictiveness is established" (p. 41) and that the behavior change program "should basically benefit the individual and should not look for its justification too far outward into society's needs or too far inward into institutional convenience" (p. 57). Recent decisions (e.g., 5.54; 5.92) have shown a trend in judicial willingness to review patients' charts and to order the release of patients who have not made progress as a result of their confinement.

On the issue of the legal distinction between "experimental" and more traditional forms of treatment, Martin conceded that it was "hard to define," but offered the following:

> Accepted treatment would encompass a broad range of approaches that
> might be followed by a majority of reasonable practitioners. The goal
> would certainly be to "cure" the problem. An experiment would be less
> tried and tested; research documentation would be part of the goal of the
> program; and "seeing what happens" for a class of people would be as
> important as solving the problem finally for any one client in particular.
> (p. 36)

In practice, many of the claims alleging negligent diagnosis and treatment by a mental health professional have at their basis a doctor–patient
fee dispute (e.g., 5.102; 5.107; 5.113). In one such case, the parents of a
child apparently brought suit against a psychologist because his diagnosis
precluded their reimbursement from an insurance carrier (5.105). In
most of the other suits alleging negligence (e.g., 5.101; 5.103; 5.118) the
basic question for the court to decide was "What would the average
professional or institution have done under the same or similar circumstances in the same or a similar community?" Case 5.120 is of interest
since it involved the potential assignment of civil liability for failure to
diagnose and report child abuse. All fifty states now have laws compelling
health professionals to officially report abused children. (Some guidelines
for detecting child abuse appear in Fontana, 1973; and Helfer, 1973; see
also Helfer, 1975; Alexander, 1974; and Burt, 1972.)

In case 5.119, a hospital was found liable for damages when the court
invoked the doctrine of *res ipsa loquitur* ("The act speaks for itself").
This doctrine is invoked when the mere fact that an injury occurred
suggests that there probably was negligence on the part of the defendant.
The injury must be the result of an accident which would not ordinarily
occur unless someone was negligent. In all cases where the doctrine is
invoked it must be shown that the defendant owed the plaintiff a duty of
due care, that the injury must have been caused by an instrumentality
under exclusive control of the defendant, that the plaintiff himself did not
cause or contribute to the injuries, and that the injury would not have
occurred if those managing the instrumentality had not been negligent.
Attempts have been made to apply this relatively liberal method of proof
to psychiatric malpractice cases. (See, for example, *Johnson v. Rodis*,
251 F.2d, 917; *Farber v. Olkon*, 254 P.2d 520; and *Meier v. Ross General Hospital*, Case 5.2).[9]

On the general subject of diagnosis and treatment, mental health
professionals should be aware of some important decisions in *medical*

---

[9]Readers interested in additional sources on the doctrine of *res ipsa loquitor* are referred to
Ybarra v. Spangard, 154 P.2d 687; *Quintal v. Laurel Grove Hospital*, 397 P.2d 161; *Clark
v. Gibbons*, 426 P.2d 525; *Vistica v. Presbyterian Hospital*, 432 P.2d 193; and "The
Application of Res Ipsa Loquitor in Medical Malpractice Cases" in the *Northwestern Law
Review*, 1966, *60*, 852.

malpractice cases with regard to misdiagnosis, missed diagnosis (not recognizing any problem), and treatment. Physicians have been held liable for failure to use a diagnostic test when it is customary and usual to do so (*Narcarato v. Grob*, 384 Mich. 248; 180 N.W.2d 788; *Smith v. Yohe*, 194 A.2d 167; *Estate of Davies*, 248 N.W.2d 344), failure to interpret test data correctly (*Green v. State, Southwest Louisiana Charity Hospital*, 309 S.2d 706), and failure to respond customarily to a patient's adverse reaction to a test (*Dill v. Miles*, 310 P.2d 896). Doctors have also been held liable for the consequences of innaccurate test results (*Johnson v. St. Paul Mercury Insurance Company*, 219 S.2d 524; *Price v. Neyland* 320 F.2d 624). In the latter context, physician/attorney John Feegel (1974) advises doctors never to assume laboratory infallibility; to do so is to be "wide open to a liability suit when, following an adverse result, the patient's attorney points out that a reasonable and prudent physician should have known that the reported lab results were inconsistent with the clinical picture" (p. 48). Physicians may avoid legal liability for misdiagnosis if the misdiagnosis does not affect treatment (*Black v. Caruso*, 9 Cal. Rptr. 634; *Romberg v. Morgan*, 218 N.W.2d 492) or if the misdiagnosis is followed by correct treatment (*McManus v. Donlin*, 127 N.W.2d 22; *Hall v. Bacon*, 453 P. 816). An interesting, academic exercise would be to speculate on how some of the decisions in the medical malpractice cases cited above would be applicable to discussions of psychodiagnosis, psychotherapy, and psychological testing.

EXPERT TESTIMONY

As stated in the California case of *Lawless v. Calaway* (147 P.2d 604), whether medical malpractice took place is usually decided upon on the basis of expert testimony: "Ordinarily, a doctor's failure to possess or exercise the requisite learning or skill can be established only by the testimony of experts." It is typically the strength of the expert testimony either for or against the parties involved that may well be the deciding factor in the assignment or nonassignment of liability in malpractice litigation (e.g., 6.5; 6.6). However, as we have seen in our discussion above of the doctrine of *res ipsa loquitur*, there are situations where "the act speaks for itself" and a court may not require expert testimony to make its decision. In such situations courts have ruled that a reasonable jury could determine whether negligence could be inferred from the circumstances of the case. Examples of such situations include cases in which a clamp was accidentally left in the abdomen of a surgical patient (*Leonard v. Watsonville Community Hospital*, 305 P.2d 306), a rectal abscess developed following a routine enema (*Davis v. Memorial Hospital*, 376 P.2d 561), and a physician failed to examine and/or x-ray a patient's hip despite repeated complaints of pain in that area (*Friedman v. Dresel*, 293

P.2d 488). As stated in *Ales v. Ryan* (64 P.2d 409), expert testimony may not be needed if, "during the performance of surgical or other skilled operations an ulterior act or omission occurs, the judgment of which does not requies scientific opinion to throw light upon the subject."

A doctrine similar to *res ipsa loquitur* is the doctrine of "common knowledge." The distinction between the two is that in *res ipsa loquitur* cases the plaintiff is required only to prove injury and not a standard of care or a specific act or omission. Generally, the common knowledge doctrine is applied after a plaintiff has already proved damage and an act or omission by the defendant professional. The effect of the invocation of the common knowledge doctrine is to obviate expert witness testimony, as it is the jury who decides what the applicable standard of care is. In essence, invocation of the doctrine of common knowledge transforms the case from one of professional malpractice into a case of ordinary negligence (see, for example, 6.8 and 6.9).

In addition to situations in which expert testimony has been deemed unnecessary, there is at least one recorded instance of a court's disregarding expert testimony and, in essence, setting its own standards. In *Helling v. Carey* (6.30), the court heard undisputed expert testimony to the fact that it was customary and usual for ophthalmologists not to give routine eye pressure tests for glaucoma to patients under forty years of age. In a somewhat atypical opinion, the Washington State Court deemed the standards of ophthalmologists *pro hac vice* to be too low, and it found the defendant ophthalmologists liable for not administering the test.[10]

One question over which there appears to be a growing amount of controversy is, Who qualifies as an expert? There is a growing minority view that holds that possession of an academic degree or professional license does not, in and of itself, make the holder of such a credential an expert (6.1). How might such a view affect litigation involving professionals in the field of mental health—a field in which most lay people believe they are "expert" anyway (cf. Cohen, Note 1). One of the questions before the court in *Sanzari* (6.8) was whether or not a physician could qualify as an expert in a trial that involved a dentist's alleged negligence. Under the circumstances of that case, the court did permit the physician's testimony to be admitted into evidence, despite the fact that expert witnesses must usually be licensed members of the profession whose standards they profess to know (*Hull v. Plume*, 37 A.2d 53 and *Rawleigh v. Donoho*, 283 Ky. 480; 38 S.W.2d 227). What circumstances might prompt a court to admit or refuse to admit into evidence the expert testimony of a member of one mental health specialty (e.g., psychiatry) in litigation involving a member of another specialty (e.g., psychology)? In *Matter of Wellington* (340 N.E.2d 31) the court observed that "the question whether

---

[10]More discussion of *Helling* appears under "Standard of Care" on pp. 244–245 below.

a nonmedical psychologist is qualified to give expert testimony of the issue of mental condition or competency has not received uniform treatment in the courts of this country.'' In this context, what treatment by the courts can psychologists and other ''nonmedical'' therapists expect from the courts in matters involving litigation? Can professionals from one state qualify as experts in another state (see, for example, 6.2)? These are only some of the numerous, complex questions with which the courts—and mental health professionals—will increasingly be faced.

Some last words on the subject of expert testimony. If you agree to act as an expert witness, make certain that you do appear at the trial. To do otherwise may incur legal liability (6.7). If you are named as a defendant in a malpractice action, make certain that when you take the stand you do not act·as an expert witness for the plaintiff (6.3; 6.4).

SUPERVISORY LIABILITY

One of the many gray areas of the law affecting mental health professionals is the law concerning the use of assistants and paraprofessionals in the private practice of psychotherapy. The rise of community psychology, behavioral treatment, and other factors has prompted an unparalleled rise in the frequency with which unlicensed persons have been utilized by licensed practitioners to aid in the treatment of psychological problems. Although mental health professionals are permitted to employ assistants, the extent of responsibility they can legally delegate to an assistant in the treatment of patients remains to be defined by law. We can say that the law does not permit mental health professionals—or any other licensed professionals—to delegate their responsibilites *in toto* to an unlicensed person. We can also say that the assistant, employee, or whatever must be competent to perform the services he is performing. This caution is based on an interpretation of Section 29.1 (9, 10) of the Rules of the New York State Board of Regents Relating to Definitions of Unprofessional Conduct (effective October 1, 1977), which reads as follows:

9. Practicing or offering to practice beyond the scope permitted by law, or accepting and performing professional responsibilities which the licensee knows or has reason to know that he or she is not competent to perform, or performing without adequate supervision professional services which the licensee is authorized to perform only under the supervision of a licensed professional, except in an emergency situation where a person's life or health is in danger.

10. Delegating professional responsibilities to a person when the licensee delegating such responsibilities knows or has reason to know that such person is not qualified by training, by experience, or by licensure to perform them.

In New York as well as other states the relationship of an assistant to a licensed professional is, legally, akin to an "extension" of the professional himself. However, a nonprofessional cannot legally function in a way so as to get the "cloak" of being a licensed professional by reason of his association with the licensed professional. If an employee of a professional is functioning in such a capacity that a reasonable person could confuse the employee with being a licensed professional, the professional is said to be "lending out" his license, and he may be subject to disciplinary action such as revocation of his license.

In his comprehensive review of the literature on supervision of psychotherapists, this author (with DeBetz, 1977) emphasized the importance of the relationship between the supervisor and the supervisee:

> Under ordinary circumstances, supervisory success stands or falls on the quality of the relationship between the participants. The most carefully prepared didactic presentation of material will fall on deaf ears if the learner is alienated from the teacher. Conversely, the least hint of theory or casual reference to the literature may suffice to motivate the inspired trainee to independently research and creatively expand on his teacher's ideas. Therefore, the *responsive mutuality*, the sensitivity and respect shared by the supervisor and the supervised is perhaps the most potent tool in the supervisory repertoire. (p. 55)

Effective supervision of your trainees, employees, and assistants is important not only for professional reasons but for legal ones as well. The legal doctrine of *respondeat superior* ("Let the master respond") is the pertinent one here. Sometimes referred to as the doctrine of "vicarious liability," *respondeat superior* holds that a "master" is responsible for the acts of his "servants" undertaken in the course and scope of the employment. In a case in which a surgeon left a sponge inside a patient's abdomen (6.16), the surgeon denied that he was responsible for the error. He argued that the hospital and not himself should be liable for the negligence of the nurses who incorrectly counted the number of sponges used. The surgeon's attempt to transfer the nurses' liability to the hospital via *respondeat superior* was successful, though the $21,000 judgment had to be paid jointly and severally[11] by the surgeon and the hospital.[12]

Schedules of supervision of employees, assistants, and other supervisees must be based on a sensitivity to the needs of the supervisee *and the*

---

[11]The terms "jointly and severally" mean that it was the plaintiff's choice as to whom he wanted to collect the total of $21,000 from and in what amounts. The plaintiff could, for example, ask for $20,000 from the surgeon and $1,000 from the hospital (presumably if he didn't like the surgeon very much!). This does not, however, mean that the surgeon could not seek a contribution from the hospital.

[12]For information on how the doctrine of *respondeat superior* has been applied to hospital attendings and chiefs of services, see Sagall and Reed (1975).

patient. Although there is no case law—yet—to reinforce this point, it seems reasonable to assume that to set up a supervision once a week or once a month *pro forma* is to ask for legal liability. A once-a-week or once-a-month supervision schedule might be all that is needed for 99 of 100 patients. However, for the 1 percent of the patients who are extraordinary in some way—or who, after the fact, turn out to have been extraordinary in some way—this routine practice of assigning supervisory hours may prove detrimental to the supervisor. A clever opposing attorney might argue, for example, that human beings are not like cars that can be routinely checked every 10,000 miles or so. Unless records document that the schedule of supervision of assistants and other employees was decided on the basis of a careful evaluation of the needs of both the supervisee and the patient, it is conceivable that a good case for malpractice could be made.

It should be clearly understood that although the doctrine of *respondeat superior* creates liability on the part of the "master" for the acts of his "servants," the servant is not totally absolved of responsibility for the consequences of his actions. All that *respondeat superior* does is give the injured party an additional person to sue; it is then up to the plaintiff to decide whether to sue the master, the servant, or both. If the master was not negligent but through *respondeat superior* must pay damages for the acts of the servant, the master has a right to bring a legal action against the servant to recover the full amount of the damages paid. Therefore, servants should not think of *respondeat superior* as insurance against liability—it is not. Each of us is responsible for our own tortious conduct.

Tangentially related to the subject of supervisory liability is the subject of partnership liability. A partner in a group professional practice is usually named as a co-defendant in legal actions taken against any of the other partners. For example, in the case of *Helling v. Carey* (6.30), Dr. Thomas Carey's partner in the medical specialty of ophthalmology, Dr. Robert C. Laughlin, was named as a co-defendant (though this fact is not evident from the standard legal citation). In this context, psychiatrist G. Wilse Robinson, Jr. (1962), recalled his involvement in four malpractice actions in which he was named as a defendant:

> A very interesting side issue in these matters is that I never saw three of these plaintiffs, nor did I talk to the families. In the other case I saw the plaintiff patient only for ½ hour. My associates and partners were not negligent in these cases, but the plaintiff thought so.
>
> The point is that as senior partner I was considered responsible for the actions of my associates, even though I had never seen the patients. This is an important point to be remembered by every senior physician. The senior officer in every organization is legally responsible for every act of his juniors, both omission and commission. (p. 780)

REFERRALS

An attorney who has written extensively on the subject of malpractice in psychiatry, Donald J. Dawidoff (1973a) has suggested that when treatment by a therapist fails to yield any demonstrable results, there may exist a legal (as well as an ethical) duty for the therapist to consult with a colleague or refer the patient to someone else. If a referral is indicated, the professional has a duty to select an appropriate professional or institution for the patient. Barring any extraordinary circumstances, the professional making the referral will not incur any liability for the acts of the person or institution that he refers the patient to, provided that the person or institution is duly licensed and equipped to meet the patient's needs (e.g., 6.19; 6.21). However, a professional who was negligent in treating a patient before referring the patient may be held liable for subsequent acts by other professionals not breaking the causality chain—such acts being seen as complicating or aggravating the effects of the original negligence (e.g., 6.20).

TEAMS

Not infrequently, patients in psychiatric hospitals and institutions are treated by psychiatric "teams." As first conceived by Healy (1915) and later popularized by Kanner (1957), the team is a group of professionals from different specialty areas, each member contributing his special expertise and unique point of view with regard to the treatment of the problem. Traditionally, the psychiatric team has consisted of a psychologist, a psychiatrist, and a social worker. When appropriate (and when they are available), psychiatric nurses, occupational therapists, school guidance counselors, educational specialists, speech therapists, and other hospital and community personnel may participate in team meetings.

Whatever the advantages and strengths of a multidisciplinary effort, though, there would appear to be an added risk of legal liability for the professional who is a member of a team. The same legal principle that has been used to hold doctors liable for the negligence of their "teammates" in physical medicine (see, for example, 6.24) could conceivably be extended to therapists rendering psychotherapy. Furthermore, as more and more persons are asked to participate in decision-making disposition conferences concerning patients, the risk of a suit alleging breach of confidentiality and/or defamation becomes greater. Conceivably, a patient might very well have a legitimate cause of action against professional team members who reveal to some "unauthorized" community member any details of his medical treatment. "Who is an 'unauthorized' team member?" This is one of those questions that needs to be answered by professional organizations—before the courts.

PAIN, SUFFERING, AND EMOTIONAL DISTRESS

Courts have traditionally been willing to award damages for physical injuries but reluctant to award damages for "emotional injuries." A widely cited decision that denied emotional distress (or "fright," in this case) to be a valid cause of action was handed down by a New York court in 1896. Annie Mitchell, the plaintiff in this case, had suffered a miscarriage as a result of fright which was caused by the negligence of the defendant trolley car company. The facts, as stated in the Northeastern Reporter (*Mitchell v. Rochester Railway Company*, 45 N.E. 354), were as follows:

> On the 1st day of April, 1891, the plaintiff was standing upon a crosswalk on Main street, in the city of Rochester, awaiting an opportunity to board one of the defendant's cars which had stopped upon the street at that place. While standing there, and just as she was about to step upon the car, a horse car of the defendant came down the street. As the team attached to the car drew near, it turned to the right, and came close to the plaintiff, so that she stood between the horses' heads when they were stopped. She testified that from fright and excitement caused by the approach and proximity of the team she became unconscious, and also that the result was a miscarriage, and consequent illness. Medical testimony was given to the effect that the mental shock which she then received was sufficient to produce that result.

The court in *Mitchell* denied fright to be a valid cause of action, holding that no damages could be awarded where there was no "immediate personal injury":

> Assuming that the evidence tended to show that the defendant's servant was negligent in the management of the car and horses, and that the plaintiff was free from contributory negligence, the single question presented is whether the plaintiff is entitled to recover for the defendant's negligence which occasioned her fright and alarm, and resulted in the injuries already mentioned. While the authorities are not harmonious upon this question, we think the most reliable and better-considered cases, as well as public policy, fully justify us in holding that the plaintiff cannot recover for injuries occasioned by fright, as there was no immediate personal injury.
> ... Assuming that fright cannot form the basis of an action, it is obvious that no recovery can be had for injuries resulting therefrom.

That the result may be nervous disease, blindness, insanity, or even a miscarriage, in no way changes the principle. These results merely show the degree of fright, or the extent of the damages.

The wording of the decision in *Mitchell* reflected concern that a veritable Pandora's Box of litigation would be opened if damages were awarded on the basis of claims of emotional distress or mental pain and suffering:

> If the right of recovery in this class of cases should be once established, it would naturally result in a flood of litigation in cases where the injury complained of may be easily feigned without detection, and where the damages must rest upon mere conjecture or speculation. The difficulty which often exists in cases of alleged physical injury, in determining whether they exist, and, if so, whether they were caused by the negligent act of the defendant would not only be greatly increased, but a wide field would be opened for fictitious or speculative claims.

For years, damages for emotional distress were awarded only if the claim of emotional distress was accompanied by evidence of some physical contact. It didn't matter if that contact was as slight as the defendant brushing against the plaintiff (*McGee v. Vanover*, 148 Ky. 737; 147 S.W. 742), so long as there was contact. In recent years, courts have increasingly acknowledged that an individual has a right to peace of mind and that the violation of that right is a tort. Thus, in *Samms v. Eccles* (11 Utah 2d 289; 358 P.2d 344), the court found the defendant liable for causing emotional distress to the plaintiff, a woman whom he had exposed himself to and propositioned. In 1972, a court awarded damages for emotional distress to a one-year-old infant (6.26), holding that the infant could recover for such injuries on the same basis as an adult.

Professionals may be sued for certifying or failing to certify that emotional distress is present. One example of a doctor being sued for certifying the existence of emotional distress was provided in the nationally televised program "60 Minutes" (CBS, aired February 13, 1977). In that report, news correspondent Mike Wallace discussed the problem of air traffic controllers who are increasingly leaving on occupational disability and receiving 75 percent of their salary in workmen's compensation. It was pointed out that the temptation is great to "punch out" (as it is called), because the employee typically earns more tax-free dollars when he does not work. Wallace pointed out that of the 550-man work force in the air traffic control center in Atlanta, 20 percent had "punched out" for reasons of anxiety and tension which had been certified by doctors as "job-related." It was reported that one insurance company has brought suit against a psychiatrist for making such certifications. More routinely, psychiatrists, clinical psychologists, and others are asked to defend their opinions in workmen's compensation cases that allege job-related emotional injury. In one such case, a Wisconsin woman working in a mail-order cheese company claimed that she had become "disorganized" as a result of her employment with the firm (*Swiss Colony, Inc. v. Department of Industry, Labor and Human Relations*, 240 N.W.2d 128).

Can a wife maintain an action in tort for emotional distress resulting from doctors' treatment of her husband? This was the question before the court hearing the case of *Ferrell v. Chesapeake and Ohio Railway Employees Hospital Association* (6.25). In that case, the widow of Thomas Ferrell alleged that the defendant hospital and doctors knew that a chicken bone was lodged in her husband's esophagus but had willfully and wantonly refused to accept that fact and willfully and wantonly diagnosed him as suffering from delirium tremens, placing him in restraints. It was also alleged that Mr. Ferrell died as a direct and proximate result of the defendants' actions and that the plaintiff (Mrs. Ferrell) suffered "unspeakable mental anguish witnessing painful and agonizing demise" of her husband as well as "unnecessary humiliation and embarrassment" by having her husband diagnosed as an alcoholic. Citing the noted authority on tort law, William L. Prosser, as well as a previous decision by the Virginia Supreme Court of Appeals, the United States District Court ruled that a valid cause of action had been stated in the complaint of Mrs. Ferrell:

[1,2]   Traditionally, the ability to recover damages for emotional distress has been limited to cases in which the plaintiff also suffered a contemporaneous physical injury. However, the trend in recent years has been to allow recovery for emotional distress which results from wilful, wanton, intentional, or vindictive conduct. Prosser, Law of Torts § 12 (4th ed. 1971). According to Professor Prosser, the rule which seems to have emerged is that there is liability for conduct, exceeding all bounds tolerated by decent society, of a nature which is especially calculated to cause, and does cause, mental distress of a very serious kind. Prosser, supra, at p. 56. Under the law of Virginia, a contemporaneous physical injury is no longer a prerequisite to recovery for emotional distress, when this distress is due to a wilful, wanton and vindictive wrong. Moore v. Jefferson Hospital, Inc., 208 Va. 438, 441, 158 S.E.2d 124, 127 (1967); Bowles v. May, 159 Va. 419, 437, 166 S.E. 550, 556 (1932). Of course, the plaintiff must prove by a preponderance of the evidence the causal connection between the tort and the injury. *Bowles,* supra, 159 Va. at 437, 166 S.E. at 556. Furthermore, the emotional distress must exist, it must be severe, and it must cause an illness or other bodily harm. *Moore,* supra, 208, Va. at 442, 158 S.E.2d at 127; Prosser, supra, at p. 59.

It has also been held that a wilful, wanton, intentional, or vindictive act against a third party which causes emotional distress to another may, under some circumstances, be actionable. In the case at bar, the alleged wilful and wanton conduct was against the plaintiff's husband rather than against the plaintiff. According to Professor Prosser, the conduct against the third party must be of such a nature that there is a high degree of probability that the mental disturbance would follow, and the defendant must have proceeded in conscious and deliberate disregard of it. Prosser, supra, at p. 61. In Moore v. Jefferson Hospital, Inc., supra, the Virginia Supreme Court of Appeals cited the following passage from the Restatement (2d) of Torts § 312 (1965) with apparent approval:

> If the actor intentionally and unreasonably subjects another to emotional distress which he should recognize as likely to result in illness or other bodily harm, he is subject to liability to the other for an illness or other bodily harm of which the distress is the legal cause, (a) although the actor has no intention of inflicting such harm, and (b) *irrespective of whether the act is directed against the other or a third person* [emphasis added]. (208 Va. at 442, 158 S.E.2d at 127)

[3] It therefore appears that under the law of Virginia, emotional distress which is directly and proximately caused by wilful, wanton, intentional, or vindictive conduct against a third person may create a cause of action in tort when the emotional distress is a foreseeable result of the wilful and wanton act. However, in measuring the foreseeability, one factor which must exist is a close relationship between the person suffering the emotional distress and the person against whom the wilful and wanton act is directed. Perhaps these possible plaintiffs would only include members of the third person's immediate family. Prosser, supra, at p. 61.

[4] It therefore appears to this court that the plaintiff in the case at bar has stated a cause of action upon which relief could be granted. This court feels that the wilful and wanton mistreatment of a patient by doctors could directly and proximately cause foreseeable emotional distress to that patient's wife.

In order for the plaintiff to prevail on the cause of action just discussed, this court must find from the evidence that the treatment of the plaintiff's husband by the defendants constituted wilful, wanton, intentional, or vindictive conduct, and if such conduct is found to have occurred then this court must find that the plaintiff suffered actual emotional distress as a direct and proximate cause thereof.

The allowance by the courts of emotional distress as a compensable injury brings upon mental health professionals a most volatile situation. Although Mrs. Ferrell did not win her case, the court did rule that her complaint of emotional distress—allegedly the result of the defendant doctors' treatment *of her husband*—stated a valid cause of action. Conceivably, therapists could be sued for causing, aggravating, or failing to relieve their patients' emotional distress and for certifying or failing to certify the existence of emotional distress. Moreover, there is the ominous possibility of being sued for emotional distress suffered by a patient's spouse (or other person in a close relationship with a patient) allegedly resulting from the patient's treatment.

STANDARD OF CARE

The concept of "standard of care" was explained in Chapter 2, and Cases 6.29 through 6.33 illustrate some interesting nonpsychiatric applications of the concept. However, it would appear that the logic expressed in the court's decisions in these cases might very well be applied to cases involving mental health professionals. For example, in *Hicks v. United States* (6.29) a patient's nausea and abdominal pain were misdiagnosed as due to a "bug" in her stomach, and she died as a result. The court's opinion regarding the requisite standard of care should be of interest to any mental health professional who has ever treated a suicidal patient. The court in *Hicks* said:

> When a defendant's negligent action or inaction has effectively terminated a person's chance of survival, it does not lie in the defendant's mouth to raise conjectures as to the measure of the chances that he has put beyond the possibility of realization. If there was any substantial possibility of survival and the defendant has destroyed it, he is answerable.

Who determines what the standard of care shall be? Does the court or does the profession? Can a court overrule the profession as to what the standard should be? In the case of *Helling v. Carey* (6.30), the Supreme Court of Washington held the defendant ophthalmologist to be negligent as a matter of law for not performing a test for glaucoma on the thirty-two-year-old patient/plaintiff who subsequently suffered a loss in vision. At the trial there was uncontradicted expert testimony stating that it was common practice for ophthalmologists not to perform routine tests for glaucoma on persons under forty years of age. This was so because glaucoma in persons under forty is a statistically rare occurrence. The question at issue in *Helling* was stated succinctly by one of the presiding justices in his opinion:

> The issue is whether the defendants' compliance with the standard of the profession of ophthalmology, which does not require the giving of a routine pressure test to persons under 40 years of age, should insulate them from liability under the facts in this case where the plaintiff has lost a substantial amount of her vision due to the failure of the defendants to timely give the pressure test to the plaintiff.

In his majority decision, Justice Hunter quoted from a 1932 decision handed down by a Justice Hand in *The Matter of T. J. Hooper*, 60 F.2d 737:

> ... a whole calling may have unduly lagged in the adoption of new and available devices ... Courts must in the end say what is required; there

are precautions so imperative that even their universal disregard will not excuse their omission.

The fact situation in *Helling* was unique, and the Supreme Court of Washington's holding was limited to that fact situation. Still, when Justice Hunter writes, "Under the facts of this case reasonable prudence required the timely giving of the pressure test to this plaintiff," is he not edging if not thrusting the court into the role of final arbiter of what is and what is not sound medical practice? Is it right for courts to decide whether standards of a profession are too low or too high? Are courts really prepared and equipped to make such decisions? Is it right for the courts to assign blame and/or assess damages against doctors and other health professionals who follow the customary standards of their profession?

Courts who do take on the role of setting standards in the health professions may find themselves embarrassed for their efforts. For example, in their decisions in *Helling*, Justices Hunter and Utter both alluded to the test for glaucoma as being harmless, reliable, and inexpensive. But as Bradford (1974) has pointed out, the test referred to is none of those things. There is a risk of damage to the eye, the test does not always reliably indicate the existence of glaucoma, and it is inexpensive only when given by itself, which it rarely is (i.e., it is given in the context of a comprehensive eye examination). Conceivably, then, if an ophthalmologist administered the test and caused harm, he may be found to be negligent for administering an unnecessary test that is not usually given. *Helling* places ophthalmologists in the State of Washington in a double bind: They may potentially incur liability for giving and for failing to give a noncustomary test.

Helling has not spurred a rash of similar standard-setting decisions by other courts. In fact, in one subsequent Washington case (*Meeks v. Max*, 550 P.2d 1158) it was reiterated that the decision in Helling was restricted to the unique fact situation of that case. A decision in 1977 by a California court agreed, *in part*, with *Helling* in holding that custom is not an absolute standard to be applied in determining negligence (*Barton v. Owen*, 139 Cal. Rptr. 494). Readers interested in pursuing other references related to this point are urged to consult the following sources: 61 Am. Jur. 2d Section 115 (p. 238); *Spears v. McKinnon*, 168 Ark. 357, 270 S.W. 524; *Ault v. Hall*, 199 Ohio St. 422, 164 N.E. 518, 60 A.L.R. 128; *Morgan v. Shepherd*, 188 N.E.2d 808; *Darling v. Charleston Community Memorial Hospital*, 33 Ill.2d 326, 211 N.E.2d 253; *Sun v. Weeks*, 7 Cal. App.2d 629; 92 P.2d 678. It can be seen from the foregoing that it is customarily the profession and not the court that determines what the applicable standard of care shall be.

An in-depth examination of what the professional standard should be and who should set it is beyond the scope of this book. Generally speaking, professionals are held to the same standard of care as other professionals in similar localities and circumstances with comparable qualifications, background, and experience. One exception to this general rule is when the requisite standard of care is prescribed by statute. Another exception has to do with students. Students acting in professional capacities have sometimes been held to the same standard of care that a duly licensed professional would be held to. This has been especially true in hospital settings, where patients have a right to expect that the services rendered by students in training are comparable to those performed by the average practitioner of that specialty.

The standard of care applied in each individual case will vary with the specialty area of the professional (e.g., in the mental health field, psychiatry, psychology, social work, psychiatric nursing, etc.) and even with subspecialty areas. For example, the standard of care applied in a case involving an industrial psychologist would not be the same as that applied in a case involving a clinical psychologist; the actions of the industrial psychologist would be judged against what other qualified industrial psychologists would have done under similar circumstances. It should be noted that a psychologist with no clinical training who took it upon himself to engage in clinical work might be judged against the same standard that a trained clinical psychologist would be judged against. This is so because when a professional represents himself as a specialist (even though he may not really be a specialist), he may be held to the same standard of care as the person he is representing himself to be. (See, for example, *Simpson v. Davis*, 219 Kan. 584, 549 P.2d 950, and *Butler v. Louisiana State Board of Education*, 331 So.2d 192.) It is also true that a professional with much training will be held to a higher standard of care than another professional with less training, even though both persons might be doing the same job. Thus a highly qualified clinical psychologist who, for lack of employment opportunities, accepts a position that is typically occupied by a masters-level school psychologist will be held to a higher standard of care than the school psychologist. Krauskopf and Krauskopf (1965) explain:

> If a client needs specialized help, the psychologist may be liable for failure to refer the client to a specialist. The counseling psychologist who should recognize that his client suffers from an abnormal, psychotic condition which he is not trained to handle is under a duty to refer the client to a clinical psychologist or psychiatrist capable of dealing with it. If he does recognize the condition but does not refer, he will be treated by the law as purporting to be as competent as a psychiatrist. In other words, he will be negligent for not exercising the same skills a psychiatrist would exercise in the case. In addition, the reasonably skilled psychologist standard will not be applied to the man who does have exceptional skill, training or knowledge. He must exercise the skill he actually has. For example, although the ordinary school psychologist may not be expected to utilize extensive projective testing, if the particular school

psychologist in question has a doctoral degree in clinical psychology, he may be required to use such diagnostic methods if others with this training would exercise them in the particular situation. . . . (p. 232)

Negative outcome in treatment or even a therapy-produced "injury" are not in and of themselves evidence of malpractice; it must be shown that the standard of care applied fell below some accepted standard. As pointed out in Chapter 2, hard and fast rules for what constitutes an acceptable standard of care in the health and mental health professions are nonexistent. Still, legal defenses based on such statements as "But I acted in good faith," will not hold up in court if a standard of care—however that standard is defined—is proved to have been violated. Generally, professionals would be well advised to administer treatments in a way that is acceptable to at least a "respected minority" of their colleagues. However, as Harris (1973, p. 419) has observed, "'respected minorities' are legion in psychotherapy" and "in several cases courts have shifted the burden to the doctor to justify the use of unorthodox methods."

THE STATUTE OF LIMITATIONS

Ask a crowd of witnesses to a car accident to describe exactly what occurred, and you may get as many different versions of the story as you have witnesses. And even if you ask the same witness for his account of the accident, his story may vary depending upon whether you ask him a minute, a month, or a year after the mishap occurred. The law takes into account the difficulty involved in fairly trying a case long after injuries are sustained. Because witnesses may relocate or die, records may be lost, and recollections may fade, plaintiffs are legally mandated to commence "timely" suits. A law that prescribes the amount of time that an injured party shall have in which to bring a lawsuit is called a statute of limitations. Each state has its own statutes of limitations for various causes of action. Thus, exactly what constitutes a "timely suit" varies from state to state and from action to action. For example, in New York State the statute of limitations for a negligence action is three years, while the statute of limitations for a medical malpractice action is two and one-half years. Exactly why that discrepancy exists is not readily apparent (though it may have something to do with the power of the physician's lobby in the New York State legislature).

Statutes of limitations are typically written with numerous provisions for their extension. For example, the "discovery rule" holds that the time limit in which to bring suit for malpractice will be extended if the plaintiff had no way of knowing within the legally prescribed time limit that the malpractice occurred. (See 6.34.) The mere fact that a plaintiff is ignorant of malpractice that occurred is not necessarily grounds for extending the statute of limitations, however. (See *Schiffman v. Hospital for Joint Diseases*, 319 N.Y.S.2d 674.)

CONTRIBUTORY NEGLIGENCE

One defense that a defendant can make to a charge of negligence is to say that the plaintiff's own negligence contributed to or caused the injury. To be deemed contributorily negligent to his own injuries, the plaintiff's acts must have fallen below the level of care that the average reasonable person would have exhibited under the same or similar circumstances. Patients have been found to be contributorily negligent to their own injuries when they have not given enough information to doctors (6.35) and when they have given false information to doctors (6.37). Horsley (1978c) strongly urges practitioners to keep careful records on what instructions patients do *not* follow as well as the ones they do. He argues that a defense of contributory negligence has been an underused strategy in the past but that this is changing:

> Although the theory of contributory negligence has long been taught in law schools, many defense attorneys ignore or overlook it in practice. They've concentrated on setting up defensive stances—in other words, trying to justify what the doctor has done—rather than launching a counterattack against the plaintiff. Fortunately, this Maginot Line mentality among defense lawyers is changing.... (p. 139)

If expert testimony or the pattern of circumstances proves that the doctor acted negligently, the fact that the patient was also negligent in carrying out the doctor's instructions will not make the doctor immune from liability, however (6.36). Also, the doctrine of contributory negligence cannot be applied to children or to adult mental incompetents.

Traditionally, the effect of a finding of contributory negligence was to bar any recovery by the plaintiff. An increasing number of states have modified this view, however, through the adoption of the relatively recent doctrine of *comparative negligence*. Simply stated, comparative negligence allows for the possibility of *partial* recovery of damages by the plaintiff even when there has been a finding of contributory negligence. Thus a court might, for example, find a plaintiff to be "80 percent contributorily negligent." In such a case the plaintiff would be awarded only 20 percent of the damages claimed.

This author's review of the literature suggested that the defense of contributory negligence has not frequently been used by mental health professionals. Given that even the seemingly most disturbed patients can act so as to manage impressions to achieve desired ends (cf. Braginsky,

Braginsky, and Ring, 1969), the defense of contributory negligence may be a most underused defense as regards allegations of negligence in psychology, psychiatry, and allied professions.

INFORMED CONSENT

A person may give his consent to a procedure or action by expressing his consent either verbally or in writing. A person's consent may also be implied in that person's behavior or implied by law. The person giving consent has the right to nullify that consent at any time. From a legal perspective, a consent may also be nullified if the action goes beyond the limits of what was consented to. In one case, for example, a woman who had consented to having sexual intercourse with a man brought suit against the man because she had contracted venereal disease; she had not consented to contracting venereal disease but only to having intercourse (*State v. Lankford*, 102 A. 63).[13] A person's consent will also be considered nullified if it was obtained under conditions of duress or fraud.

A consent is said to be "informed" if all of the risks and possible consequences of the procedure in question along with alternatives to it have been explained to the consenter and the consenter has given evidence that he understands all that has been explained to him. Meisel, Roth, and Lidz (1977) note that the consent must be voluntary and "free from coercion and from unfair persuasions and inducements" (p. 286). As discussed in Chapter 3, deciding upon the amount of information that should be required for a consent to be "informed" can be a complex task. If a doctor knows (or should know) of a possible complication of treatment, he is under a legal duty to disclose that information to his patient (6.38). In *Jeffries v. McCague*, case cited by Speaker (1977), the plaintiff became incontinent after surgery and sued his urologist for failing to inform him that incontinency was a possible risk of the procedure. The doctor admitted knowing that incontinency was a risk of the procedure but had no recollection of warning the patient. He did meet with the patient before the operation and routinely discussed the nature of the procedure as well as possible alternatives and results. The trial court granted a summary judgment against the doctor, but the verdict was reversed by the higher court, which asked in essence whether any "reasonable man" would have let the possibility of incontinence stand in the way of the operation:

---

[13]A similar case was reported in an article entitled "Misery Worth Millions" in *Time*, May 31, 1976, p. 45. An affair between a Washington secretary and the son of a former ambassador resulted in the secretary's contracting gonorrhea. After doctors told her that she probably would not be able to have children as a result of the disease, she brought suit against her former lover. A jury awarded the venereal disease victim $1.3 million in damages.

After hearing evidence concerning whether incontinence was a meaningful or only a slight possibility of the procedure used by [the doctor], the jury must decide whether, in the light of the severity of the [patient's] condition, a reasonable man would have considered the possibility of incontinence material to his decision to undergo treatment.

An earlier precedent had been established that "a physician must appraise a patient of possible results of a surgical procedure." However, the court noted here that "this duty has not been construed to mean that the physician must disclose every conceivable result, no matter how remote." Instead, doctors are bound to disclose "only those risks which a reasonable man would consider material to his decision whether or not to undergo treatment." The court further held as follows:

The rule that the issue is to be decided by the jury, not on a medical standard, but on a reasonable man standard, reflects concern for two problems: on the one hand, the rule preserves the patient's dignity in choosing his own course; on the other hand, by requiring only that information that would be relevant to a reasonable man, a doctor is not required to give every patient a complete course in anatomy and to explain every risk, no matter how remote, before a consent would be valid. (*Jeffries v. McCague*, 363 A.2d 1167)

This "reasonable man" test of informed consent would appear to be the more enlightened view, but there are problems with it, too, as it may be applied to mental health professionals. For example, what does a "reasonable man" need to know before undertaking psychotherapy? The judgment of who is and who is not competent or "reasonable" enough to apply the reasonable man test to is also something that is unclear and resolved on a case-by-case basis. For example, one court held that involuntary patients did not have the right to consent to treatment because they "live in an inherently coercive institutional environment" (*Kaimowitz v. Michigan Department of Mental Health*, 42 U.S.L. Week 2063). Also, what must a doctor do to ascertain that his patient understands his disclosure? Meisel et al. (1977) have observed that patients don't always articulate a decision to consent to or refuse treatment but "may be said to imply consent to treatment through their conduct rather than verbally" (p. 287). Needless to say, proving in a court of law that a mental patient's act was indicative of consent may be a frustrating experience. Finally, there are problems with the reasonable man test when it comes to the question of the informed consent of minors. (See the discussion of *Bartley v. Kremens* in *Law and Behavior*, Summer 1976, pp. 1–2.)

The duty to disclose the risks of treatment to a patient in a manner that conforms to prevailing medical practice standards and to obtain a patient's consent to treatment may legally be breached under two conditions. If there is an emergency situation and the patient's consent cannot be obtained for some reason (for example, the patient is unconscious or cannot comprehend the disclosure, or time is of the essence in treatment), then treatment can proceed without it. Perhaps of greater interest to mental health professionals is the second situation—in which the doctor may breach his duty of disclosure if he can "reasonably" conclude that informing the patient might be detrimental to the well-being of the patient. With reference to the *Emory Law Journal* (1974, *23*, 503–522), Meisel et al. (1977) noted that "if disclosure of certain information—especially the risks of treatment—is likely to upset the patient so seriously that he or she will be unable to make a rational decision, then the physician has the 'therapeutic privilege' to withhold such information" (p. 286). Therapists who choose to invoke such "therapeutic privilege" should be advised that if they do so the burden of proof will fall on them. That is, the therapist withholding information from a patient must be prepared to prove that full and proper disclosure would have in some way hurt the patient.

As emphasized by Balliet (1974), however, obtaining informed consent to treatment should be standard operating procedure for all practitioners:

> Many an old-fashioned doctor may advise you in your early days of private practice to go right ahead and do whatever you think is best for the patient. The trouble is, the old-timer's attitude was formed long before the doctrine of informed consent became a working reality in courtrooms across the country. Its meaning is exceedingly clear: A competent individual has the right to say what's to be done with his body, under what circumstances it's to be poked or traumatized, and by whom. Many a doctor who has plunged ahead without an informed consent has lived to rue the day. They have been the victims of some of the largest malpractice judgments handed down to date. (p. 72)

One final word on informed consent: It will not remove liability for actual negligence in performance of the doctor's responsibilities. A patient may give his informed consent to treatment, but if the treatment is rendered negligently, the doctor will be held liable.

BREACH OF CONTRACT

Courts have allowed injured parties to sue health professionals under either tort law or contract law. This is so because when a health professional undertakes the treatment of a patient an implied contract arises; that contract holds that the professional has the requisite training, experience, and skill to render such treatment and that he will render such treatment with at least average care and skill.[14] Although doctor–patient reassurances and opinions do not typically constitute guarantees or warranties (6.40), there is sometimes a fine line between what will be considered a "reassurance" and what will be considered a "contract to cure the patient" (6.41; see also *Rogala v. Silva*, 305 N.E.2d 571). Generally, when a doctor expressly guarantees a specific result he may be held liable for his failure to achieve that specific result—even if ordinary and reasonable care were used in the treatment. A doctor may also be held liable under a theory of breach of contract if he agrees to use one method of treatment and then uses another (6.42).

INVASION OF PRIVACY

Most states recognize an individual's "right to be let alone" either in statutes or in case law. To prove that privacy has been wrongfully invaded, it is necessary to prove that the defendant's action caused (in the factual and legal sense) some invasion of the plaintiff's privacy and that this invasion caused the plaintiff to suffer injury. Wrongful invasion of privacy is a cause of action that may be undertaken against a defendant for either his intentional acts (e.g., peeping, wiretapping) or his unintentional acts (e.g., negligent disclosure of private information to unauthorized sources). In Chapter 2 the concept of "strict liability" was briefly discussed, and it was noted that it had application to invasion of privacy. Its application here is that a defendant may be held liable for invading a plaintiff's privacy for an act that was *neither* an intentional invasion nor a negligent invasion—just so long as it was an invasion of privacy. In *Kerby v. Hal Roach Studios* (127 P.2d 577), for example, the plaintiff Marion Kerby brought suit against a movie company for the use of her name in a publicity stunt advertising the studio's forthcoming film *Topper*. In that film, a character named "Marion Kerby" was a sexy ghost. It was alleged and proven that the publicity stunt had caused extreme embarrassment and emotional distress to the plaintiff Marion Kerby.

One rather unique set of circumstances involving a mental health professional and an allegation of invasion of privacy appears in *Schwartz v. Thiele* (5.23). In that case, psychiatrist David Thiele had occasion to meet Judith Schwartz in a restaurant parking lot. After their meeting (which lasted less than three minutes), Thiele sent a letter to the psychiatric department of the Superior Court stating that Schwartz was mentally ill and she was likely to injure herself or others if she was not hospitalized immediately.

Invasion of privacy should be distinguished from defamation, in that

---

[14]See *Wolfe v. Virusky*, 306 Fed. Supp.2d 519 (Georgia, 1960).

in the former tort there is not necessarily any injury to the plaintiff's reputation.[15] In fact, even when the invasion of privacy stems from a publication of *complimentary* material, damages may be recovered. Similarly, truth is no defense to invasion of privacy, and neither is good faith or lack of malice. Thus, despite the best intentions of a doctor who wanted to take pictures of a patient in the interest of medical science (6.43), the individual's "right to be let alone" superceded that interest. (Interestingly, "newsworthiness" and "legitimate, current public interest" have been deemed to be valid defenses, thus protecting Hollywood gossip columnists, among others, from litigation.) Mental health professionals should be aware, however, that one certain defense to a charge of invasion of privacy is consent.

UNDUE INFLUENCE

Health professionals and their patients have been held to be in a fiduciary relationship. The nature of this relationship was defined in Chapter 2 (see p. 41). It is precisely because doctors and patients are fiduciaries that actions as seemingly innocent as the purchase of a patient's land (6.44) may be considered suspect and a legitimate matter for legal scrutiny.

INSURANCE

It is good professional practice to fill out patients' insurance forms promptly (6.46) and to inform insurers of an impending malpractice suit (if not of an "alleged injury"—see 6.45) as soon as possible. In this context, it is also important for health professionals to read their own insurance policies carefully with an eye toward delineating the kinds of suits they will and will not be protected against. For example, the professional liability insurance offered to American Psychological Association members by the American Professional Agency does not protect psychologists from office or property liability. That is, any damages that result from a patient's slipping on the office carpet will not be reimbursed. The policy offered to psychologists also does not insure supervisors against damages caused by their negligent supervision of supervisees who hold less than a master's degree or by the acts of such supervisees. Most professional liability insurance policies stipulate that awards arising out of acts that are nonprofessional in character will not be paid. Consider

---

[15]For an extended discussion of the concept of privacy (and of defamation) the reader is urged to consult *Gertz v. Robert Welch, Inc.*, 94 S.Ct. 2997 (Supreme Court, 1974).

how this stipulation could have been invoked in *Zipkin* (5.82), where one of the concurring judges wrote as follows:

> In my opinion many of the acts of Dr. Freeman did not constitute malpractice, nor did they have any true relationship with services performed or omitted. Some of them were willful, malicious acts, such as: ... putting on swimming parties in the nude ... the promoting of an actual and acted-out hostility between her and her husband. ...
>
> Regardless of all psychiatric theories, whether of transference, withdrawal, or otherwise, this relationship (and the doctor's acts) passed the point at which anyone could logically believe that they had any services, or that they were being performed in the course of any legitimate treatment. In other words, the "treatment" ceased, and an ordinary person-to-person invasion of plaintiff's rights, civil or criminal or both, began.

Despite the fact that the judge writing the above decision suggested that Freeman and not the insurance carrier should be responsible for the damages, it was ruled that Freeman's actions stemmed from his mishandling of the transference and were thus professional in nature and so payable by the insurance company.

Some mental health professionals who work in institutional settings do not engage in independent practice. These professionals are typically informed by officials at the hospital, university, or other institution they are employed at that their needs for professional liability insurance coverage have been taken care of by the employer. Such professionals would do well to carry their own private malpractice insurance in addition to whatever the employer is offering. The reason is that in any action against the professional the institution is likely to be named as a codefendant. The institution may then provide only one lawyer to argue for its interests as well as those of its employees. Needless to say, you will probably be better off if you have your own lawyer, representing your interests exclusively.

If you are in a group practice, your insurance needs should be updated with every addition or subtraction of personnel. If you are in independent practice and are a professional corporation (P.C.), you should discuss the insurance needs of the corporation with your insurance company representative and/or your attorney. Although there would appear to be obvious advantages to the incorporated practitioner in paying the additional premiums, some have argued against insurance for the corporation:

> ... [M]any solo professional corporations have relatively limited assets. Therefore, it is absurd to pay an additional premium for professional liability coverage for the corporation when that premium may approach, equal, or exceed the total practice assets. ...

> We believe as a matter of law that the person actually and primarily responsible for the malpractice bears the ultimate liability. Therefore, if the corporation were held liable by a court of law, it would have a cause of action against its only physician employee (who was primarily responsible for the malpractice). This could result in the insurer of the corporation really having no ultimate liability at all, with the total burden falling upon the physician and/or his *personal* malpractice coverage. (Beck, Kalogredis, and Cynwyd, 1977, p. 23)

To Beck et al.'s misgivings must be added the recent decision of the Supreme Court of Kentucky which found an orthopedic surgeon *personally* liable for the negligence of his corporation's employees. In that case, test reports mislaid by the doctor's office staff delayed the plaintiff's surgery for nine months. Suit was brought against the surgeon for the pain suffered by the plaintiff during the period of the delay. Overturning a lower court ruling, Justice John S. Palmore held that if a jury was to award damages to the plaintiff, that money would be collected from the surgeon and not from his professional corporation. Palmore wrote that if the surgeon "had been an old-fashioned country doctor without any office help and had mislaid his notes on this lady's care and then put her off and forgotten her, there can be little doubt that he could have been held responsible had she died as a consequence of that neglect." Palmore went on to hold that "placing a layer of other people, by whomsoever they may be employed, between a physician and his patient does not alter the situation, because the physician's professional duties are not susceptible of being delegated or diffused" (cited in *Medical World News*, April 17, 1978, p. 88).

Some health professionals have unrealistically attempted to sidestep the rapidly rising cost of insurance by "going bare"—i.e., not carrying any insurance. One strategy has been to put assets into an irrevocable trust. Besides the immediate problem of having assets tied up in such a trust, there is an additional problem with such a strategy: courts can disallow the transfer of assets if it can be proven that the action was taken to avoid payment to a pre-existing creditor. Another equally unrealistic strategy some have used to avoid the payment of malpractice premiums is the "malpractice war chest" plan. By regularly saving a sizable amount of money in an interest-earning savings account, some doctors believe they are protecting themselves against damages incurred from a malpractice suit. Such a plan is most risky, as one large settlement for compensatory damages may not only bankrupt the doctor but keep him in a perpetual state of bankruptcy as well, through liens on future earnings. It must strongly be recommended, therefore, that all mental health professionals carry professional liability insurance. It should also be stressed that although insurance alone will not cover all of the "costs" of a malpractice suit in the broad sense of the word (i.e., time, reputation, peace of mind, etc.), it will certainly help.

MEDICAL PRACTICE AND RELIGION

An Israeli surgeon at the University of Tel Aviv Medical School transplanted the heart of a sixty-year-old Jewish man (who had willed his body to science) into the chest of a twenty-three-year-old Arab man who was dying of congestive heart failure. The heart was subsequently rejected by the recipient's body, and he died weeks after the operation. Heart transplantation is forbidden by both Orthodox Jewish and Moslem religious laws. The political and religious outcry that resulted from the surgery prompted the Israeli attorney general to begin collecting data on this case of so-called "double murder"—as it was described in an article entitled "Israeli Heart Graft Causes Religious and Medical Storm" (*Medical World News*, April 17, 1978, pp. 22–23):

> The charge that taking out two hearts constituted double murder stems from the orthodox belief that the heart is the organ of life. A religious Jew, therefore, would view the removal of two beating hearts as a double killing. After the Chief Rabbi reiterated this tenet, ultrareligious members of the Knesset called for manslaughter prosecution.

As this author has stated elsewhere,

> [a]lthough the intermingling of religion with science is not to be encouraged, such enmeshment is bound to occur from time to time. When dilemmas are raised by such overlapping and conflicting interests, I believe that the solution that sides with life, human welfare, and physical/mental well-being must be sought. (Cohen, 1977b, p. 1170)

Courts have come to similar conclusions. In Case 6.48, for example, where a blood transfusion was indicated on medical grounds but prohibited according to the patient's religious beliefs, the court found in favor of the defendant hospital, holding that "there is no constitutional right to choose to die" and that "religious beliefs are absolute, but conduct in pursuance of religious beliefs is not wholly immune from governmental restraint." In somewhat less extreme circumstances, such as in the case of abortions and sterilizations, courts have allowed hospitals administered by religious sects somewhat more leeway (6.47; see also *Doe v. Billin Memorial Hospital*, 479 F.2d 756).

PHYSICAL MINISTRATIONS

In *Corey* (6.49), a city ordinance prohibiting administration of massage to a member of the opposite sex was struck down by a federal court.

Although it is a safe presumption that the ordinance was passed to outlaw "massage parlors" (within which massage is the most innocuous of the goings-on), the existence of such an ordinance should give cause for reflection to "Rolfers," "orgonomists," and others associated with the field of mental health: How much therapist–patient touching should be carried out in the name of "therapy"?

8

Protecting Your Practice

> No man sued for malpractice ever wins completely. . . . You can't know
> what it's like to go through such an ordeal—until you do it. One day
> you're a respected, confident professional man. The next day your
> ability is being debated in court, with all your friends and patients
> looking on—and wondering. (Balliet, 1974, p. 73)

An oral surgeon who was sued for malpractice after a patient swallowed one of his tools is the source of the above quote. The surgeon's
words serve to remind health professionals that there is no such thing as a
"winner" once courtroom proceedings have begun. The key to "winning"
at malpractice litigation is to successfully prevent it. In this chapter I shall
provide a checklist for avoiding legal jeopardy. Additionally, some suggestions for dealing with a claim of malpractice have been included.

PROTECTING YOUR PRACTICE: A CHECKLIST OF GENERAL CONSIDERATIONS

Communication, Relationship, and Treatment

- Don't practice beyond your competence.
- Be familiar with the current literature on the treatment you offer, and
  have a knowledge of alternative modes of treatment. If you work in an
  institutional setting it is especially important that you employ the "least
  restrictive alternative" form of treatment.

- Obtain consent for all forms of treatment, and make certain that that consent is "informed." Specifically, make certain that you have explained to the patient possible outcomes and risks of treatment (as best as you can foresee them), as well as possible alternatives to treatment. Ascertain that the patient has understood what you have told him and that he has knowingly (and voluntarily) agreed to treatment.

- Keep in mind that any statement you make regarding the effectiveness of your therapy might be construed by the patient as a guarantee of cure or a warranty of success.

- Keep confidential matters confidential, and take reasonable precautions to safeguard the confidentiality of your files and records.

- Although there may arise some extreme situations where a breach of confidentiality appears warranted, it would seem to be a good idea to discuss any such prospective situation with a respected colleague before taking action.

- Remember that the "privilege" in privileged communication lies with the patient and not with you.

- Be cautious about statements you make to patients regarding their treatment, as your most casual remarks may come back to haunt you in the courtroom as expert testimony—*for the plaintiff!*

- Avoid any hint of social or sexual involvement with patients by acting thoroughly professionally in your interactions with them.

Record Keeping

- Take a careful history of all patients, and pay particular attention to events pertinent to homicidal or suicidal attempts, gestures, and/or ideation.

- Keep all evaluations up to date, and pay particular attention to the evaluations of patients about to be discharged.

Supervision, Referrals, and Teams

- Supervise your supervisees closely and "responsively" (i.e., on a basis of mutual sensitivity and respect).

- If a referral to another professional or agency is necessary, make certain that the person or institution is duly licensed and equipped to handle the patient's needs.

- Monitor the actions of the "teammates" on your psychiatric team, as it is conceivable that you could be held liable for the negligence of another member of the team.

Institutional Treatment and Commitment

- Supervise closely those patients who are at high risk of suicide or assaultive behavior, or be prepared to document why the therapeutic value of minimal supervision or an open ward outweighed the need for such supervision (and outweighed the risk of suicide or assault).

- In institutional treatment (as well as in private group treatment), keep in mind that the articulation of goals and the assessment of patient progress should allow for tailoring of treatment to the patients' unique needs.

- Exercise due caution and care in executing papers for commitment, and faithfully and comprehensively reevaluate the condition of committed patients.

Medication and Lab Work

- Write prescriptions for medication carefully and legibly. Be familiar with the literature on every drug prescribed, and inform patients about the consequences of the drug's use.

- If you prescribe medication that is classified by the FDA as "investigational," be sure to have your patients' informed consent and written permission.

- Closely follow the guidelines of professional organizations when administering controversial treatments (e.g., electroshock therapy) and/or ask the advice of your county medical society.

- Exercise care in writing requests for laboratory work and in reading the returned reports; never assume "laboratory infallibility".

Legal Education

- Keep up with recent legislation, administrative regulations, and judicial decisions by reading appropriate journals, attending meetings of professional organizations, and in other ways ensuring your continuing education in legal as well as professional matters.

Insurance

- Read the professional liability insurance policies offered by several insurance companies before buying. Periodically review your insurance needs as your practice grows or changes in scope.

- It is a good idea to carry your own professional liability insurance even if the hospital, clinic, or other institution that employs you offers such insurance as a benefit of employment. This is important in ensuring that your individual interests (and not only those of the State of New

York or whoever your employer is) will be vigorously protected should litigation arise.

PROTECTING YOUR PRACTICE: AN ELABORATION

Don't Practice Beyond Your Competence

A practicing attorney and faculty member at a graduate school of social work, Barton Bernstein (1978), cautioned that not all mental health professionals are equipped to handle all kinds of problems:

> The social worker is not equipped to treat all cases. Often, a particular client's problems will require the expertise of a psychologist or psychiatrist. The social worker should be aware of the limitations of his ability and training and, when appropriate, should seek the aid of a consultant or should refer the patient to a professional with more specialized knowledge. (p. 110)

At the most basic level, the caution against not practicing beyond your level of competence means "Do not do what you are not legally entitled to do." Thus, for example, psychologists and other nonphysicians should not under any circumstances prescribe drugs to patients, attempt to titrate medication, or in any conceivable way practice medicine. But that is rather commonsensical, and the issue of competency in relation to the delivery of psychotherapeutic services is far more complex—not only because of the very real problems involved in measuring psychotherapeutic competency but also owing to the unfounded belief on the part of an untold number of therapists (legally licensed and otherwise) that they are competent to handle "anything that walks through the office door."

For years, the proper definition of the term "competency" as regards psychotherapy-related activities has plagued those who would assess psychotherapeutic competency. The problems attendant to the licensing and credentialing of psychotherapists have led to a nationwide "almost anything goes" state of affairs when it comes to who may legally engage in the practice of psychotherapy and use such titles as "psychotherapist," "therapist," "counselor," etc. The problem is woefully complicated by the fact that even "legitimate" mental health professionals—such as licensed psychologists and board-certified psychiatrists—are not necessarily "competent" to render the services they offer to the public, owing to wide disparities in training backgrounds and inadequacies in formal credentialing procedures.[1]

---

[1] A detailed treatment of the problems of measuring competency in the mental health profession, and the unfortunate consequences thereof, appears in Cohen (Note 1).

From a practical standpoint, psychologists who are licensed and psychiatrists who are board-certified would be wise not to view their professional credentials as legal licenses to practice any and all psychotherapy-related activities. Specifically, if a professional holds himself out to the public as an expert, for example, in marital or sex therapy, he will be held to the same standard of care as expert marital or sex therapists. The couple that consults a board-certified psychiatrist for marital problems has a right to expect that that individual has not spent the overwhelming majority of his professional life writing medication orders for back-ward schizophrenics in a state hospital. The couple seeking sex therapy from a licensed psychologist has a right to expect that that individual has not spent his entire professional life administering the Stanford–Binet Intelligence Scale and other psychological tests to grade-school children. The point here is simply that the mental health professional who holds himself out to the public as an expert in a specific mode of treatment incurs correspondingly greater legal obligations; of course, this injunction against professionals' practicing beyond their competence is grounded not only in legal but in moral/ethical considerations as well.

Practice Effective Communication

> Even in later stages of the analysis one must be careful not to communicate the meaning of a symptom or the interpretation of a wish until the patient is already close upon it, so that he has only a short step to take in order to grasp the explanation himself. In former years I often found that premature communication of interpretations brought the treatment to an untimely end, both on account of the resistances suddenly aroused thereby and also because of the relief resulting from the insight so obtained. (Freud, 1913/1959, p. 361)

Styles of therapist–patient communication have undergone quite a bit of change since the days of the father of psychotherapy, Sigmund Freud. Today, many consumer-oriented patients demand therapy contracts that specify in detail what symptoms they desire to be rid of in what time period. If a patient had come to Freud and said, "If only you will relieve me of this, I will put up with the rest," Freud would have observed:

> They exaggerate the selective capacity of the analysis in this. The analyst is certainly able to do a great deal, but he cannot determine beforehand exactly what results he will effect. (p. 350)

Mental health professionals practicing in a society where the specter of malpractice litigation looms must acquire the communication skills necessary for keeping their patients' expectations reality-based. It is a good idea not to accept a new patient for treatment without first scheduling an initial consultation to discuss the scope of the presenting problem and your forthright assessment of whether or not you can be of assistance. The initial consultation—depending of course on the circumstances—is also a good time to clarify the patient's goals in initiating therapy as well as your own in accepting him, to inform him of some special techniques you may be using in therapy (e.g., video or audiotape, biofeedback, hypnosis), to outline the kinds of "homework assignments" the patient may be expected to do in therapy (e.g., keep records of behaviors, recall dreams, etc.), and to agree on the fees for therapy (including what the arrangement will be for missed sessions and for therapist as well as patient vacations) and related services such as psychological assessment.

Depending upon the terms of the initial agreement, the theoretical predilections of the therapist, and the psychological state of the patient, periodic therapist–patient communication concerning the patient's progress may be in order. It is a good idea to keep your patients informed well in advance of any planned absences from your practice, and to tell them something about the suitable replacement who will be "covering" while you are away. Dawidoff (1973b) suggests that it is important, in doctor–patient communication,

> to be certain that suggestions are suggestions and prescriptions are prescriptions. When a psychiatrist tells a patient that a little sex would do him good or that he should stand up to his boss, the physician should be certain that the patient is capable of taking his advice as a suggestion rather than as medical direction. Failure to do so may invite a lawsuit where the patient blindly follows advice to his own or a third party's detriment. (p. 700)

Mental health professionals who regularly give their patients "deep" interpretations had better be prepared to defend the "depth" of such interpretations to a judge and a jury. Imagine what a clever attorney might have done in cross-examination to a witness who gave the following testimony:

> The first . . . chance actions of the patient . . . will betray one of the governing complexes of the neurosis. A clever young philosopher, with leanings towards aesthetic exquisiteness, hastens to twitch the crease in his trousers into place before lying down for the first sitting; he reveals himself as an erstwhile coprophiliac of the highest refinement, as was to be expected of the developed aesthete. A young girl on the same occasion hurriedly pulls the hem of her skirt over her exposed ankle; she has betrayed the kernel of what analysis will discover later, her narcissistic pride in her bodily beauty and her tendencies to exhibitionism.

Our hypothetical attorney—regardless whether he practiced in Victorian or modern times—would probably have little difficulty in challenging the credibility of the witness, this despite the fact that the "testimony" above was provided by no less an authority on psychotherapy than Sigmund Freud (1913/1959, p. 359). As any attorney experienced in defending mental health professionals will advise you, judges and juries tend to be rather "concrete" when it comes to evaluating the credibility of patient/plaintiffs and therapist/defendants. If a patient argues to a jury that he is "happy" and in fact looks "happy" to a jury, you will have your work cut out for you if you wish to convince the jury that the patient is actually depressed. Psychotherapists must stand prepared to defend their interpretations of patients' verbal and nonverbal behaviors *in terms that lay people can understand and appreciate.*

As psychotherapy progresses, the therapist–patient relationship becomes a potent tool for helping the patient reach his goal in therapy. Moreover, as Slawson (1970) has suggested, the single most important factor in protecting one's practice is

> the integrity of the doctor–patient relationship. It sounds obvious, but apparently it is not. This is an area in which psychiatrists are acknowledged experts and yet, when the unexpected arises, they may react in a tactless and defensive manner. (p. 139)

The communication skills necessary to initiate and build a psychotherapeutic relationship are no less important than those needed to successfully terminate the process. Not infrequently, transient feelings of abandonment or even rejection plague the patient whose treatment is drawing to a close. Ideally, the psychotherapeutic skills necessary to deal with such feelings have already been acquired in professional preparatory training and have been sharpened with each year of clinical practice.

Only Treat Minors with Parental Consent

Mental health professionals who regularly treat children and adolescents should be cognizant of the laws in their state regarding the treatment of minors. Notwithstanding suggestions that minors of age fifteen and above are, as a group, no less competent than adults to consent to treatment (see Grisso and Vierling, 1978), the general rule is "Don't treat minors without the consent of the parent or guardian." No matter how effective, appropriate, or needed your intervention is, you are setting yourself up for legal liability if you treat a minor without parental consent.

There are many exceptions to the above rule, and you should check the laws of your particular state to find out which are applicable. For example, in some states parental consent is *not* necessary if the minor is:

1. 12 or older and either has venereal disease or uses depressant or stimulant drugs;

2. a parent, pregnant, or married;

3. referred by a physician, clergyman, or agency for birth control counseling; or

4. in need of emergency care. (Note that psychological counseling is not
   usually considered to be emergency care, though it may be in the case
   of a suicide attempt).

It should also be noted that in treating minors, any waiver of privilege
should come from the parent or guardian. Mental health professionals are
also reminded here that they have a legal obligation in all fifty states to
report suspected cases of child abuse. Professionals who regularly have
occasion to place children in residential treatment facilities should also be
aware of a new judicial trend toward ensuring that "adolescents who
protest their hospitalization may obtain court review and representation
by appointed attorneys" (Miller and Burt, 1977, p. 153).

Child psychologists, child psychiatrists, and other mental health professionals who have occasion to treat children on a regular basis should be
familiar with the statute of limitations as it applies to minors. In the
treatment of adults, most states' statutes of limitations provide that a
malpractice action must be brought within some time period (e.g., two to
three years) from the date the malpractice occurred, from the date the
patient should have known of the malpractice, or from the date the malpractice was discovered (it depends how the statute is written). However,
for minors the time limit for bringing a malpractice action, as with any
negligence action, does not begin to run until they come of age legally.
This means that professionals treating minors are not only susceptible to a
suit taken by the patient's parents, but they are additionally subject to a
suit brought by the patient himself some five or ten years after treatment
may have been terminated.

Keep Careful Records

The value of good record-keeping habits in everyday practice—for
facilitating treatment, for training purposes, and for administrative
convenience—cannot be overemphasized (cf. Zaro et al., 1977). But in
addition to all of the practical reasons for developing good record-keeping
habits, there is one very good legal reason for doing so: Carefully
documented records may well mean the difference between a court judgment for you and a court judgment against you. Clear, concise statements
summarizing your contacts with the patient are looked upon favorably by
judges and juries. Conversely, the professional who comes into court with
a confused jumble of notes and who testifies in a like manner (e.g., "On
that day we talked about. . . . No, wait now, I think it was two weeks
before that we got into something like that . . .") will certainly not make a

very convincing witness. Slawson (1970) has advised that "good clinical
records are the keystone" of a defendant's case and that "in those cases
that go to trial, sloppy and incomplete records count heavily against the
litigant who relies upon them" (p. 139). Hamilton (1970) recalled the
importance of sound record keeping being emphasized to him in the
course of his own training:

> In many conferences in the department, I, along with other residents,
> would frequently describe procedures which had been done and the
> results which had been achieved only to have the professor call for a look
> at the record, following which we would receive a lecture revolving
> around why we had not reduced this previous recitation to writing. His
> maxim about this was simply, "Work not written is work not done." In
> essence, this is the importance of records. We have little to fear in the
> malpractice area, generally, if we have meticulously prepared written
> accounts of our professional behavior in relation to the particular pa-
> tient involved. (p. 71)

What should patients' charts contain? At a minimum, charts should
contain a descriptive summary of all contacts; progress notes and regular
summaries of progress (e.g., three-month summaries); previous and present psychological test data, if available; medication history; notations of
informed consent to all aspects of treatment (including therapy, medication, tests, etc.); notations of phone contacts and conversations with "significant others" in the patient's life; and copies of all correspondence
with the patient. Dawidoff (1973b) advised that records should also contain citations to the relevant literature and added that

> it may be helpful in the cases of patients with severe perceptual incapac-
> ity to obtain consent of a parent, guardian, or spouse so that the issue of
> capacity to consent to treatment may be favorably resolved. Recording
> the treatment rendered and making memoranda of the cooperation of
> parent or spouse can prove helpful so that any resistance to treatment
> from such sources may be memorialized and the blame placed where it
> ought to lie should litigation arise. (p. 699)

I have found a pre-treatment questionnaire I devised (Cohen, Note
11) to be useful as a screening device for the detection and assessment of
psychopathology. Potentially useful in private practice as well as in hospital and teaching settings, the Cognition/Behavior Survey (C/BS) is an
eleven-page form that is designed to survey cognitive and behavioral problem areas. The form is completed by the patient, on his own time, after the
first or second psychotherapy session. Because the form contains both
"objective" and "projective" questions, it can potentially provide the
clinician with a wealth of "leads" in therapy. Moreover, the C/BS represents a valuable addition to the patient's chart as it contains information

on the patient's self-report of his perception of the events currently taking place in his life, his past history, and future expectations. The form can thus be useful in bringing to light deficiencies that may exist in the patient's judgment and insight. Section III of the C/BS (reproduced below) is designed to reflect the patient's report of severe psychopathology:

Has any of the following been a problem for you?   YES   NO

1. Hearing, smelling, seeing, or feeling something that wasn't really there?   ____   ____

2. Feeling possessed by a demon, spirit, or the like?   ____   ____

3. Feeling as if you are out of control, or that another person is controlling your thoughts or actions?   ____   ____

4. Feeling as if someone is out to get you?   ____   ____

5. Feeling as if you want to hurt yourself, with or without intent to commit suicide?   ____   ____

6. Feeling as if you could seriously consider harming another?   ____   ____

7. If you answered "Yes" to items 1, 2, 3, or 4, please elaborate in the space below or on a separate sheet of paper.

8. If you answered "Yes" to item 5 (or if you answered "No" to item 5 but believe that answering any of the following questions will be useful to your therapist in your treatment), please respond to the following:

What is it about you that needs to be punished through self-hurt?

Have you ever seriously considered suicide? When? How frequently?

Have you ever attempted suicide?

Do you believe that you have the capability to commit suicide?

How would you commit suicide?

What would the consequences of your suicide be?

What has kept you from committing suicide?

How can your therapist and those around you be most responsive to your needs in this regard?

9. If you answered "Yes" to item 6 (or if you answered "No" to item 6 but believe that answering any of the following questions will be useful to your therapist in your treatment), please respond to the following:

Whom have you seriously considered harming?

What have you considered doing to this person (or persons), and why?

Have you ever attempted to inflict injury or serious harm on another?

Do you believe that you have the capability of inflicting serious harm on another?

What would be the consequences of such acts?

What has kept you from committing such acts?

How can your therapist and those around you be most responsive to your needs in this regard?

Records become especially important if you are dealing with a patient who you think is a potential litigant. If you have such a patient, you should note your concerns in writing and describe precisely what you did to remedy the situation: e.g., "I called Dr. Johnson at University Medical Center to discuss this matter and to plan a course of treatment." Do not, however, include statements that are highly subjective or opinionated with regard to how difficult the patient is; such statements will probably reflect poorly on you in court. Contrariwise, statements admitting legal liability should not be included in the record either.

Should a patient be institutionalized in the course of treatment, regular entries on the hospital progress notes should be made if you are continuing to render treatment. Remember to sign these notes, and do not hesitate to remark in writing on any aspect of the house staff's treatment of the patient that displeases you. Also with regard to institutional record keeping, Hamilton (1970) has advised that records validating the commitment status of a patient (e.g., commitment certificates, court orders, voluntary requests for commitment and treatment) are important to keep, as are psychiatric and social-work case studies, progress notes by medical and nonmedical staff, staff conference notes and summaries, special-incident reports, laboratory test data, and discharge summaries.

Use Behavioral Descriptions with Psychiatric Diagnoses. As judges and lawyers become increasingly sophisticated with respect to the unreliability of psychiatric diagnoses and as insurance companies increasingly challenge doctors' certifications of "emotional distress," "anxiety neurosis," and the like, mental health professionals would do well to supplement or, if possible, exchange their psychiatric diagnoses for clear behavioral descriptions, complete with concrete behavioral vignettes that support their conclusions. A good example of an intake report that provides a behavioral description in no uncertain terms can be found in Goldfried and Davison (1976, pp. 52–53). Mental health professionals who are compelled (by either the institution where they work, the insurance company they are requesting reimbursement from, or force of habit) to apply a psychiatric diagnostic lable when none of the existing categories appears to be appropriate should use the DSM–II (American Psychiatric Association, 1968) diagnosis # 317, "Non-specific conditions." The comparable diagnosis (for non-psychotic individuals) in the operational criteria draft for DSM–III (American Psychiatric Association, 1977) is diagnosis # 307.99, "Unspecified mental disorder (non-psychotic)."

Practice Office Safety

The growing number of activities undertaken in the name of "psychotherapy" has prompted the appearance of aversive stimulation machinery, biofeedback gadgetry, and numerous other therapeutic aids where once a table and a box of tissues stood. Clinicians who intend to purchase such equipment should do so only after thorough investigation as to the quality of the product they are considering. They should know that skimping on costs before purchasing may cost them a lot more than they bargained for in legal fees later. Of course, they should also have a working familiarity with the potential hazards of the particular approaches they use. For example, those who employ electric shock as an aversive stimulus should know that shocking devices tend to produce both intended shock (that which the therapist/experimenter wants to be produced) and leakage current (accidental shock caused by equipment components such as the transformers, motors and coils, or resisters). Butterfield (1975) cautions that "if sufficiently large, leakage currents pose a serious danger to both patient and operator" (p. 1).

If a dentist drills the wrong tooth, it is clearly not the drill which is at fault. However, if while he is drilling the right tooth the dentist's drill breaks, causing permanent damage to the patient, who is liable? The dentist? The manufacturer of the drill? As pointed out earlier in this book, the law expects only the ordinary and usual amount of expertise from professionals. If it could be shown that the dentist had taken the usual precautions in purchasing the drill (whatever those precautions are) and if he did nothing unusual while drilling, there would be no reason to suspect that the patient in this hypothetical case would be able to successfully sue for malpractice. The law compels professionals to provide services which are only as good as the average level of service; it does not guarantee that patients will not have their health impaired as a result of a visit to a health professional. In fact, the hypothetical patient in the example above would probably have more of a chance of collecting from the dentist if he tripped over a denture which was negligently left on the floor by the dentist. The point with regard to the use of machinery is that there is a difference between malpractice and malfunction. If it can be shown that all of the necessary and usual precautions were taken before an instrument was used, then most likely the manufacturer of the instrument and not the professional will be held legally liable.

In considering charges of malpractice resulting from the use of faulty instruments, courts will also seek to determine whether the defect was patent (outwardly noticeable to an observer) or latent (not readily observable). Clearly, if it can be shown that a professional used an instrument with a patent defect, the chances are that that professional did not exercise reasonable care. If it is determined that the instrument contained a latent defect, liability may revert back to the manufacturer, depending upon the circumstances of the case.

Beyond using mechanically sound and safe instruments in a reasonable manner, professionals need to keep abreast of legal developments concerning the use of such equipment (e.g., a biofeedback apparatus is now classified by the Food and Drug Administration as a "medical device"). Readers interested in further exploring legal/ethical issues attendant to the use of devices in treatment are referred to the writings of R. Kirk Schwitzgebel (1976; 1977; 1978). Whether or not devices are used, office safety also entails "reasonable" maintenance of your premises. This means, for example, that nothing is inadvertently left around the office for patients to trip on, that a policy of not leaving children unattended in the waiting room is enforced, and that there are no sharp edges anywhere in the office that patients can accidentally cut themselves on.

Group Practice Is Preferable to Private Practice

Psychologists, psychiatrists, and other mental health professionals engaged in applied work would do well to join together in group practice if they are unaffiliated with teaching or service institutions. The opportunity for formal and informal meeting with colleagues to discuss treatment approaches is indispensable and is to be much preferred to sequestering oneself professionally. Group practice also facilitates the provision of twenty-four-hours-a-day, seven-days-a-week coverage for the patient who may have an emergency or a crisis. Another advantage of group practice is the advantage it offers if a malpractice action does arise. The competent professional whose work is respected by colleagues will have no difficulty in finding sympathetic expert witnesses should that need arise.

If you do decide to form a group practice you should discuss with an attorney the specific type of structure and organization that will best suit your needs. Like individual practice, group practice is looked upon by the law as a *business* and must be governed as such. Some of the forms this business can take, as well as some suggestions for avoiding liability, appear below.

Types of Group Practice.   In New York as well as other states, the term "group practice" has, in and of itself, no clear legal definition. It is the nature of the relationship between the professionals in the "group practice" that determines whether the practice is, or should be called an office-space-sharing agreement, a partnership, or a professional corporation. There are also privately maintained teaching/research entities (e.g., institutes), which are chartered by the State Department of Education or Board of Regents. Although the laws may vary from jurisdiction to jurisdiction, you may find, after checking with an attorney, that the principals in a partnership or a professional corporation may not be from different professions—that is, that a psychologist may not enter into a partnership with a psychiatrist or a social worker, but only with another psychologist. You may find it attractive that personnel can be more easily changed in a professional corporation than in a partnership. These are all matters to be discussed before the group practice is set up.

Titles.   Another consideration in the formation of a group practice is the title each principal and employee, consultant, and advisor is given. In New York and other states, it is illegal to describe as "psychological" the services of a psychiatrist, a social worker, or anyone other than a licensed psychologist. (It should be noted, however, that certain institutions have been held to be exempt from this law and are allowed to use derivatives of the word "psychology" to describe the title of nonlicensed psychologists, e.g., "psychology intern.") Psychologists should avoid the use of any title that could be confused with a title held by one licensed to practice medicine. For example, if a psychologist and a physician started a group practice and were codirectors of that practice, the psychologist could, depending upon the name of the group and other factors, be held to be holding himself out to practice medicine without a license and in violation of law. All licensed persons need to be wary of the titles they give to unlicensed persons and the way in which unlicensed persons are listed on a group practice letterhead. Licensed practitioners are not allowed to "lend out" their licenses to unlicensed persons. That is, mixing an unlicensed person's name with licensed persons' names on the letterhead may be confusing and misleading to the public and may subject the licensed persons to disciplinary action.

Assignment of Patients.   Given the fact that psychologists, psychiatrists, social workers, psychiatric nurses, occupational therapists, and other mental health professionals have varied backgrounds in terms of education, training, supervision, and clinical experience; different rights as regards privileged communication; and different privileges as regards third party reimbursement, how are patients to be assigned to one or another therapist in a group practice?

Legal and ethical guidelines on this question are lacking. All that can be said here is that assignment of a patient to a therapist must be made on the basis of the patient's individual needs. All patients should be screened for the purpose of assigning them to the appropriate therapist and the appropriate therapy modality (e.g., individual or group treatment). What should *not* occur is the routine assignment of patients on a rotational or "next up" basis among the members of the group. Particularly in a partnership, each partner's caseload is usually kept about equal; new patients get assigned to the partner who is "next up" for a referral. But suppose the partner who is due for the next referral is a social worker, and suppose the patient to be referred is a depressed patient. Further, let us suppose that the social worker, for whatever reason, never refers the patient to a psychiatrist for evaluation for medication. Finally, let us suppose that some time later the patient is seen by an outside psychiatrist and responds favorably and achieves symptom remission after adminis- tration of a drug (e.g., lithium). The patient in this hypothetical example might have grounds for a malpractice action against the group.

Fee-splitting. Fee-splitting—no matter how it is cloaked—is un- ethical and illegal, and may result in the revocation of licenses if it is found to have occurred. Consider the situation in which Dr. Jones (or "Mr." Jones, as he need not be a professional) refers a patient, Mrs. Schwartz, to Dr. Smith. After the referral is made, Dr. Jones has no participation whatever in Mrs. Schwartz's treatment. However, Doctor Jones receives a portion of the fees Mrs. Schwartz pays to Dr. Smith. In this case, Jones and Smith are clearly guilty of fee-splitting. If Jones was supervising Smith or otherwise participating in the treatment of Mrs. Schwartz, a court might rule that fee-splitting was not taking place, de- pending on the amount of the fees paid to Jones and other circumstances unique to the case.

Think Twice about "Putting Down"
Colleagues

Defense attorneys Burr Markham of Minneapolis, Minnesota, and Kenneth Weyl of Phoenix, Arizona, have strongly criticized the practice of doctors speaking out against colleagues. When interviewed on the sub- ject of how malpractice litigation could be reduced, Markham and Weyl (cited in "Six Ways," 1977) emphasized that one doctor making remarks critical of another doctor's treatment can trigger a malpractice suit. Markham went so far as to say that doctors who criticize colleagues are the single largest cause of malpractice litigation. He noted that patients may interpret one doctor's open discussion and honest questioning of a case as an indication of negligence on the part of the doctor being dis- cussed. Weyl observed that critical remarks tend to result in patients' loss of confidence in their doctors and therefore predispose them to taking legal action. It should be remembered that the professional who is con- stantly pointing out the failings of his fellow professionals is subtly en- couraging them to do the same with respect to him.

Follow Through for Each Patient, with Treatment or Referral

No doctor in private practice is legally compelled to accept any patient for treatment. The mental health professional may feel that he does not have the expertise to deal with a particular problem; he may not have the number of hours needed to provide adequate services; he may not see himself as able to establish a good enough rapport with the patient; the patient may not be able to pay the doctor's fee, etc. But while there are any number of perfectly acceptable reasons for refusing to treat a patient, there is *no* reason to justify abandonment of a patient once treatment begins. Before accepting a new patient, the mental health professional would be wise to schedule an initial consultation for the purpose of a mutual evaluation of suitability. If a doctor accepts a patient but some time later believes he can no longer be of value (because, for example, he has discovered factors operating that are beyond his competence to deal with), "following through" would mean advising this patient of the state of affairs and referring him to an appropriate mental health professional.

Recognize the "High Risk" Patient

The "high risk" patient referred to here is the patient who is at high risk of suing you. Patients may express dissatisfaction with (and resistance to) their treatment in many ways, including oral and written statements, nonverbal communication, and nonpayment or late payment of bills. Each of these expressions of dissatisfaction should, at the clinician's discretion, be explored when it occurs. Oral and nonverbal communications may be dealt with on a face-to-face basis in the office, while a letter or a nonpayment of bill from a patient no longer being seen might best be dealt with by a sympathetic phone call. If the patient is dissatisfied and voices dissatisfaction in terms that lead the doctor to suspect that litigation may be on the way, the doctor might avoid a potential lawsuit by telling the patient that he's sorry about the dissatisfaction but has done his best. He might also add that he wouldn't want the patient to pay for services with which he was not happy.

This is *not* to say that doctors need be intimidated by patients. Exactly how such situations should be handled varies greatly with the circumstances of the individual case. One thing doctors should never do, however, is routinely turn late accounts over to collection agencies. Collection agencies can be coarse in their treatment of patients, and they might push patients thinking about litigation into actually contacting an attorney.

Persons in the insurance business tend to agree that a patient's nonpayment of bill is one of the first and surest "warning signs" of dissatisfaction and a possible malpractice suit. Although no formal psychiatric profiles of litigants are available, the person considered to be at high risk of bringing suit is one who is, first of all, concerned with fees to a rather exaggerated degree. The high-risk patient has also been identified by persons in the professional liability field as one who is critical of previous doctors' treatment and has unrealistically high expectations of therapeutic gain. To protect your practice, these warning signs should be noted and tactfully dealt with as they arise.

DEALING WITH A MALPRACTICE SUIT

Given the increasingly litigious times we live in, even the mose careful clinician may find himself named as a defendant in a malpractice action. If you hold a malpractice insurance policy, the insurance company will appoint a lawyer to act on your behalf. If you do not hold such a policy you will have to find a defense counsel on your own. Chief Justice Warren E. Berger has expressed his belief that as many as half of this country's trial lawyers are incompetent. Although Horsley (1978b) believes that figure to be somewhat inflated, he does concede that he has personally seen "hundreds of briefcase-toters stumbling around in court when they just don't have the knowledge, experience, or temperament to try cases . . . most get away with their bungling because clients aren't aware of what went wrong" (p. 154). Horsley cautions those shopping for attorneys to interview candidates carefully:

> If you have to hire a lawyer to try a case, how can you tell a good one from a bad one? First of all, don't pay too much attention to the certificates on the reception-room wall; they can be obtained for a lot of things besides trial work. Question the lawyer. Ask him how many cases he's actually tried in the past year. If he says, "Oh, a couple or so," he's probably not the man for you. If he says he's tried 50, he's spouting hot air; no trial lawyer who does his homework properly can try that many cases in 52 weeks. If he tells you he tries 10 to 14 significant cases a year, it's likely that he's properly experienced.
>
> But cases vary. Ask him about the types he's tried; make sure your sort is included. Also get the names of some recent cases, and explain that you may want to check them in the courthouse files. (p. 154)

Horsley (1978b) also cautions that approximately half of all *legal* malpractice suits are based on failures to meet some specific deadline. It may therefore be a good idea to monitor your attorney's actions by asking him for a calendar of events including final dates for which certain actions must be executed (e.g., summonses, depositions, etc.). Generally, you would do well to avoid retaining an attorney who is already representing a party with an interest that is conflicting to your own (lawyers are permitted to represent parties with conflicting interests provided it is with the full knowledge and consent of the parties). For example, if the state is named as a co-defendant in an action in which you too are named as a defendant you may not want to be represented by the same attorney who is representing the state. Summarizing, the rule of thumb in shopping for a defense counsel is to seek out a competent, experienced, lawyer who has no competing commitments.

Obtaining a lawyer to represent you is, of course, only the first step in dealing with a malpractice suit. In the following pages we offer some additional suggestions designed to guide the professional who has become involved in litigation.

Before the Trial

You will probably find out that you are being sued when you receive a letter on legal stationery from the plaintiff's attorney. Patients seldom call to personally inform you that they are bringing suit. But regardless of whether you get a lawyer's letter or a phone call or are informed in some other way, your initial reaction will probably be the same: anger. The important thing to remember is not to act on the anger. Some doctors may be tempted to telephone the patient forthwith to argue that no negligence has been committed. Other doctors (fewer, we suspect) may be tempted to telephone the patient and apologetically admit they made a mistake. Neither of these responses is appropriate. Once you are notified of a suit, the only person to contact immediately is your insurer, by a phone call and a certified letter in which you have enclosed a copy of the plaintiff's attorney's letter. Do not discuss the case with the patient, the patient's relatives, the local media—*anyone*. Refer all questions about the case to your attorney.

At some time during the pretrial discovery process (see Chapter 2), you may be asked for copies of personal or hospital records. Some professionals foolishly attempt to "tighten up" or alter the records so that the records will show them in a better light in court. What these professionals do not know is that the plaintiff's attorney may have somehow gotten to the records and copied them long before the letter advising the doctor of the litigation was sent. In such a case, the "doctored" records will then reflect quite poorly on the health professional.[2] One need only look at the course of events in recent American history to be reminded that the consequences of attempting to "cover up" can be dramatic.

---

[2]Those who doctor records may incur criminal as well as civil liability. In a recent malpractice case in Maryland, some crucial medical evidence (x-rays) was lost under mysterious circumstances. The case prompted a bill which provided for a fine of up to $5,000 and/or imprisonment of up to one year for the tampering, altering, or destruction of records by medical personnel.

All of the plaintiff's requests for information should be referred to your attorney. It is emphasized that if you have not carried your own malpractice insurance and have been dependent on the attorney for your employer (e.g., the state) to protect your interests as well, you would be well advised to retain your own counsel if possible.

At some point in the pretrial proceedings (or even well into the trial, for that matter), the attorneys for all of the parties involved may agree on a dollar amount for which they will settle the claim out of court. As the professional being sued, you may want to "go the distance" to clear your name, and you may view the insurance company's willingness to settle out of court as a "cop-out." As we pointed out in Chapter 2, however, out-of-court settlements do not impute blame; they merely state that the claim is being dropped for unspecified reasons in return for a fixed dollar amount. If you want to proceed with the trial, you may have to do so at your own cost or risk.

Thorough preparation for trial is a must. This means that all information pertinent to the case must be physically (and mentally) ordered and at your disposal. Thorough preparation for trial means going over your progress notes, summaries, and psychological assessment data and making certain that you can justify each and every statement you have made. If you administered psychological tests, it is a good idea to go through the raw data as well as the test report. This is especially important if you administered tests in which arithmetic calculations were required (e.g., the Wechsler tests, the Stanford–Binet, etc.). Errors in arithmetic are relatively easy for an opposing attorney to spot (an experienced attorney will look for them in the raw data) and, if found, will reflect very poorly on your thoroughness and competence as a clinician. Keep in mind that amending psychological reports should not be confused with "doctoring" official records and documents. You have the right to amend a report before a trial, but you do not have the right to "doctor" records.

During the pretrial discovery process the plaintiff's attorney may invite you to his office or somewhere else for the purpose of obtaining a deposition. A deposition is a sworn statement that has been taken and recorded before the trial. Depositions are taken for the purpose of obtaining your version of the facts and for discovering leads to other evidence pertinent to the case. Depositions may also be taken to record the testimony of an individual who may not be available when the case is tried. If you are asked to make a deposition, make certain that you allow yourself enough time to prepare for it. You should have the facts of the case at your fingertips by the time you walk into the deposition room. Nothing in your deposition should contradict what you are planning to say in court. Your attorney will probably accompany you to the deposition and will prepare you for it. Additionally, the following guidelines may be helpful.

1. The first rule is to be honest. You are under oath and should be telling the truth at all times. If you do not tell the truth you may be subject to criminal charges. Additionally, if it can be demonstrated that there are falsehoods in your sworn testimony on any point (however minor), then your credibility on other points will be called into question.

2. Do not answer any question unless you are absolutely certain that you understand it fully. Do not be embarrassed to ask for as much clarification as you need or to say "I don't know."

3. If you are certain of your facts, state them as forthrightly as possible. On the other hand, if you are asked a question to which you really are not 100 percent certain of the facts it is all right to use qualifiers such as, "My best recollection is . . ."; "As best as I can recall . . ."; and "I believe. . . ."

4. If you are concerned about how to answer the examiner on some sensitive aspect of the case, or you believe that your answer might prove to be embarrassing, discuss the issue fully with your attorney before the deposition. Together you can decide if the matter is relevant to the case and, if so, what position to take.

5. The examiner may ask you what patient charts, documents, textbooks, or other sources you have consulted in preparing for your deposition. If you are a witness appearing on someone else's behalf he will probably ask you about the financial arrangements that have been made concerning your appearance at the deposition and your participation in the case. Be prepared for such questions by discussing them in advance with your attorney.

6. At any time during the deposition you may ask to have a private conference with your attorney. Similarly, you may at any time ask for a break if you are becoming fatigued or uncomfortable.

7. The well-known Army rule "never volunteer" is most appropriate as regards to making a deposition. Do not volunteer any information that you are not specifically asked. Short answers—"yes" or "no" when possible—are best.[3] Do not volunteer to look anything up, obtain any records, or do anything at all unless your attorney has advised you to do so. Do not volunteer the name of someone who might know the answer to a question, and do not volunteer opinions if you are not asked for them.

8. Be cautious about deciding on which patient charts, notes, documents, or other memoranda you wish to bring with you into the deposition room, as the examiner may ask to look at such materials. It is therefore a good idea to have your attorney approve whatever it is you wish to bring in with you.

---

[3]However, if an answer you give to a question would be misleading if you simply answered "yes" or "no," you have a right to clarify your answer and explain what the "yes" or "no" means.

9. If the examiner has in his possession a patient's chart or some other document and he asks you questions about it, read it over carefully before replying.

10. It is usually a good idea to wait a moment or two before answering any question during the deposition (as opposed to the trial). The brief pause will provide you with additional time to get your answer the way you want it, and it will provide your attorney with the time to raise any objections he might have to the question. If your attorney instructs you not to answer the question do not answer it, even if you think it will help your case to do so.

11. Speak slowly when answering all questions, and stop talking if your attorney interrupts. You may ask for some time to think about an answer to a question if the question is particularly difficult or complicated. Remember, the written transcript of your deposition will not reflect how long it took you to answer any questions, so do not feel pressured into giving quick answers.

12. If the opposing lawyers get into an argument, stay out of it. You should, however, listen carefully to what is being said and be particularly attentive to the point that your own counsel is trying to make. Such disagreements may alert you to an aspect of the case to which you may not have given due consideration before the deposition.

13. Some examiners may try to provoke you to the point where your judgment and memory is somewhat clouded. Methods of rattling you will vary, but a common technique is to accuse you of being inconsistent in your testimony. Alternatively, the examiner may refer to some document or record that your testimony supposedly contradicts. Be prepared for such contingencies, and do not let the examiner succeed in his goal. Be courteous and professional at all times.

14. Some examiners may appear to be exceptionally concerned, friendly, and understanding. In some instances this is a ploy designed to obtain more from you than you are willing to give. The examiner is not your buddy. During the deposition the examiner will probably be sizing you up in terms of where your weak spots are as a witness on the stand. Therefore, you should be cordial but not overly friendly or anxious to please. If you are there to impress the examiner with anything, it is your credibility and self-confidence as a witness.

15. At some point in the deposition the examiner may attempt to summarize what you have said. Listen carefully to what he says when he is supposedly paraphrasing your testimony. Do not let him put words in your mouth. If what he is saying is not what you meant to say, do not hesitate to say so. Also, be aware of the fact that you can have any portion of your testimony read back to you at your request.

The importance of the deposition cannot be overemphasized. However, you should remember that it is only a deposition and not the trial itself. Not all of the facts may come out during a deposition, and certain examiners will hear only what they want to. You will have the opportunity to remedy any misinterpretations the examiner has made when he examines you at the trial and when your own attorney cross-examines.

At the Trial

Experienced trial lawyers will tell you that the skills necessary to be an impressive trial witness are somewhat different from those needed to be a successful examinee at a deposition. Perhaps the primary difference is that *appearances* count so much more in court than they do in the deposition room. For example, when you are giving your deposition, it is not crucially important that you impress the examiner with your candor. Many attorneys specifically encourage their clients to be guarded in their responses (i.e., pause before answering each question, speak slowly, etc.) to the examiner at the deposition. However, candor on the courtroom witness stand—or at least the appearance thereof—is looked upon quite favorably by judges or juries. Conversely, responses that are consistently guarded, highly qualified, or roundabout will not win friends and influence jurors. This point has been made elsewhere:

> Juries determine facts both by what is said and by the manner in which it is said. As soon as a person takes the witness stand, the jurors . . . begin to formulate impressions on his credibility. There are many factors underlying these impressions:
>
> - whether the witness answers promptly or hesitates;
> - whether he exaggerates;
> - whether he is overbearing;
> - whether he appears insincere;
> - whether he is crude; and
> - whether he is obviously prejudiced toward one side.
>
> In addition, juries judge a witness by his physical appearance. (US News and World Report Books, 1973, pp. 26–27)

Generally, your testimony should be kept as objective as possible and as grounded in sound psychological theory and research as you can make it. If you are asked a question to which you honestly do not know the answer, the courtroom is not the place to attempt a guess. Rather, a candid, "I don't know" with an appropriate qualifier (e.g., "The question presupposes a knowledge of psychoanalytic theory and my training was in behavior therapy") is to be preferred. Admitting your limitations and conceding what you do not know can be as important as impressing the court with what you do know. If your answers stray too far from your area of expertise, the opposing attorney may sense your weakness and zoom in on it to expose you.

To be able to be as candid as possible, you should discuss with your attorney the difference between what constitutes "reasonable" error and what constitutes legal liability. Barring decisions such as that made in the case of *Helling* (6.30) you will not be held liable for engaging in practices that are usual and customary in terms of the standard of the profession. However, the court will take a dim view of candid admissions of legal liability. When testifying in court, unlike making a deposition, you may want to volunteer anecdotal material to bolster a point you wish to make. Do so only with the prior approval of counsel and be sure that the material speaks to the point you wish to make. The idea is to impress the trier of fact with your candor and sincerity, not your talent as a storyteller.

Needless to say, you will be under oath at the trial, and everything you say must be what you honestly believe to be true. Qualifiers such as "my best recollection" may be used as needed. But it is best to try to enter the courtroom with an overlearned familiarity with the details of the case. If there are references in the psychological literature germane to what will unravel in the courtroom, you should be familiar with them too. If it is possible to use these references in presenting your own defense, do so. The plaintiff's attorney may cite such references and ask you whether you agree or disagree with them. Most important, if *you* have written anything that touches on the matter to be debated in court, be certain that your testimony does not contradict your published opinion (or be prepared to tell why). Enter the courtroom having in your possession copies of all the pertinent records (e.g., consultant's notes, psychological test data, etc.). Finally, having discussed with your attorney all aspects of the case (including any and all "sensitive" areas) that are likely to come up at the trial, you should know what information to volunteer and what not to volunteer. Your preparedness to testify in court may reflect somewhat on the judge's and jury's perception of your preparedness to render treatment.

Many mental health professionals, to their detriment, make what might be termed "What's–wrong–with–that? (WWT)" errors in their court testimony. When a supposedly revealing statement about a patient's pathology compels the majority of the jury to ask themselves, "What's wrong with that?" a WWT error has been made. For example, suppose "Mr. Citizen," the patient, is forcibly taken from his home by the police, handcuffed, and packed into a police car in full view of his friends and neighbors. And suppose "Dr. Smith," a psychiatrist, testifies that the patient was verbally abusive and hostile to the therapist on admission. Jury members are likely to ask themselves, "What's wrong with that? Who wouldn't be verbally abusive and hostile under such conditions?" This is especially true if Mr. Citizen appears to be composed and "normal" in the courtroom. Smith may compound his WWT error by going on to say something like, "Further, Mr. Citizen denied that he was mentally ill." Again, jury members—who are more likely to identify with a patient than a psychiatrist—are likely to ask themselves, "What's wrong with that? I would deny it under the same circumstances." To weaken his testimony still further, Smith might testify that the patient's denial of mental illness demonstrated lack of insight, which was evidence of mental illness. Although all of Smith's statements might make sense to experienced mental health professionals, they will probably not make much sense to the lay people of the jury. WWT errors can be avoided with some forethought, factual documentation, and practice in presenting professional opinion to lay audiences.

Trial lawyers are experts at calming down or riling up witnesses. As in the deposition, you may run across an attorney whose *modus operandi* includes an attempt to irritate you or make you so defensive that you become careless and say something that you really would have preferred not to say. When any health professional loses his composure on the stand, it does not look good for him. When a mental health professional loses his composure on the stand it probably looks all the worse. This is so because judges and juries, like much of the public at large, may harbor unrealistically high expectations about how those in the mental health profession should look and carry themselves (cf. Cohen, Note 1). A popular expectation, for example, has it that one must be "together himself" before one can treat others.[4] At any rate, be prepared to deal with the attorney who is out to rattle you, and guard against having your composure or your professional demeanor shaken.

After the Trial

If the trial court's decision is not to your liking, the case can, on the advice of your attorney, be appealed to a higher court. Another course of action open to a defendant doctor at any time from the initiation of litigation is a countersuit. In one Illinois case, a patient filed a malpractice action against a radiologist claiming that the radiologist improperly administered x-rays and failed to detect a fracture in her hand. The patient claimed that the radiologist's negligence had led to her hand becoming "permanently disabled." The radiologist admitted that the fracture was not revealed in the x-rays taken under his supervision, but he argued that the plaintiff received the same care that she would have gotten if the x-ray had revealed the fracture. He then filed a countersuit charging that the plaintiff had "wantonly and willfully" involved him in litigation without reasonable cause and that the standards of the lawyers who accepted the case were "below the legal standards of the community" because they had failed to investigate the case properly. Both cases were to be heard simul-

---

[4]As discussed in detail elsewhere (Cohen, Note 1), the "together himself" expectation paradoxically coexists with another popular fallacy that "you have to be a little crazy yourself to go into that field."

taneously by the same judge, though the woman who had brought suit against the doctor withdrew her claim before the trial date. The doctor decided to go ahead with his suit against the patient and her attorneys. The jury found in the doctor's favor, and after only fifteen minutes of deliberation awarded him $2,000 in compensatory damages and $6,000 in punitive damages ("Illinois Doctor," 1976).

Another kind of successful countersuit involved a plaintiff neurosurgeon who brought suit against the defense attorney who had defended him some years before in a malpractice suit that had been brought against himself and another doctor (an orthopedist). Both the orthopedist and the neurosurgeon had been represented by the same defense attorney, and they had been found to be liable for damages in the amount of $400,000. The neurosurgeon's malpractice suit against his defense attorney alleged that had the defense been more vigorous, only the orthopedist would have had to pay damages to the plaintiff. The suit was successful, and the court awarded the neurosurgeon $130,000 in damages (case cited in *Legal Aspects of Medical Practice*, March 1978, pp. 4–5).

After cardiologist Sidney Burness prevailed in what he viewed as a frivolous malpractice action against him, he considered the possibility of a countersuit against the attorneys for the plaintiff who had sued him. As related by Rosenberg (1978), the doctor was reluctant to enter the legal arena again but felt compelled to do so:

> Scorched as he was by his recent legal experience, Burness was wary about jumping into the fire all over again. What finally persuaded him to take the plunge, he says, was that "nobody, not even our prestigious professional organizations, seemed to be doing anything about the malpractice situation, which was lousy for doctors all over the country. I figured it was time that *somebody* showed turkey lawyers they can't get away with this forever." (p. 36)

A complaint against the attorneys claiming legal malpractice, malicious prosecution, malicious misuse of process, and $2 million in damages was filed. After pretrial discovery proceedings the defendant attorneys sought to settle with an "offer of judgment"[5] in the amount of $15,000. A settlement was made for $15,000 plus court costs.

Like Dr. Burness, many doctors may be angered by "turkey lawyers" (p. 36) who litigate frivolously. However, anger and a desire for vengence are very poor reasons for initiating counterlitigation. In his complaint, Burness had charged the defendant attorneys with not conducting an investigation concerning the alleged negligence, a charge that was supported by statements made by one of the defendant attorneys in a pretrial deposition. The point here is that Burness had a strong case against the

---

[5]This specialized form of plea is legal in the State of Florida as well as in other states.

defendant attorneys—not simply anger. *The countersuit was not filed frivolously.*

Before considering the initiation of a countersuit you should be aware that there are very serious risks involved in doing so (cf. Reilly, 1977; Lavin, 1978). Countersuits can be costly (many lawyers will not accept one on a contingency basis), and their initiation may make you liable for still another suit. Specifically, if you claim that an attorney was negligent in not properly investigating the merits of a case before accepting it, you are making a very serious charge which you had better be able to document with "hard" evidence.

The deterrent value of a countersuit alleging defamation, barratry, or abuse of the process of law must be weighed against the potentially considerable expenditure of time and money that such suits are likely to incur. You and your lawyer will have to carefully weigh the amount and quality of the evidence on which you will base your countersuit. For example, you will have to ask yourself whether you have enough evidence to legally prove that there was "malevolent intent" on the part of the party who initiated the litigation. Documenting such intent, along with the other elements of proof that will be necessary for your countersuit to succeed, may be no easy matter.

Another course of action open to the professional who feels that he is the victim of frivolous litigation is to write the county bar association to which the plaintiff's attorney belongs, charging that the lawyer violated his profession's code of ethics by accepting the case.[6] Such a letter should be accompanied by all of the evidence and documentation available to justify the rather serious charge that the lawyer for the plaintiff knew or should have known that the charges lodged against the defendant were unfounded, frivolous, or filed in bad faith. Of course, the writing of such a letter should be done only at the advice of an attorney—otherwise, the letter itself may become grounds for a countersuit by the plaintiff's attorney, who may charge character defamation.

Some jurisdictions make provision for persons who are victims of frivolous litigation to recover the cost of defending themselves in that litigation. Within some time period (e.g., thirty days) after the verdict is handed down, the defendant in the action may request the court to assess court costs and attorney fees. Exactly how much you will recover from the plaintiff for defense costs (if indeed you will recover anything at all) may be totally at the discretion of the trial judge. Your attorney will be able to tell you if your state makes provision for recovering defense costs and if a motion for recovery of these costs is advisable in your case.

---

[6]The would-be letter writer is also encouraged to read an article entitled "Our Irresponsible Bar Associations" by internist Philip Alper (1978), in order to prepare himself for the potentially disappointing and frustrating consequences of that letter.

HAS AN ILL WIND BLOWN GOOD?

One of the Stanford–Binet Intelligence Scale proverbs used to determine if a person is a "Superior Adult III" is "It's an ill wind that blows nobody good" (Terman and Merrill, 1960, p. 119). To obtain full credit for interpreting the meaning of the proverb correctly, the respondent must say something to the effect that "someone usually benefits even by a calamity which brings general misfortune." At this juncture in our study of malpractice and the mental health profession, it seems appropriate to ask if the "ill wind" of the increasingly litigious society has "blown anybody good." Specifically, has anything beneficial to the profession or to society as a whole emerged from an atmosphere in which lay people are predisposed to litigate and professionals have heightened defenses to such litigation? The answer, I would suggest, is yes.

The malpractice crisis has prompted critical examination of the legal theory of negligence as that theory applies to medical malpractice litigation. Scholarly analyses of the role of the law in the maintenance of quality health care have been written as the result of individual and collaborative efforts of concerned lawyers, legislators, and health professionals (e.g., Epstein, 1976; Schwartz and Komesar, 1978). Many reports on the subject of malpractice in professional journals and the popular media have been helpful in acquainting both professionals and patients with their legal rights and obligations.

In an article entitled "The Implications of Malpractice Suits," Middleton (1970) argued that one of the positive effects of the litigious atmosphere of our day was that patients were now much better informed than ever before and were much more active participants in the health care they receive. Additionally, health professionals have been prompted to question their own competency to do the things they are licensed to do. The prevailing atmosphere has, perhaps, pushed more private practitioners to attend professional meetings than ever before and has "forced us into a greater realization of our responsibilities as professional people" (Middleton, 1970, p. 79). Beyond the effect the current state of affairs has had on the popularity of continuing education, Middleton cited still another advantage:

> Certainly, malpractice has been a boon to preventive medicine. Today, I can say to my patient, "I suggest and advise you to have a certain series of x-rays." She says, "Well, doctor, I can't afford it; I don't want to do it." I could say, "Okay, I can only advise you; you have to do it; you have to make an effort; I will make the arrangements." And she may say, "Well, I don't want to do this." Again I say, "Well, I will write it down here in the note, and if something happens six months from now, you can't come back and say I didn't warn you." This causes many people to take the care which they would otherwise not take, because

frequently when it becomes the patient's responsibility, he will accept it. We are no longer the father figures of the past. (p. 79)

Doctors have traditionally been somewhat reluctant to testify against other doctors. Not only do they fear possible reprisals from the other doctors or their friends or insurance company, but preparing for courtroom testimony takes time from their own day-to-day schedules. Accompanying the medical malpractice crisis has been a heightened need for expert witnesses and, perhaps, an increase in the number of health professionals who are willing to compromise themselves as "professional witnesses":

> When good doctors shun the courtroom, they create a vacuum on the witness stand, and professional witnesses quickly fill it. Few of the physicians come forward because they want to see justice done in cases of medical negligence. They are simply ready, willing, and eager to harpoon another doctor for the right price.
>
> They attend all the trial lawyers' conventions, where they are to be found caucusing in the corridors. They write "medical" articles in legal journals, and they register with agencies that run ads in the very same journals offering to supply medical experts for lawyers. Reviewing cases is a sizable part of their income, and testifying for the plaintiff an even greater part. They conceal their financial arrangements with the plaintiff to the point of testifying under oath that they have not discussed a fee, or that they will bill at a reasonable hourly rate, when we all know that the agency firms up the deal before they open their mouths.
>
> The worst of it is that they don't come to court to testify dispassionately and honestly. They come to say whatever has to be said to get the plaintiff's case to a jury. (Griffith, 1978, pp. 87–88)

It is possible that the malpractice crisis, with its proliferation of "professional witnesses," might have the positive effect of motivating reputable doctors to become involved in litigation. And if doctors do not begin to come forward from a sense of what is ethically proper, they may be legally compelled to do so. The new Federal Rules of Evidence contains a rule that provides for the court's appointment of impartial experts (Fed. R. Evid. 706), a rule that already has a counterpart in some states. Even if the malpractice crisis subsides, once doctors are no longer ostracized by other doctors for testifying—are even encouraged to testify—against colleagues, the days of the "professional witness" will be numbered. The demise of the professional witness could potentially bring with it fairer trials, more accurate expert input into matters concerning what constitutes standard and substandard practice, and a lasting reduction in the number of unjustified suits brought. As doctors become more involved in litigation there may also be a rise in public trust and confidence in the medical profession:

The more that doctors try to keep colleagues from testifying, the more they pump up public distrust. If people become convinced that medicine is out to deny expert witnesses to the plaintiff, then why believe the medical witnesses the defendant himself calls? The only way to win credibility is to stand up and be counted when you see a patient who's been injured through what you believe to be the neglect of a colleague. (Griffith, 1978, pp. 90; 95)

The malpractice pall has probably encouraged mental health professionals to ask more questions than ever before about themselves and their modes of treatment. The malpractice pall has motivated psychologists, psychiatrists, social workers and other mental health professionals to better educate themselves with respect to the legal/ethical issues attendant to professional practice. It is unfortunate that this unprecedented degree of "professional soul searching" had to be precipitated by a malpractice crisis, but professionals and lay people alike can share the hope that the result will be both immediate and long-term benefits to those under the care of mental health professionals.

One group that the "ill wind" of rapidly increasing malpractice litigation has most conspicuously profited is an organization of lawyers called the Inner Circle of Advocates. To qualify for membership in the Inner Circle, a lawyer must have won a jury settlement in a personal injury suit of one million dollars or more. The organization was founded in 1972, and by mid-1976, seventy-two attorneys had qualified for membership (*Time*, May 31, 1976, p. 45). By continuing to serve their patients in the best traditions of their professions and by keeping abreast of current legal/ethical developments and issues, mental health professionals will be doing their part to keep membership in the Inner Circle very exclusive.

Appendix: *Tarasoff v. Regents of University of California*

MAJORITY AND DISSENTING OPINIONS*

Justice Tobriner (for the majority):

On October 27, 1969, Prosenjit Poddar killed Tatiana Tarasoff.[1] Plaintiffs, Tatiana's parents, allege that two months earlier Poddar confided his intention to kill Tatiana to Dr. Lawrence Moore, a psychologist employed by the Cowell Memorial Hospital at the University of California at Berkeley. They allege that on Moore's request, the campus police briefly detained Poddar, but released him when he appeared rational. They further claim that Dr. Harvey Powelson, Moore's superior, then directed that no further action be taken to detain Poddar. No one warned Tatiana of her peril.

Concluding that these facts neither set forth causes of action against the therapists and policemen involved, nor against the Regents of the University of California as their employer, the superior court sustained defendants' demurrers to plaintiffs' second amended complaints without leave to amend.[2] This appeal ensued.

---

*Excerpted from *Tarasoff v. Regents of University of California*, 529 P.2d 553.

[1]The criminal prosecution stemming from this crime is reported in People v. Poddar (1974) 10 Cal.3d 750, 111 Cal.Rptr. 910, 518 P.2d 342.

[2]The therapist defendants include Dr. Moore, the psychologist who examined Poddar and decided that Poddar should be committed; Dr. Gold and Dr. Yandell, psychiatrists at Cowell Memorial Hospital who concurred in Moore's decision; and Dr. Powelson, chief of the department of psychiatry, who countermanded Moore's decision and directed that the staff take no action to confine Poddar. The police defendants include Officers Atkinson, Brownrigg and Halleran, who detained Poddar briefly but released him; Chief Beall, who received Moore's letter recommending that Poddar be confined; and Officer Teel, who, along with Officer Atkinson, received Moore's oral communication requesting detention of Poddar.

Plaintiffs' complaints predicate liability on two grounds: defendants' failure to warn plaintiffs of the impending danger and their failure to use reasonable care to bring about Poddar's confinement pursuant to the Lanterman-Petris-Short Act (Welf. & Inst.Code, § 5000ff.) Defendants, in turn, assert that they owed no duty of reasonable care to Tatiana and that they are immune from suit under the California Tort Claims Act of 1963 (Gov. Code, § 810 ff.).

We shall explain that defendant therapists, merely because Tatiana herself was not their patient, cannot escape liability for failing to exercise due care to warn the endangered Tatiana or those who reasonably could have been expected to notify her of her peril. When a doctor or a psychotherapist, in the exercise of his professional skill and knowledge, determines, or should determine, that a warning is essential to avert danger arising from the medical or psychological condition of his patient, he incurs a legal obligation to give that warning. Primarily, the relationship between defendant therapists and Poddar as their patient imposes the described duty to warn. We shall point out that a second basis for liability lies in the fact that defendants' bungled attempt to confine Poddar may have deterred him from seeking further therapy and aggravated the danger to Tatiana; having thus contributed to and partially created the danger, defendants incur the ensuing obligation to give the warning.

We reject defendants' asserted defense of governmental immunity; no specific statutory provision shields them from liability for failure to warn, and Government Code section 820.2 does not protect defendants' conduct as an exercise of discretion. We conclude that plaintiffs' complaints state, or can be amended to state, a cause of action against defendants for negligent failure to warn.

Defendants, however, may properly claim immunity from liability for their failure to *confine* Poddar. Government Code section 856 bars imposition of liability upon defendant therapists for their determination to refrain from detaining Poddar and Welfare and Institutions Code section 5154 protects defendant police officers from civil liability for releasing Poddar after his brief confinement. We therefore conclude that plaintiffs cannot state a cause of action for defendants' failure to detain Poddar. Since plaintiffs base their claim to punitive damages against defendant Powelson solely upon Powelson's failure to bring about such detention, not upon Powelson's failure to give the above described warnings, that claim likewise fails to state a cause of action.

1. *Plaintiffs' complaints*

[1] Plaintiffs, Tatiana's mother and father, filed separate but virtually identical second amended complaints. The issue before us on this appeal is whether those complaints now state, or can be amended to state,

causes of action against defendants. We therefore begin by setting forth the pertinent allegations of the complaints.[3]

Plaintiffs' first cause of action, entitled "Failure to Detain a Dangerous Patient," alleges that on August 20, 1969, Poddar was a voluntary outpatient receiving therapy at Cowell Memorial Hospital. Poddar informed Moore, his therapist, that he was going to kill an unnamed girl, readily identifiable as Tatiana, when she returned home from spending the summer in Brazil. Moore, with the concurrence of Dr. Gold, who had initially examined Poddar, and Dr. Yandell, assistant to the director of the department of psychiatry, decided that Poddar should be committed for observation in a mental hospital. Moore orally notified Officers Atkinson and Teel of the campus police that he would request commitment. He then sent a letter to Police Chief William Beall requesting the assistance of the police department in securing Poddar's confinement.

Officers Atkinson, Brownrigg, and Halleran took Poddar into custody, but, satisfied that Poddar was rational, released him on his promise to stay away from Tatiana. Powelson, director of the department of psychiatry at Cowell Memorial Hospital, then asked the police to return Moore's letter, directed that all copies of the letter and notes that Moore had taken as therapist be destroyed, and "ordered no action to place Prosenjit Poddar in 72-hour treatment and evaluation facility."

Plaintiffs' second cause of action, entitled "Failure to Warn On a Dangerous Patient," incorporates the allegations of the first cause of action, but adds the assertion that defendants negligently permitted Poddar to be released from police custody without "notifying the parents of Tatiana Tarasoff that their daughter was in grave danger from Posenjit Poddar." Poddar persuaded Tatiana's brother to share an apartment with him near Tatiana's residence; shortly after her return from Brazil, Poddar went to her residence and killed her.

Plaintiffs' third cause of action, entitled "Abandonment of a Dangerous Patient," seeks $10,000 punitive damages against defendant Powelson. Incorporating the crucial allegations of the first cause of action, plaintiffs charge that Powelson "did the things herein alleged with intent

---

[3]Plaintiffs' complaints allege that defendants failed to warn Tatiana's parents of the danger to Tatiana from Poddar. The complaints do not specifically state whether defendants warned Tatiana herself. Such an omission can properly be cured by amendment. As we stated in Minsky v. City of Los Angeles: "It is axiomatic that if there is a reasonable possibility that a defect in the complaint can be cured by amendment or that the pleading liberally construed can state a cause of action, a demurrer should not be sustained without leave to amend. (3 Witkin, Cal.Procedure, Pleading, § 844, p. 2449; accord La Sala v. American Sav. & Loan Assn. (1971), 5 Cal.3d 864, 876, 97 Cal. Rptr. 849, 489 P.2d 1113; Lemoge Electric v. County of San Mateo (1956) 46 Cal.2d 659, 664, 297 P.2d 638; Beckstead v. Superior Court (1971) 21 Cal.App.3d 780, 782, 98 Cal.Rptr. 779.) We believe a cause of action has been stated here." (11 Cal.3d 113, 118–119, 113 Cal.Rptr. 102, 107, 520 P.2d 726, 731).

to abandon a dangerous patient, and said acts were done maliciously and oppressively."

Plaintiff's fourth cause of action, for "Breach of Primary Duty to Patient and the Public" states essentially the same allegations as the first cause of action, but seeks to characterize defendants' conduct as a breach of duty to safeguard their patient and the public. Since such conclusory labels add nothing to the factual allegations of the complaint, the first and fourth causes of action are legally indistinguishable.

2. Plaintiffs can state a cause of action for negligent failure to warn

The second cause of action in plaintiffs' complaints alleges that Tatiana's death proximately resulted from defendants' negligent failure to warn plaintiffs of Poddar's intention to kill Tatiana and claims general and special damages. Ordinarily such allegations of negligence, proximate causation, and damages would establish a cause of action. (See Dillon v. Legg (1968) 68 Cal.2d 728, 733–734, 69 Cal.Rptr. 72, 441 P.2d 912.) Defendants, however, contend that in the circumstances of the present case they owed no duty of care to Tatiana or her parents and that, in the absence of such duty, they were free to act in careless disregard of Tatiana's life and safety.

In analyzing this contention, we bear in mind that legal duties are not discoverable facts of nature, but merely conclusory expressions that, in cases of a particular type, liability should be imposed for damage done. As stated in Dillon v. Legg, *supra*, at page 734, 69 Cal.Rptr. at page 76, 441 P.2d at page 916: "The assertion that liability must . . . be denied because defendant bears no 'duty' to plaintiff 'begs the essential question— whether the plaintiff's interests are entitled to legal protection against the defendant's conduct. . . . [Duty] is not sacrosanct in itself, but only an expression of the sum total of those considerations of policy which lead the law to say that the particular plaintiff is entitled to protection.' (Prosser, Law of Torts [3d ed. 1964] at pp. 332–333.)" Rowland v. Christian (1968) 69 Cal.2d 108, 113, 70 Cal.Rptr. 97, 100, 443 P.2d 561, 564, listed the principal considerations: "the foreseeability of harm to the plaintiff, the degree of certainty that the plaintiff suffered injury, the closeness of the connection between the defendant's conduct and the injury suffered, the moral blame attached to the defendant's conduct, the policy of preventing future harm, the extent of the burden to the defendant and consequences to the community of imposing a duty to exercise care with resulting liability for breach, and the availability, cost, and prevalence of insurance for the risk involved."[4]

Although under the common law, as a general rule, one person owed

---

[4]See Merrill v. Buck (1962) 58 Cal.2d 552, 562, 25 Cal.Rptr. 456, 375 P.2d 304; Biakanja v. Irving (1958) 49 Cal.2d 647, 650, 320 P.2d 16; Walnut Creek Aggregates Co. v. Testing Engineers Inc. (1967) 248 Cal.App.2d 690, 695, 56 Cal.Rptr. 700.

no duty to control the conduct of another[5] (Richards v. Stanley (1954) 43 Cal.2d 60, 65, 271 P.2d 23; Wright v. Arcade School Dist. (1964) 230 Cal.App.2d 272, 277, 40 Cal.Rptr. 812; Rest.2d Torts (1965) 315), nor to warn those endangered by such conduct (Rest.2d Torts, supra, § 314, com. c; Prosser, Law of Torts (4th ed. 1971) § 56, p. 341), the courts have noted exceptions to this rule. In two classes of cases the courts have imposed a duty of care: (1) cases in which the defendant stands in some special relationship to either the person whose conduct needs to be controlled or in a relationship to the foreseeable victim of that conduct (see Rest.2d Torts, *supra*, §§ 315–320); and (2) cases in which the defendant has engaged, or undertaken to engage, in affirmative action to control the anticipated dangerous conduct or protect the prospective victim. (See Rest.2d Torts, *supra*, §§ 321–324a.)[6] Both exceptions apply to the facts of this case.

Turning, first, to the special relationships present in this case, we note that a relationship of defendant therapists to either Tatiana or to

[5]This rule derives from the common law's distinction between misfeasance and nonfeasance, and its reluctance to impose liability for the latter. (See Harper & Kime, The Duty to Control the Conduct of Another (1934) 43 Yale L.J. 886, 887.) Morally questionable, the rule owes its survival to "the difficulties of setting any standards of unselfish service to fellow men, and of making any workable rule to cover possible situations where fifty people might fail to rescue. . . ." (Prosser, Torts (4th ed. 1971) § 56, p. 341.) Because of these practical difficulties, the courts have increased the number of instances in which affirmative duties are imposed not by direct rejection of the common-law rule, but by expanding the list of special relationships which will justify departure from that rule. (See Prosser, *supra*, § 56; at pp. 348–350.)

[6]A line of cases discussing the liability of a defendant who negligently provides an instrumentality by which a third person injures the plaintiff presents issues similar to the present case, although distinguishable in that such cases require the defendant only to take reasonable precautions to safeguard his own property. In Richards v. Stanley (1954) 43 Cal.2d 60, 271, P.2d 23, defendant left the ignition keys in her car; a thief stole the car and, driving negligently, injured the plaintiff. Relying on the rule that "Ordinarily, . . . in the absence of a special relationship between the parties, there is no duty to control the conduct of a third person so as to prevent him from causing harm to another" (43 Cal.2d at p. 65, 271 P.2d at p. 27), the court affirmed a judgment for defendant. A year later, however, in Richardson v. Ham (1955) 44 Cal.2d 772, 285 P.2d 269, the court held that defendants who left a bulldozer unlocked could be held liable for damage caused after trespassers started the vehicle and then abandoned it to run amuck. Distinguishing Richards v. Stanley, the court stated that the "extreme danger created by a bulldozer in uncontrolled motion and the foreseeable risk of intermeddling fully justify imposing a duty on the owner to exercise reasonable care to protect third parties from injuries arising from its operation by intermeddlers." (44 Cal.2d at p. 776, 285 P.2d at p. 271.) In Hergenrether v. East (1964) 61 Cal.2d 440, 39 Cal.Rptr. 4, 393 P.2d 164, the court further limited the scope of Richards v. Stanley, and imposed liability upon a defendant, who parked his truck in a "skid row" area with the ignition keys in the truck, for damages caused by the reckless driving of a thief. Again the court distinguished *Richards* on the ground that "[S]pecial circumstances which impose a greater potentiality of foreseeable risk of more serious injury, or require a lesser burden of preventative action, may be deemed to impose an unreasonable risk on, and a legal duty to, third persons." (61 Cal.2d at p. 444, 39 Cal.Rptr. at p. 6, 393 P.2d at p. 166.) The cases thus exemplify an evolution from a rule of "no duty" to a rule in which imposition of a duty of care depends upon the foreseeability of serious injury and the burden of precautions. (See Schwartz v. Helms Bakery Limited (1967) 67 Cal.2d 232, 240–242, 60 Cal.Rptr. 510, 430 P.2d 68.)

Poddar will suffice to establish a duty of care; as explained in section 315 of the Restatement Second of Torts, a duty of care may arise from either "(a) a special relation... between the actor and the third person which imposes a duty upon the actor to control the third person's conduct, or (b) a special relation... between the actor and the other which gives to the other a right to protection."

[2] Although plaintiffs' pleadings assert no special relation between Tatiana and defendant therapists, they establish as between Poddar and defendant therapists the special relation that arises between a patient and his doctor or psychotherapist.[7] Such a relationship may support affirmative duties for the benefit of third persons. (See Fleming & Maximov, The Patient or His Victim: The Therapist's Dilemma (1974) 62 Cal.L.Rev. 1025, 1027–1032.) Thus, for example, a hospital must exercise reasonable care to control the behavior of a patient which may endanger other persons.[8] A doctor must also warn a patient if the patient's condition or medication renders certain conduct, such as driving a car, dangerous to others.[9]

Although the California decisions that recognize this duty have involved cases in which the defendant stood in a special relationship *both* to the victim and to the person whose conduct created the danger,[10] we do not think that the duty should logically be constricted to such situations. Decisions of other jurisdictions hold that the single relationship of a doctor to his patient is sufficient to support the duty to use reasonable care to

---

[7]The pleadings establish the requisite relationship between Poddar and both Dr. Moore, the psychotherapist who treated Poddar, and Dr. Powelson, who supervised that treatment. Plaintiffs also allege that Dr. Gold personally examined Poddar, and that Dr. Yandell, as Powelson's assistant, approved the decision to arrange Poddar's commitment. These allegations are sufficient to raise the issue whether a doctor-patient or psychotherapist-patient relationship, giving rise to a possible duty by the doctor or therapist reasonably to warn threatened persons of danger arising from the patient's mental illness, existed between Gold or Yandell and Poddar. (See Harney, Medical Malpractice (1973) p. 7.)

[8]When a "hospital has notice or knowledge of facts from which it might reasonably be concluded that a patient would be likely to harm himself *or others* unless preclusive measures were taken, then the hospital must use reasonable care in the circumstances to prevent such harm." (Vistica v. Presbyterian Hospital (1967) 67 Cal.2d 465, 469, 62 Cal. Rptr. 577, 580, 432 P.2d 193, 196.) (Emphasis added.) A mental hospital may be liable if it negligently permits the escape or release of a dangerous patient (Underwood v. United States (5th Cir. 1966) 356 F.2d 92; Fair v. United States (5th Cir. 1956) 234 F.2d 288). Greenberg v. Barbour (E.D.Pa. 1971) 322 F. Supp. 745, upheld a cause of action against a hospital staff doctor whose negligent failure to admit a mental patient resulted in that patient assaulting the plaintiff.

[9]Kaiser v. Suburban Transp. System (1965) 65 Wash.2d 461, 398 P.2d 14, 401 P.2d 350; see Freese v. Lemmon (Iowa 1973) 210 N.W.2d 576 (concurring opinion of Uhlenhopp, J.)

[10]Ellis v. D'Angelo (1953) 116 Cal.App.2d 310, 253 P.2d 675, upheld a cause of action against parents who failed to warn a baby-sitter of the violent proclivities of their child; Johnson v. State of California (1968) 69 Cal.2d 782, 73 Cal.Rptr. 240, 447 P.2d 352, upheld a suit against the state for failure to warn foster parents of the dangerous tendencies of their ward; Morgan v. County of Yuba (1964) 230 Cal.App.2d 938, 41 Cal.Rptr. 508, sustained a cause of action against a sheriff who had promised to warn decedent before releasing a dangerous prisoner, but failed to do so.

warn of dangers emanating from the patient's illness. The courts hold that a doctor is liable to persons infected by his patient if he negligently fails to diagnose a contagious disease (Hofmann v. Blackmon (Fla.App.1970) 241 So.2d 752), or, having diagnosed the illness, fails to warn members of the patient's family (Wojcik v. Aluminum Co. of America (1959) 18 Misc.2d 740, 183 N.Y.S.2d 351, 357–358; Davis v. Rodman (1921) 147 Ark. 385, 227 S.W. 612; Skillings v. Allen (1919) 143 Minn. 323, 173 N.W. 663; see also Jones v. Stanko (1938) 118 Ohio St. 147, 160 N.E. 456.)

More closely on point, since it involved a dangerous mental patient, is the decision in Merchants Nat. Bank & Trust Co. of Fargo v. United States (D.N.D.1967) 272 F.Supp. 409. The Veterans Administration arranged for the patient to work on a local farm, but did not warn the farmer of the man's background. The farmer consequently permitted the patient to come and go freely during nonworking hours, the patient borrowed a car, drove to his wife's residence and killed her. Notwithstanding the lack of any "special relationship" between the Veterans Administration and the wife, the court found the Veterans Administration liable for the wrongful death of the wife.

[3] As the present case illustrates, a patient with severe mental illness and dangerous proclivities may, in a given case, present a danger as serious and as foreseeable as does the carrier of a contagious disease or the driver whose condition or medication affects his ability to drive safely. We conclude that a doctor or a psychotherapist treating a mentally ill patient, just as a doctor treating physical illness, bears a duty to use reasonable care to give threatened persons such warnings as are essential to avert foreseeable danger arising from his patient's condition or treatment.

[4] As we stated previously, a duty to warn may also arise from a voluntary act or undertaking by a defendant. Once the defendant has commenced to render service, he must employ reasonable care; if reasonable care requires the giving of warnings, he must do so. Numerous cases hold that if a defendant's prior conduct has created or contributed to a danger, even if that conduct itself is non-negligent or protected by government immunity, the defendant bears a duty to warn affected persons of such impending danger. (See Johnson v. State of California (1968) 69 Cal.2d 782, 796–797, 73 Cal.Rptr. 240, 447 P.2d 352, and cases there cited; Rest.2d Torts, supra, § 321 and illus. to com. (a), § 323 and com. (c).)

The record in People v. Poddar (1974) 10 Cal.3d 750, 111 Cal.Rptr. 910, 518 P.2d 342 indicates, and plaintiffs' complaints could be amended to assert, that following Poddar's encounter with the police, Poddar broke off all contact with the hospital staff and discontinued psychotherapy. From those facts one could reasonably infer that defendants' actions led Poddar to halt treatment which, if carried through, might have led him to abandon his plan to kill Tatiana, and thus that defendants, having contributed to the danger, bear a duty to give warning.

Defendant therapists advance two policy considerations which, they suggest, justify a refusal to impose a duty upon a psychotherapist to warn third parties of danger arising from the violent intentions of his patient. We explain why, in our view, such considerations do not preclude imposition of the duty in question.

First, defendants point out that although therapy patients often express thoughts of violence, they rarely carry out these ideas. Indeed the open and confidential character of psychotherapeutic dialogue encourages patients to voice such thoughts, not as a device to reveal hidden danger, but as part of the process of therapy. Certainly a therapist should not be encouraged routinely to reveal such threats to acquaintances of the patient; such disclosures could seriously disrupt the patient's relationship with his therapist and with the persons threatened. In singling out those few patients whose threats of violence present a serious danger and in weighing against this danger the harm to the patient that might result from revelation, the psychotherapist renders a decision involving a high order of expertise and judgment.

[5] The judgment of the therapist, however, is no more delicate or demanding than the judgment which doctors and professionals must regularly render under accepted rules of responsibility. A professional person is required only to exercise "that reasonable degree of skill, knowledge, and care ordinarily possessed and exercised by members of [his] profession under similar circumstances." (Bardessono v. Michels (1970) 3 Cal.3d 780, 788, 91 Cal. Rptr. 760, 764, 478 P.2d 480, 484.) As a specialist, the psychotherapist, whether doctor or psychologist, would also be "held to that standard of learning and skill normally possessed by such specialist in the same or similar locality under the same or similar circumstances." (Quintal v. Laurel Grove Hospital (1964) 62 Cal.2d 154, 159-160, 41 Cal.Rptr. 577, 580, 397 P.2d 161, 164.) But within that broad range in which professional opinion and judgment may differ respecting the proper course of action, the psychotherapist is free to exercise his own best judgment free from liability; proof, aided by hindsight, that he judged wrongly is insufficient to establish liability.

In other words, the fact that a decision calls for considerable expert skill and judgment means, in effect, that it be tested by a standard of care which takes account of those circumstances; the standard used in measuring professional malpractice does so. But whatever difficulties the courts may encounter in evaluating the expert judgments of other professions, those difficulties cannot justify total exoneration from liability.

Second, defendants argue that free and open communication is essential to psychotherapy (see In re Lifschutz (1970) 2 Cal.3d 415, 431-432, 85 Cal.Rptr. 829, 467 P.2d 557); that "Unless a patient . . . is assured that . . . information [revealed by him] can and will be held in utmost confidence, he will be reluctant to make the full disclosure upon which diagnosis and treatment . . . depends." (Sen. Committee on the Judiciary, comments on Evid. Code, § 1014.) The giving of a warning, defendants contend, constitutes a breach of trust which entails the revelation of confidential communications.

We recognize the public interest in supporting effective treatment of mental illness and in protecting the rights of patients to privacy (see In re Lifschutz, *supra*, 2 Cal.3d at p. 432, 85 Cal.Rptr. 829, 467 P.2d 557), and the consequent public importance of safeguarding the confidential character of psychotherapeutic communication. Against this interest, however, we must weigh the public interest in safety from violent assault. The Legislature has undertaken the difficult task of balancing the countervailing concerns. In Evidence Code section 1014, it established a broad rule of privilege to protect confidential communications between patient and psychotherapist. In Evidence Code section 1024, however, the Legislature created a specific and limited exception to the psychotherapist-patient privilege: "There is no privilege ... if the psychotherapist has reasonable cause to believe that the patient is in such mental or emotional condition as to be dangerous to himself or to the person or property of another and that disclosure of the communication is necessary to prevent the threatened danger."[11]

[6] The revelation of a communication under the above circumstances is not a breach of trust or a violation of professional ethics; as stated in the Principles of Medical Ethics of the American Medical Association (1957) section 9: "A physician may not reveal the confidences entrusted to him in the course of medical attendance ... *unless he is required to do so by law or unless it becomes necessary in order to protect the welfare of the individual or of the community.*" (Emphasis added.) We conclude that the public policy favoring protection of the confidential character of patient-psychotherapist communications must yield in instances in which disclosure is essential to avert danger to others. The protective privilege ends where the public peril begins.

Our current crowded and computerized society compels the interdependence of its members. In this risk-infested society we can hardly tolerate the further exposure to danger that would result from a concealed knowledge of the therapist that his patient was lethal. If in the exercise of

---

[11]Fleming and Maximov note that "While [section 1024] supports the therapist's less controversial *right* to make a disclosure, it admittedly does not impose on him a *duty* to do so. But the argument does not have to be pressed that far. For if it is once conceded ... that a duty in favor of the patient's foreseeable victims would accord with general principles of tort liability, we need no longer look to the statute for a source of duty. It is sufficient if the statute can be relied upon ... for the purpose of countering the claim that the needs of confidentiality are paramount and must therefore defeat any such hypothetical duty. In this more modest perspective, the Evidence Code's 'dangerous patient' exception may be invoked with some confidence as a clear expression of legislative policy concerning the balance between the confidentiality values of the patient and the safety values of his foreseeable victims." (Emphasis in original.) Fleming & Maximov, The Patient or His Victim: The Therapist's Dilemma (1974) 62 Cal.L. Rev. 1025, 1063.

reasonable care the therapist can warn the endangered party or those who can reasonably be expected to notify him, we see no sufficient societal interest that would protect and justify concealment. The containment of such risks lies in the public interest.

[7, 8] For the foregoing reasons, we find that plaintiffs' complaints can be amended to state a cause of action against defendants Moore, Powelson, Gold, and Yandell and against the Regents as their employer, for breach of a duty to warn Tatiana arising from the relationship of these defendants to Poddar.[12] The complaints can also be amended to assert causes of action against the police defendants for failure to warn on the theory that the officers' conduct increased the risk of violence. The judgment of the superior court, sustaining defendants' demurrers without leave to amend must therefore be reversed.

3. Defendants are not immune from liability for failure to warn

We turn to the issue of whether defendants are protected by governmental immunity for having failed to warn Tatiana or those who reasonably could have been expected to notify her of her peril. We focus our analysis on section 820.2 of the Government Code.[13] That provision declares, with exceptions not applicable here, that "a public employee is not liable for an injury resulting from his act or omission where the act or omission was the result of the exercise of the discretion vested in him, whether or not such discretion [was] abused."[14]

Noting that virtually every public act admits of some element of discretion, we drew the line in Johnson v. State of California (1968) 69 Cal.2d 782, 73 Cal.Rptr. 240, 447 P.2d 352, between discretionary policy decisions which enjoy statutory immunity and ministerial administrative acts which do not. We concluded that section 820.2 affords immunity only for "*basic* policy decisions." (Emphasis added.) (See also Elton v. County of Orange (1970) 3 Cal.App.3d 1053, 1057–1058, 84 Cal.Rptr. 27; 4

---

[12]Moore argues that after Powelson countermanded the decision to seek commitment for Poddar, Moore was obliged to obey the decision of his superior and that he therefore should not be held liable for any dereliction arising from his obedience to superior orders. Plaintiffs in response argue that Moore's duty to members of the public endangered by Poddar should take precedence over his duty to obey Powelson. Since plaintiffs' complaints do not set out the date of Powelson's order,the specific terms of that order, or Powelson's authority to overrule Moore's decisions respecting patients under Moore's care, we lack sufficient factual background to adjudicate this conflict.

[13]No more specific immunity provision of the Government Code appears to address the issue.

[14]Section 815.2 of the Government Code declares that "[a] public entity is liable for injury proximately caused by an act or omission of an employee of the public entity within the scope of his employment if the act or omission would, apart from this section, have given rise to a cause of action against that employee or his personal representative." The section further provides, with exceptions not applicable here, that "a public entity is not liable for an injury resulting from an act or omission of an employee of the public entity where the employee is immune from liability." The Regents, therefore, are immune from liability only if all individual defendants are similarly immune.

Cal.Law Revision Com.Rep. (1963), p. 810; Van Alstyne, Supplement to Cal. Goverment Tort Liability (Cont.Ed.Bar 1969) § 5.54, pp. 16–17; Comment, California Tort Claims Act: Discretionary Immunity (1966) 39 So.Cal.L.Rev. 470, 471; cf. James, Tort Liability of Governmental Units and their Officers (1955) 22 U.Chi. L.Rev. 610, 637–638, 640, 642, 651.)

We also observed that if courts did not respect this statutory immunity, they would find themselves "in the unseemly position of determining the propriety of decisions expressly entrusted to a coordinate branch of government." (Johnson v. State of California, *supra*, 69 Cal.2d at p. 793, 73 Cal.Rptr. at p. 248, 447 P.2d at p. 360.) It therefore is necessary, we concluded, to "isolate those areas of quasi-legislative policy-making which are sufficiently sensitive to justify a blanket rule that courts will not entertain a tort action alleging that careless conduct contributed to the governmental decision." (Johnson v. State of California, *supra*, at p. 794, 73 Cal.Rptr. at p. 248, 447 P.2d at p. 360.) After careful analysis we rejected, in *Johnson*, other rationales commonly advanced to support governmental immunity,[15] and concluded that the immunity's scope should be no greater than is required to give legislative and executive policymakers sufficient breathing space in which to perform their vital policymaking functions.

[9] Relying on *Johnson*, we conclude that defendants in the present case are not immune from liability for their failure to warn of Tatiana's peril. *Johnson* held that a parole officer's determination whether to warn an adult couple that their prospective foster child had a background of violence "present[ed] no . . . reasons for immunity" (Johnson v. State of California, *supra*, at p. 795, 73 Cal.Rptr. 240, 447 P.2d 352), was "at the lowest, ministerial rung of official action" (*id.* at p. 794, 73 Cal.Rptr. at p. 250, 447 P.2d at p. 362), and indeed constituted "a classic case for the imposition of tort liability." *Id.*, p. 797, 73 Cal.Rptr. at p. 251, 447 P.2d at p. 363; cf. Morgan v. County of Yuba (1964) 230 Cal.App.2d 938, 942–943, 41 Cal.Rptr. 508.) Although defendants in *Johnson* argued that the decision whether to inform the foster parents of the child's background required the exercise of considerable judgmental skills, we concluded that the state was not immune from liability for the parole officer's failure to warn because such a decision did not rise to the level of a "basic policy decision."

---

[15]We dismissed, in *Johnson*, the view that immunity continues to be necessary in order to insure that public employees will be sufficiently zealous in the performance of their official duties. The California Tort Claims Act of 1963 provides for indemnification of public employees against liability, absent bad faith, and also permits such employees to insist that their defenses be conducted at public expense. (See Gov. Code, §§ 825–825.6, 995–995.2.) Public employees thus no longer have a significant reason to fear liability as they go about their official tasks. We also, in *Johnson*, rejected the argument that a public employee's concern over the potential liability of his or her employer serves as a basis for immunity. (Johnson v. State of California, *supra*, 69 Cal.2d at pp. 790–793, 72 Cal.Rptr. 240, 447 P.2d 352.)

We also noted in *Johnson* that federal courts have consistently categorized failures to warn of latent dangers as falling outside the scope of discretionary omissions immunized by the Federal Tort Claims Act.[16] (See United Air Lines, Inc. v. Weiner (9th Cir. 1964) 335 F.2d 379, 397–398, cert. den. sub nom. United Air Lines Inc. v. United States, 379 U.S. 951, 85 S. Ct. 452, 13 L.Ed.2d 549 (decision to conduct military training flights was discretionary but failure to warn commercial airline was not); United States v. Washington (9th Cir. 1965) 351 F.2d 913, 916 (decision where to place transmission lines spanning canyon was assumed to be discretionary but failure to warn pilot was not); United States v. White (9th Cir. 1954) 211 F.2d 79, 82 (decision not to "dedud" army firing range assumed to be discretionary but failure to warn person about to go onto range of unsafe condition was not); Bulloch v. United States (D. Utah 1955) 133 F.Supp. 885, 888 (decision how and when to conduct nuclear test deemed discretionary but failure to afford proper notice was not); Hernandez v. United States (D.Hawaii 1953) 112 F.Supp.·369, 371 (decision to erect road block characterized as discretionary but failure to warn of resultant hazard was not).

[10] We conclude, therefore, that the defendants' failure to warn Tatiana or those who reasonably could have been expected to notify her of her peril does not fall within the absolute protection afforded by section 820.2 of the Government Code. We emphasize that our conclusion does not raise the specter of therapists employed by government indiscriminately held liable for damages despite their exercise of sound professional judgment. We require of publicly employed therapists only that quantum of care which the common law requires of private therapists, that they use that reasonable degree of skill, knowledge, and conscientiousness ordinarily exercised by members of their profession. The imposition of liability in those rare cases in which a public employee falls short of this standard does not contravene the language or purpose of Government Code section 820.2.

4. *Defendant therapists are immune from liability for failing to confine Poddar*

[11] We sustain defendant therapists' contention that Government

---

[16]By analogy, section 830.8 of the Government Code furnishes additional support for our conclusion that a failure to warn does not fall within the zone of immunity created by Section 820.2. Section 830.8 provides: "Neither a public entity nor a public employee is liable . . . for an injury caused by the failure to provide traffic or warning signals, signs, markings or devices described in the Vehicle Code. Nothing in this section exonerates a public entity or public employee from liability by such failure if a signal, sign, marking or device . . . was necessary to warn of a dangerous condition which endangered the safe movement of traffic and which would not be reasonably apparent to, and would not have been anticipated by, a person exercising due care." The Legislature thus concluded at least in another context that the failure to warn of a latent danger is not an immunized discretionary omission. (See Hilts v. County of Solano (1968) 265 Cal.App.2d 161, 174, 71 Cal.Rptr. 275.)

Code section 856 insulates them from liability for failing to confine Poddar. Section 856 affords public entities and their employees absolute protection from liability for "any injury resulting from determining in accordance with any applicable enactment . . . whether to confine a person for mental illness."[17] The section includes an exception to the general rule of immunity, however, "for injury proximately caused by . . . negligent or wrongful act[s] or omission[s] in carrying out or failing to carry out . . . a determination to confine or not to confine a person for mental illness. . . ."

Turning first to Dr. Powelson's status with respect to section 856, we observe that the actions attributed to him by plaintiffs' complaints fall squarely within the protections furnished by that provision. Plaintiffs allege Powelson ordered that no detention action be taken. This conduct definitionally reflected Powelson's "determining . . . [not] to confine [Poddar]." Powelson therefore is immune from liability for any injuries stemming from his decision. (See Hernandez v. State of California (1970) 11 Cal.App.3d 895, 90 Cal.Rptr. 205.)

Section 856 also insulates Dr. Moore for his conduct respecting confinement, although the analysis in his case is a bit more subtle. Clearly, Moore's decision that Poddar *be* confined was not a proximate cause of Tatiana's death, for indeed if Moore's efforts to bring about Poddar's confinement had been successful, Tatitna might still be alive today. Rather, any confinement claim against Moore must rest upon Moore's failure to overcome Powelson's decision and actions opposing confinement.

Such a claim, based as it necessarily would be upon a subordinate's failure to prevail over his superior, obviously would derive from a rather onerous duty. Whether to impose such a duty we need not decide, however, since we can confine our analysis to the question whether Moore's failure to overcome Powelson's decision realistically falls within the protections afforded by section 856. Based upon the allegations before us, we conclude that Moore's conduct is protected.

Plaintiffs' complaints imply that Moore acquiesced in Powelson's countermand of Moore's confinement recommendation. Such acquiescence is functionally equivalent to "determining . . . [not] to confine" and thus merits protection under section 856. At this stage we are unaware, of course, precisely how Moore responded to Powelson's actions; he may

---

[17]Section 5201 of the Welfare and Institutions Code provides: "Any individual may apply to the person or agency designated by the county for a petition alleging that there is in the county a person who is, as a result of mental disorder a danger to others, or to himself, or is gravely disabled, and requesting that an evaluation of the person's condition be made." We believe that defendant therapists' power to recommend confinement as provided by section 5201 suffices to place them within the class of persons protected by section 856 of the Government Code. They are persons who can "determin[e] in accordance with [section 5201] whether to confine a person for mental illness."

have debated the confinement issue with Powelson, for example, or taken no initiative whatsoever, perhaps because he respected Powelson's judgment, feared for his future at the hospital, or simply recognized that the proverbial handwriting was on the wall. None of these possibilities constitutes, however, the type of careless or wrongful behavior subsequent to a decision respecting confinement which is stripped of protection by the exceptionary language in section 856. Rather, each is in the nature of a decision not to continue to press for Poddar's confinement. No language in plaintiffs' original or amended complaints suggests that Moore determined to fight Powelson but failed successfully to do so due to negligent or otherwise wrongful acts or omissions. Under the circumstances, we conclude that plaintiffs' second amended complaints allege facts which trigger immunity for Dr. Moore under section 856.[18]

5. *Defendant police officers are immune from liability for failing to continue Poddar in their custody*

[12] Confronting, finally, the question whether the defendant police officers are immune from liability for releasing Poddar after his brief confinement, we conclude that they are. The source of their immunity is section 5154 of the Welfare and Institutions Code, which declares that "[t]he professional person in charge of the facility providing 72-hour treatment and evaluation, his designee, *and the peace officer responsible for the detainment of the person* shall not be held civilly or criminally liable for any action by a person released at or before the end of 72 hours . . ." (Emphasis added.)

Although defendant police officers technically were not "peace officers" as contemplated by the Welfare and Institutions Code,[19] plaintiffs' assertion that the officers incurred liability by failing to continue Poddar's confinement clearly contemplates that the officers were "responsible for the detainment of [Poddar]." We could not impose a duty upon the officers to keep Poddar confined yet deny them the protection furnished by a statute immunizing those "responsible for . . . [confinement]." Because plaintiffs would have us treat defendant officers as persons who were capable of performing the functions of the "peace officers" contemplated by the Welfare and Institutions Code, we must accord defendant officers the protections which that code prescribes for such "peace officers."

---

[18]Because Dr. Gold and Dr. Yandell were Dr. Powelson's subordinates, the analysis respecting whether they are immune for having failed to obtain Poddar's confinement is similar to the analysis applicable to Dr. Moore.

[19]Welfare and Institutions Code section 5008, subdivision (i), defines "peace officer" for purposes of the Lanterman-Petris-Short Act as a person specified in sections 830.1 and 830.2 of the Penal Code. Campus police do not fall within the coverage of section 830.1 and were not included in section 830.2 until 1971.

6. Plaintiffs' complaints state no cause of action for examplary damages

[13, 14] Plaintiffs' third cause of action seeks punitive damages against defendant Powelson. Incorporating by reference the factual allegations of the first cause of action, plaintiffs assert that Powelson "did the things herein alleged with intent to abandon a dangerous patient, and said acts were done maliciously and oppressively."[20] The incorporated allegations speak only of Powelson's failure to bring about Poddar's commitment; they do not refer to his failure to warn Tatiana or her parents. Since we have concluded that Powelson is protected by governmental immunity from liability for his decision not to commit Poddar, plaintiffs' complaints state no basis for recovery of exemplary damages against Powelson.

7. Conclusion

For the reasons stated, we conclude that plaintiffs can assert the elements essential to a cause of action for breach of a duty to warn. The judgment of the superior court dismissing plaintiffs' action is reversed, and the cause remanded for further proceedings consistent with the views expressed herein.

WRIGHT, C. J., and MOSK, SULLIVAN and BURKE,* JJ., concur.

Justice Clark (dissenting):

The majority's opinion correctly holds that when a psychiatrist, in terminating treatment to a patient, increases the risk of his violence, the psychiatrist must warn the potential victim. However, I do not agree with the majority's conclusion that the psychiatrist must also disclose threats of violence based solely on his prior psychiatrist-patient relationship. Further, I do not agree with the majority's holding that police officers shall become subject to the same duty.

1. Duty to disclose based on psychiatrist–patient relationship

Generally, one person owes no duty to control the conduct of another.

---

[20]Defendant Powelson points out that plaintiffs do not allege that Powelson knew Tatiana or plaintiffs, nor that his alleged malice or oppression was directed toward them. Such an allegation, however, is not essential to a cause of action for punitive damages. In Toole v. Richardson-Merrell Inc. (1967) 251 Cal.App.2d 689, 60 Cal.Rptr. 398, the court upheld an award of punitive damages against the manufacturer of a dangerous drug. Rejecting the contention that proof of a deliberate intention by the manufacturer to injure the users was essential to punitive damages, the court stated that "malice in fact, sufficient to support an award of punitive damages on the basis of malice as that term is used in Civil Code section 3294, may be established by a showing that the defendant's wrongful conduct was wilful, intentional, and done in reckless disregard of its possible results." (251 Cal.App.2d at p. 713, 60 Cal.Rptr. at p. 415.)

*Retired Associate Justice of the Supreme Court sitting under assignment by the Chairman of the Judicial Council.

(Richards v. Stanley (1954) 43 Cal.2d 60, 65, 271 P.2d 23; Wright v. Arcade School Dist. (1964) 230 Cal.App.2d 272, 277, 40 Cal.Rptr. 812; Rest.2d Torts (1965) § 315.) Exceptions arise only in limited situations where (1) a special relationship exists between the defendant and the injured party giving the latter a right to protection, or (2) a special relationship exists between the defendant and the active wrongdoer imposing a duty on the defendant to control the wrongdoer's conduct. The majority does not contend the first exception is applicable to this case.

Overriding considerations of policy compel the conclusion that the duty to warn a potential victim may not be founded on the mere existence of a psychiatrist-patient relationship.

The imposition of a duty depends on policy considerations. (Dillon v. Legg (1968) 68 Cal.2d 728, 734, 69 Cal.Rptr. 72, 441 P.2d 912.) The principal considerations include the burden on the defendant, the consequence to the community, the prevention of future violence, and the foreseeability of harm to the plaintiff. (Rowland v. Christian (1968) 69 Cal.2d 108, 113, 70 Cal.Rptr. 97, 443 P.2d 561.)

Although the majority fleetingly acknowledges these considerations, it neglects applying them to our case. More specifically, the majority opinion fails to realistically evaluate the devastating impact their new duty will have on the field of mental health—and the repercussions resulting to society.

The importance of psychiatric treatment is well-recognized in California, reflected in this court's recent statement, "We recognize the growing importance of the psychiatric profession in our modern, ultracomplex society. The swiftness of change—economic, cultural, and moral—produces accelerated tensions in our society, and the potential for relief of such emotional disturbances offered by psychological therapy undoubtedly establishes it as a profession essential to the preservation of societal health and well-being." (In re Lifschutz (1970) 2 Cal.3d 415, 421–422, 85 Cal.Rptr. 829, 832, 467 P.2d 557, 560.)

Successful psychotherapy demands confidentiality. (In re Lifschutz, *supra*, 2 Cal.3d 415, 422, 85 Cal.Rptr. 829, 467 P.2d 557.) "It is clearly recognized that the very practice of psychiatry vitally depends upon the reputation in the community that the psychiatrist will not tell." (Slovenko, Psychiatry and a Second Look at the Medical Privilege (1960) 6 Wayne L. Rev. 175, 188.)

Assurance of confidentiality is important in three ways.

First, without a substantial guarantee of confidentiality, people requiring treatment will be deterred from seeking assistance. (See Senate Judiciary Committee's comment accompanying section 1014 of the Evid. Code; Slovenko, *supra*, 6 Wayne L. Rev. 175, 187–188; Goldstein and Katz, Psychiatrist-Patient Privilege: The GAP Proposal and the Connecticut Statute (1962) 36 Conn.Bar J. 175, 178.) It remains an unfortunate fact in our society that a stigma attaches to people seeking psychiatric guidance (apparently increased by the propensity of people considering treatment to see themselves in the worst possible light) creating a well-recognized reluctance to seek aid. (Fisher, The Psychotherapeutic Professions and the Law of Privileged Communications (1964) 10 Wayne L.Rev. 609, 617; Slovenko, *supra*, 6 Wayne L.Rev. 175, 188; see also Rappeport, Psychiatrist-Patient Privilege (1963) 23 Md.L.J. 39, 46–47.) This reluctance is alleviated by the psychiatrist's assurance of confidentiality.

Second, the guarantee of confidentiality is important in eliciting the full disclosure necessary for effective treatment. To carry out the cure, the doctor must first diagnose the disease. Candor is essential to psychiatric diagnosis. This diagnostic process requires "a searching evaluation of the given personality in the light of his past experiences and current relationships" (Heller, Some Comments to Lawyers of the Practice of Psychiatry (1957) 30 Temp. L.Q. 401), requiring intensive examination of "innate and constitutional factors, the history of the individual's emotional, educational, cultural, vocational and medical backgrounds, the influence of sexual and aggressive instincts, so-called ego or personality strength, judgment and reality-testing." (*Id.* at p. 402.) Summarily stated, "The process involves a prying into the most hidden aspects of personality, a prying which discloses matters theretofore unknown even to the conscious mind of the patient." (Slovenko, *supra*, 6 Wayne L. Rev. 175, 185.)

The assurance of confidentiality is essential to bringing about full disclosure since the psychiatric patient approaches treatment with conscious and unconscious inhibitions to revealing his innermost thoughts. (Goldstein and Katz, *supra*, 36 Conn.B.J. 175, 178; Guttmacher and Weihofen, Privileged Communications Between Psychiatrist and Patient (1952) 28 Ind.L.J. 32, 34.) "Every person, however well-motivated, has to overcome resistances to therapeutic exploration. These resistances seek support from every possible source and the possibility of disclosure would easily be employed in the service of resistance." (Goldstein and Katz, *supra*, 36 Conn. Bar J. 175, 179; see also, 118 Am.J.Psych. 734, 735.) Until a patient can trust his psychiatrist not to violate their confidential relationship, "the unconscious psychological control mechanism of repression will prevent the recall of past experiences." (Butler, Psychotherapy and Griswold: Is Confidentiality a Privilege or a Right? (1971) 3 Conn.L.Rev. 599, 604.)[1]

Third, even if full disclosure is accomplished, assurance that the confidential relationship will not be breached is necessary to maintain the

---

[1]One survey indicated that five of every seven people interviewed said they would be less likely to make full disclosure to a psychiatrist in the absence of assurance of confidentiality. (See, Comment, Functional Overlap Between the Lawyer and Other Professionals: Its Implications for the Doctrine of Privileged Communications (1962) 71 Yale L.J. 1226, 1255.)

patient's trust of his psychiatrist, the very means by which treatment is effected. "[T]he essence of much psychotherapy is the contribution of trust in the external world and ultimately in the self, modelled upon the trusting relationship established during therapy." (Dawidoff, The Malpractice of Psychiatrists, 1966 Duke L.J. 696, 704.) Patients will be helped only if they can form a trusting relationship with the psychiatrist. (*Id.* at p. 704, fn. 34; Burnham, Separation Anxiety (1965) 13 Arch.Gen.Psychiatry 346, 356; Heller, *supra*, 30 Temp. L.Q. 401, 406.) Conversely, all authorities appear to agree treatment will be frustrated if the trust relationship cannot be developed because of collusive communication between the psychiatrist and others. (See, e.g., Ralph Slovenko (1973) Psychiatry and Law, p. 61; Cross, Privileged Communications Between Participants in Group Psychotherapy (1970) Law and the Social Order, 191; 199; Hollender, The Psychiatrist and the Release of Patient Information (1960) 116 Am.J.Psychiatry 828, 829.)

Therefore, given the importance of confidentiality to the practice of psychiatry, it becomes clear the duty to warn imposed by the majority will cripple the use and effectiveness of psychiatry: many people, potentially violent—yet susceptible to treatment—will be deterred from seeking it; those seeking aid will be inhibited from making the self-revelation necessary to effective treatment; finally, requiring the psychiatrist to violate the patient's trust by forcing the doctor to disseminate confidential statements will destroy the interpersonal relationship by which treatment is effected.

The law recognized the psychiatrist's ability to lessen a patient's propensity for violence. Indeed, this ability is so well-established that the majority, in its second reason for imposing a duty to warn, concludes that because the psychiatrists' conduct caused Poddar to discontinue treatment, the psychiatrists actually "contributed to the danger" that Poddar would act violently. (*Ante*, p. 135 of 118 Cal.Rptr., p. 135 of 529 P.2d.)

By imposing such duty on psychiatrists, the majority contributes to society's danger. Given the majority's recognition that under existing psychiatric procedures only a relatively few receiving treatment will ever present a serious risk of violence (*ante*, p. 136 of 118 Cal.Rptr., p. 560 of 529 P.2d.), the newly imposed duty will likely result in a *net increase* in violence—inconsistent with the policies of preventing future violence and of weighing the consequence to the community.

The majority overlooks the widespread impact of its new duty by pointing out that only a few psychiatric patients will ever really create a serious risk of violence and by assuming that the number of necessary warnings will similarly be few. (*Ante*, p. 136 of 118 Cal.Rptr., p. 560 of 529 P.2d.), This assumption strays from reality.

The psychiatric community recognizes that the process of determining potential violence in a patient is far from exact, being wrought with complexity and uncertainty. (See, Rector, *Who Are the Dangerous?* (July 1973) Bull. of the Amer. Acad. of Psych. and the Law 186; Kozol,

Boucher, and Garofalo, *The Diagnosis and Treatment of Dangerousness* (1972) 18 Crime and Delinquency 371; Justice and Birkman, *An Effort to Distinguish the Violent From the Nonviolent* (1972) 65 So. Med.J. 703.) In fact, precision has not ever been attained in predicting who of those having already committed violent acts will again become violent, a task recognized to be of simpler proportion. (Kozol, Boucher, and Garofalo, *supra*, 18 Crime and Delinquency 372, 384.)

This predictive uncertainty is fatal to the majority's underlying assumption that the number of disclosures will necessarily be small. As noted, above psychiatric patients are encouraged to discuss all thoughts of violence. And, as the majority concedes, they often express such thoughts. However, unlike this court, the psychiatrist does not enjoy the benefit of hindsight in seeing which few, if any, of his patients will ultimately become violent. Now, operating under the majority's duty, the psychiatrist—with each patient and each visit—must instantaneously calculate potential violence. The difficulties researchers have encountered in accurately predicting violence will be heightened for the practicing psychiatrist dealing for brief periods in his office with heretofore nonviolent patients. And, given the decision not to warn must always be made at the psychiatrist's civil peril, one can expect all doubts will be resolved in favor of warning.

Relying on sections 1013, 1014, and 1924 of the Evidence Code, the majority suggests that, in any event, the new duty's harmful impact on the community has already been balanced by the Legislature in favor of warning. However, this conclusion is faulty, failing to differentiate between the *permissive* language of section 1024 and the *mandatory* duty of the majority.

Section 1014 of the Evidence Code provides that "the patient, whether or not a party, has a privilege to refuse to disclose, and to prevent another from disclosing, a confidential communication between patient and psychotherapist . . . ." Section 1013 expressly provides that the patient is the holder of the privilege. Section 1024 provides, "There is no privilege under this article if the psychotherapist has reasonable cause to believe that the patient is in such mental or emotional condition as to be dangerous to himself or to the person or property of another and that disclosure of the communication is necessary to prevent the threatened danger."

Section 1024 is solely permissive. When a psychiatrist has determined to his satisfaction that some sort of formal disclosure must be made to protect the patient or others, section 1024 precludes the patient from invoking the section 1014 privilege to prevent him from doing so.[2] Clearly,

---

[2]This purpose is made simplistically clear in the Law Revision Commission's comment accompanying section 1024: "Although this exception might inhibit the relationship between the patient and his psychotherapist to a limited extent, it is essential that appropraite action be taken if the psychotherapist becomes convinced during the course of treatment that the patient is a menace to himself or others *and the patient refuses to permit the psychotherapist to make the disclosure necessary to prevent the threatened danger.*" (Italics added.)

section 1024 neither imposes—nor contemplates—a legal duty mandating the psychiatrist to warn, and the impact of *requiring* him to warn is much greater than that of *allowing* him to do so.

Our sympathy for the victim of violent acts of the mentally ill should not blind us to the needs of the mentally ill or to the ultimate goal of reducing the level of violence. Because the majority's holding will severely impair the ability of the doctor to treat effectively, resulting in a net increase in violence, I cannot concur in the majority's new rule.

2. Duty of police to warn

Although the police defendants get lost in the course of the majority's opinion, the holding concludes the officers may also be liable for failing to warn.

The ground for imposing liability on the police officers is unclear. The holding is so broad it may be understood, in light of the facts of this case, as meaning that the mere release of Poddar gave rise to the duty to warn. The majority not only imposes a new duty on police officers, but may also have held that jail and prison officials must now warn of potential violence whenever a prisoner is released pursuant to bail order, parole, or completion of sentence.

It is disturbing that the majority should take, by ambiguous statement and without discussion, the very broad step of imposing on a peace officer the near impossible duty to notify potential victims of threatened violence. The majority states that duty is dependent on considerations of policy— but the policy goes unexplained.

3. Conclusion

It appears the tragedy of Tatiana Tarasoff has led the majority of our court to unfairly penalize the professions of psychiatry and law enforcement, to the detriment of society.

I would permit plaintiffs to proceed against the psychiatrists for failure to warn on the theory the psychiatrist's conduct in terminating treatment increased the risk of violence. Absent such conduct, I would disallow a cause of action for failure to warn based solely on the existence of the prior psychiatrist-patient relationship. Finally, I conclude no justification has been shown for imposing the inordinate duty to warn on the police officers.

McCOMB, J., concurs.

DR. MOORE'S LETTER TO POLICE CHIEF BEALL[1]

Mr. Poddar was first seen at Cowell Hospital by Dr. Stuart Gold June 5, 1969, on an emergency basis. After receiving medication he was referred to the outpatient psychiatry clinic for psychotherapy. Since then I have seen him here seven times.

His mental status varies considerably. At times he appears to be quite rational, at other times he appears quite psychotic. It is my impression that currently the appropriate diagnosis for him is paranoid schizophrenic reaction, acute and severe. He is at this point a danger to the welfare of other people and himself. That is, he has been threatening to kill an unnamed girl[2] who he feels has betrayed him and has violated his honor. He has told a friend of his . . . that he intends to go to San Francisco to buy a gun and that he plans to kill the girl. . . .

I have discussed this matter with Dr. Gold and we concur in the opinion that Mr. Poddar should be committed for observation in a mental hospital. I request the assistance of your department in this matter.

---

[1]Excerpted from the Brief for Respondent Moore in *Tarasoff v. Regents of University of California*, on file with Clerk of the Supreme Court of California, 1 Civil No. 31, 168.
[2]Dr. Moore did not know the name of the girl Poddar planned to murder at the time he wrote this letter. However, the police found out it was Tatiana Tarasoff after questioning Poddar. See *Tarasoff v. Regents of University of California*, 108 Cal.Rptr. 878 at p. 889.

Reference Notes

1. Cohen, R. J. *Professional psychology in the public eye.* Chicago: University of Chicago Press. Book in preparation.
2. St. Paul Fire and Marine Insurance Company. *Preserving a medical malpractice insurance marketplace: Problems and remedies.* St. Paul, Minn.: Author, 1975.
3. Wiggins, J. Insuring your practice. In A. H. Canter (Chair), *Insurance crisis and psychotherapy.* Symposium presented at the 84th annual convention of the American Psychological Association, Washington, D.C., 1976.
4. "Mal-psychotherapy" suits may soon beset psychiatrists. *Roche Report Frontiers of Psychiatry,* March 1, 1978, pp. 1–2.
5. Knerr, C. R. Compulsory disclosure to the courts of research data and sources. In S. T. Margulis (Chair), *Privacy, the law, and the practice of psychology.* Symposium presented at the 84th annual convention of the American Psychological Association, Washington, D.C., 1976.
6. Kovacs, A. Implications of the malpractice crisis for training of graduate students. In A. H. Canter (Chair), *Insurance crisis and psychotherapy.* Symposium presented at the 84th annual convention of the American Psychological Association, Washington, D.C., 1976.
7. McLemore, C. W. When worlds collide: Psychotherapy and religion. In C. W. McLemore (Chair), *Religion and psychotherapy.* Symposium presented at the 86th annual convention of the American Psychological Association, Toronto, Ontario, Canada, 1978.
8. Ellis, A. Religion and psychopathology. In C. W. McLemore (Chair), *Religion and psychotherapy.* Symposium presented at the 86th annual convention of the American Psychological Association, Toronto, Ontario, Canada, 1978.
9. Cohen, R. J. The case of Mary and the issue of control. In C. W. McLemore (Chair), *Religion and psychotherapy.* Symposium presented at the 86th annual convention of the American Psychological Association, Toronto, Ontario, Canada, 1978.
10. Greenwald, H. Psychotherapy as fun. In R. A. Harper (Chair), *Humor, play and absurdity in psychotherapy.* Symposium presented at the 84th annual convention of the American Psychological Association, Washington, D.C., 1976.
11. Cohen, R. J. *The cognition/behavior survey.* New York: Author, 1978.

References

Alexander, J. Protecting the children of life-threatening parents. *Journal of Clinical Child Psychology*, 1974, *3*(2), 53–54.

Alper, P. R. Our irresponsible bar associations. *Private Practice*, April 1974, pp. 31; 34; 36; 41; 42.

American Psychiatric Association. The principles of medical ethics, with annotations especially applicable to psychiatry. *American Journal of Psychiatry*, 1973, *130*, 1057–1064.

American Psychiatric Association. *Diagnostic and statistical manual of mental disorders* (2nd ed.). Washington D.C.: Author, 1968.

American Psychiatric Association. *DSM–III: Operational criteria draft*. Washington, D.C.: Author, 1977.

American Psychological Association. *Ethical standards of psychologists* (1977 Revision). Washington, D.C.: Author, 1977.

Andren, H. E. Treatment or mistreatment in psychiatry (observations on electroconvulsive therapy). *Diseases of the Nervous System*, 1976, *37*, 605–609.

Appleman, J. A. Professional liability of psychologists. *American Psychologist*, 1953, *8*, 686–690.

Appleton, W. S. Legal problems in psychiatric drug prescription. *American Journal of Psychiatry*, 1968, *124*, 877–882.

Arnhoff, F. N. Some factors influencing the unreliability of clinical judgments. *Journal of Clinical Psychology*, 1954, *10*, 272–275.

Arnot, R. E. Observations on the effects of electric convulsive treatments in man—psychological. *Diseases of the Nervous System*, 1975, *36*, 499–502.

Asher, J. Confusion reigns in APA malpractice plan. *APA Monitor*, March 1976, pp. 1; 11.

Asnis, G. M., Fink, M., and Saferstein, S. ECT in metropolitan New York hospitals: A survey of practice, 1975–1976. *American Journal of Psychiatry*, 1978, *135*, 479–482.

Atkinson, R. C. Reflections on psychology's past and concerns about its future. *American Psychologist*, 1977, *32*, 205–210.

Atthowe, J. M., Jr. Legal and ethical accountability in everyday practice. *Behavioral Engineering*, 1975, *3*, 25–38.

Ayd, F. J., Jr. Fatal hyperpyrexia during chlorpromazine therapy. *Journal of Clinical Psychopathology*, 1956, *22*, 189–192.

Ayd, F. J., Jr. A survey of drug-induced extrapyramidal reactions. *Journal of the American Medical Association*, 1961, *175*, 1054–1060.

Baker, R. Terminal jurisprudence, *New York Times Magazine*, March 20, 1977, p. 12.

Ball, T. S. Issues and implications of operant conditioning: The re-establishment of social behavior. *Hospital and Community Psychiatry*, 1968, *19*, 230–232.

Balliett, G. 13 ways to protect yourself against malpractice suits. *Resident and Staff Physician*, 1974 *20*(4), 70–73; 75.

Bandura, A. *Principles of behavior modification.* New York: Holt, Rinehart, and Winston, 1969.

Beck, L. C., Kalogredis, V. J., and Cynwyd, B. Should the solo physician insure his corporation? *Pennsylvania Medicine*, 1977, *80*(1), 23–24.

Bellamy, W. A. Malpractice risks confronting the psychiatrist: A nationwide fifteen-year study of appellate court cases, 1946 to 1961. *American Journal of Psychiatry*, 1962, *118*, 769–779.

Bernard, J. L. The significance for psychology of O'Connor v. Donaldson. *American Psychologist*, 1977, *32*, 1085–1088.

Bernstein, B. E. Legal and social interface in counseling homosexual clients. *Social Casework*, 1977, *58*, 36–40.

Bernstein, B. E. Malpractice: An ogre on the horizon. *Social Work*, 1978, *23*, 106–112.

Bernstein, I. C., Bernstein, D. M., and Adzick, G. R. Electrotherapy and renal transplantation: Impediment to treatment. *Minnesota Medicine*, 1977, *60*, 410–411.

Bernstein, I. C., Bernstein, D. M., and Adzick, G. R. Legal aspects of electrotherapy in a catatonic renal transplant patient. *The Journal of Clinical Psychiatry*, 1978, *39*, 252–253.

Bersoff, D. N. Professional ethics and legal responsibilities: On the horns of a dilemma. *Journal of School Psychology*, 1975, *13*, 359–376.

Bersoff, D. N. Therapists as protectors and policemen: New roles as a result of *Tarasoff? Professional Psychology*, 1976, *7*, 267–273.

Bersoff, D. N. Representation for children in custody decisions: All that glitters is not *Gault. Journal of Family Law*, 1976–77, *15*, 27–49.

Bersoff, D. N. and Prasse, D. Applied psychology and judicial decision making: Corporal punishment as a case in point. *Professional Psychology*, 1978, *9*, 400–411.

Bieber, I. A discussion of "Homosexuality: The ethical challenge." *Journal of Consulting and Clinical Psychology*, 1976, *44*, 163–166.

Bindrim, P. A report on a nude marathon. *Psychotherapy: Theory, Research and Practice*, 1968, *5*, 180–188.

Black, H. C. *Black's law dictionary* (Rev. 4th ed.). St. Paul: West Publishing, 1968. Revised by the publisher's editorial staff.

Boderman, A., Freed, D. W., and Kinnucan, M. T. "Touch me, like me": Testing an encounter group assumption. *Journal of Applied Behavioral Science*, 1972, *8*, 527–533.

Bradford, R. T. A unique decision. *Journal of Legal Medicine*, 1974, *2*, 52–55.

Bragg, R. A. and Wagner, M. K. Issues and implications of operant conditioning: Can deprivation be justified? *Hospital and Community Psychiatry*, July 1968, *19*, 229–230.

Braginsky, B. M., Braginsky, D. C., and Ring, K. *Methods of madness.* New York: Holt, Rinehart and Winston, 1969.

Breger, L. and McGaugh, J. L. Critique and reformulation of "learning theory" approaches to psychotherapy and neurosis. *Psychological Bulletin*, 1965, *63*, 338–358.

Burt, R. A. Protecting children from their families and themselves: State laws and the Constitution. *Journal of Youth and Adolescence*, 1972, *1*, 91–111.

Butler, S. *Sexual contact between therapists and patients.* Unpublished doctoral dissertation, California School of Professional Psychology (Los Angeles), 1975.

Butler, S. and Zelen, S. L. Sexual intimacies between therapists and patients. *Psychotherapy: Theory, Research, and Practice*, 1977, *14*, 139–145.

Butterfield, W. H. Electric shock—hazards in aversive shock conditioning of humans. *Behavioral Engineering*, 1975, *3*, 1–28.

Byrne, D. *An introduction to personality*. Englewood Cliffs, N.J.: Prentice-Hall, 1974.

Cahoon, D. C. Issues and implications of operant conditioning: Balancing procedures against outcomes. *Hospital and Community Psychiatry*, 1968, *19*, 228–229.

Carstairs, G. M. A land of lotus eaters? *American Journal of Psychiatry*, 1969, *125*, 1576–1580.

Carter, L. F., Brim, O. G., Stalnaker, J. M., and Messick, S. Psychological tests and public responsibility. *American Psychologist*, 1965, *20*, 123–142.

Cases Unlimited, Inc. Is a surgeon an expert in radiology? *Resident and Staff Physician*, 1975, *21*(6), 32; 35. (a)

Cases Unlimited, Inc. The need for expert testimony. *Resident and Staff Physician*, 1975, *21*(7), 44. (b)

Cases Unlimited, Inc. Must you guarantee a tubal ligation? *Resident and Staff Physician*, 1976, *22*(1), 101.

Cassidy, P. S. The liability of psychiatrists for malpractice. *University of Pittsburgh Law Review*, 1974, *36*, 108–137.

Chairman addresses regulators. *MLC Commentary*, 1975, *2*(7), 3–4.

Chapman, L. and Chapman, J. Genesis of popular but erroneous psychodiagnostic observations. *Journal of Abnormal Psychology*, 1967, *72*, 193–204.

Childers, R. T. Hyperpyrexia, coma, and death during chlorpromazine therapy. *Journal of Clinical and Experimental Psychopathology*, 1961, *22*, 163–164.

Cline, E. J. Viewpoints: The malpractice problem. *Michigan Medicine*, 1973, *72*, 67–68.

Cohen, R. J. Loyalty or legality in obedience: Note on the Watergate proceedings. *Psychological Reports*, 1973, *33*, 964.

Cohen, R. J. Comments on the "cattle-prod controversy." *Perceptual and Motor Skills*, 1976, *42*, 146. (a)

Cohen, R. J. Is dying being worked to death? *American Journal of Psychiatry*, 1976, *133*, 575–577. (b)

Cohen, R. J. Dr. Cohen replies. *American Journal of Psychiatry*, 1976, *133*, 1348–1349. (c)

Cohen, R. J. Reich, antipodal legitimacy, and communication in psychology. *American Psychologist*, 1977, *32*, 985–986. (a)

Cohen, R. J. Socially reinforced obsessing: A reply. *Journal of Consulting and Clinical Psychology*, 1977, *45*, 1166–1171. (b)

Cohen, R. J. and DeBetz, B. Responsive supervision of the psychiatric resident and clinical psychology intern. *American Journal of Psychoanalysis*, 1977, *37*, 51–64.

Cohen, R. J. and Smith, F. J. Socially reinforced obsessing: Etiology of a disorder in a Christian Scientist. *Journal of Consulting and Clinical Psychology*, 1976, *44*, 142–144.

Cooper, C. L. and Bowles, D. Physical encounter and self-disclosure. *Psychological Reports*, 1973, *33*, 451–454.

Corpus juris secundum. New York: American Law Book Company, 1955.

Coyne, J. C. The place of informed consent in ethical dilemmas. *Journal of Consulting and Clinical Psychology*, 1976, *44*, 1015–1017.

Curran, W. J. Confidentiality and the prediction of dangerousness in psychiatry. *New England Journal of Medicine*, 1975, *293*, 285–286.

Curran, W. J. The lawyers' role in medical malpractice claims. *The New England Journal of Medicine*, 1977, *296*, 24–25.

Dahlberg, C. Sexual contact between patient and therapist. *Contemporary Psychoanalysis*, 1970, *6*, 107–124.

Davidson, H. A. Legal and ethical aspects of psychiatric research. *American Journal of Psychiatry*, 1969, *126*, 237–240.

Davidson, V. Psychiatry's problem with no name: Therapist–patient sex. *American Journal of Psychoanalysis*, 1977, *37*, 43–50.

Davison, G. C. Homosexuality: The ethical challenge. *Journal of Consulting and Clinical Psychology*, 1976, *44*, 157–162.

Dawidoff, D. J. *The malpractice of psychiatrists.* Springfield, Ill.: Charles C Thomas, 1973. (a)

Dawidoff, D. J. Some suggestions to psychiatrists for avoiding legal jeopardy. *Archives of General Psychiatry*, 1973, *29*, 699–701. (b)

DeLeon, P. H. and Borreliz, M. Malpractice: Professional liability and the law. *Professional Psychology*, 1978, *9*, 467–477.

Demac, D. Masters blasts innumerable patient rapes. *Hospital Tribune*, 1975, *9*(13), 1.

DeMarco, C. T. *Pharmacy and the law.* Germantown, Md.: Aspen Systems Corporation, 1975.

Dies, R. R. and Greenberg, B. Effects of physical contact in an encounter group context. *Journal of Consulting and Clinical Psychology*, 1976, *44*, 400–405.

Drude, K. P. Psychologists and civil commitment: Review of state statutes. *Professional Psychology*, 1978, *9*, 499–506.

Dubey, J. Confidentiality as a requirement of the therapist: Technical necessities for absolute privilege in psychotherapy. *American Journal of Psychiatry*, 1974, *131*, 1093–1096.

Duty to warn vs. confidentiality is conflict that can be resolved. *Clinical Psychiatry News*, April 1978, pp. 2; 38.

Eisberg, J. F. Doctor must pay damages, child-rearing expenses for failed vasectomy. *Legal Aspects of Medical Practice*, 1978, *6*(3), 48–49.

Ellenberger, H. *The discovery of the unconscious.* New York: Basic Books, 1970.

Epstein, R. A. Medical malpractice: The case for contract. *American Bar Foundation Research Journal*, 1976, *1*, 87–149.

Feegel, J. F. Malpractice and lab tests. *Resident and Staff Physician*, 1974, *20*(4), 47–50.

Feldman, W. S. Who decides admission—judge or physician? *Legal Aspects of Medical Practice*, 1978, *6*(3), 8.

Few suits arising from congenital defects have factual basis. *Pediatric News*, 1976, *10*(6), 7.

Finney, J. C. Therapist and patient after hours. *American Journal of Psychotherapy*, 1975, *29*, 593–602.

Flemenbaum, A. Pavor nocturnus: A complication of single daily tricyclic or neuroleptic dosage. *American Journal of Psychiatry*, 1976, *133*, 570–572.

Fontana, V. J. When to suspect parental assault. *Resident and Staff Physician*, 1973, *19*(8), 48.

Foster, H. H. The conflict and reconciliation of the ethical interests of therapist and patient. *Journal of Psychiatry and Law*, 1975, *3*, 39–61.

Freedman, A. M. and Kaplan, H. I. *Comprehensive textbook of psychiatry.* Baltimore: Williams and Wilkins, 1967.

Freeman, L. and Roy, J. *Betrayal.* New York: Stein and Day, 1976.

Freud, S. [Further recommendations in the technique of psycho-analysis] In E. Jones (Ed.) and J. Riviere (trans.), *Collected Papers*, (Vol. 2). New York: Basic Books, 1959. (Originally published, 1913.)

Gauron, E. F. and Dickinson, J. K. Diagnostic decision making in psychiatry. *Archives of General Psychiatry*, 1966, *14*, 225–232.

Gergen, K. F. The codification of research ethics: Views of a doubting Thomas. *American Psychologist*, 1973, *28*, 907–912.

"Going bare" becomes popular in South, West. *MLC Commentary*, 1976, *3*(3), 2–3.

Goldfarb, A. Reliability of diagnostic judgments by psychologists. *Journal of Clinical Psychology*, 1959, *15*, 392–396.

Goldfried, M. R. and Davison, G. C. *Clinical behavior therapy.* New York: Holt, Rinehart and Winston, 1976.

Gordon, H. L. Fifty shock therapy theories. *Military Surgeon*, 1948, *103*, 397–401.

Gottlieb, R. M., Nappi, T., and Strain, J. J. The physician's knowledge of psychotropic drugs: Preliminary results. *American Journal of Psychiatry*, 1978, *135*, 29–32.

Green, R. K. and Cox, G. Social work and malpractice: A converging course. *Social Work*, 1978, *23*, 100–105.

Greenblatt, D. J., Shader, R. I., and Koch-Weber, J. Psychotropic drug use in the Boston area. *Archives of General Psychiatry*, 1975, *32*, 518–521.

Greene, P. W. Viewpoints: The malpractice problem. *Michigan Medicine*, 1973, *72*, 67.

Griffith, J. L. Malpractice: The one sure way to shut "hired mouths." *Medical Economics*, July 24, 1978, pp. 84–85; 87–88; 90; 95; 98.

Grisso, T. and Vierling, L. Minors' consent to treatment: A developmental perspective. *Professional Psychology*, 1978, *9*, 412–427.

Gross, M. L. *The brain watchers.* New York: Random House, 1962.

Gross, M. L. *The psychological society.* New York: Random House, 1978.

Grossman, M. Insurance reports as a threat to confidentiality. *American Journal of Psychiatry*, 1971, *128*, 96–100.

Gurevitz, H. *Tarasoff:* Protective privilege versus public peril. *American Journal of Psychiatry*, 1977, *134*, 289–292.

Halleck, S. L. Discussion of "Socially Reinforced Obsessing." *Journal of Consulting and Clinical Psychology*, 1976, *44*, 146–147.

Hamilton, J. M. Malpractice from the private practice and institutional psychiatric viewpoint. *Maryland State Medical Journal*, January 1970, *19*, 69–74.

Harris, M. Tort liability of the psychotherapist. *University of San Francisco Law Review*, 1973, *8*, 405–436.

Hart, J., Corriere, R., and Binder, J. *Going sane.* New York: Delta, 1975.

Healy, W. *The individual delinquent.* Boston: Little, Brown, 1915.

Helfer, R. E. Seven guidelines in child abuse cases. *Resident and Staff Physician*, 1973, *19*, 8; 57.

Helfer, R. E. Why most physicians won't get involved in child abuse and what to do about it. *Children Today*, 1975, *4*(3), 28–32.

Herron, W. G., Green, M., Guild, M., Smith, A., and Kantor, R. E. *Contemporary school psychology.* Scranton, Pa.: Intext, 1970.

Hershey, N. and Miller, R. D. *Human experimentation and the law.* Germantown, Md.: Aspen Systems Corporation, 1976.

Hoch, P. H. Clinical and biological interrelations between schizophrenia and epilepsy. *American Journal of Psychiatry*, 1943, *99*, 507–511.

Hoffman, P. J. *The tyranny of testing.* New York: Crowell–Collier, 1962.

Hollender, M. H. Privileged communication and confidentiality. *Diseases of the Nervous System*, 1965, *26*, 169–175.

Hollingshead, A. B., and Redlich, F. C. *Social class and mental illness.* New York: Wiley, 1958.

Hollister, L. E. and Kosek, J. C. Sudden death during treatment with phenothiazine derivatives. *Journal of the American Medical Association*, 1965, *192*, 1035–1038.

Holroyd, J. C. and Brodsky, A. M. Psychologists' attitudes and practices regarding erotic and nonerotic physical contact with patients. *American Psychologist*, 1977, *32*, 843–849.

Horsley, J. E. Here's the nth degree of malpractice liability. *Medical Economics*, April 17, 1978, p. 89. (a)

Horsley, J. E. How to protect yourself against *legal* malpractice. *Medical Economics*, August 7, 1978, pp. 149; 153–154; 156; 158. (b)

Horsley, J. E. Malpractice: An old line of defense gains new strength. *Medical Economics*, September 4, 1978, pp. 137; 139; 143–145; 149. (c)

Illinois doctor wins countersuit. *MLC Commentary*, 1976, *3*(7), 4.

Illinois Medical Journal. Editorial comment. Author, 1977, *151*, 134.

Impastato, D. J. The story of the first electroshock treatment. *American Journal of Psychiatry*, 1960, *116*, 1113–1114.

Ingelfinger, F. J. The unethical in medical ethics. *Annals of Internal Medicine*, 1975, *83*, 264–269.

Insurance industry cites cultural trends as problem. *MLC Commentary*, 1976, *3*(1), 3–4.

Jagim, R. D., Wittman, W. D., and Noll, J. O. Mental health professionals' attitudes toward confidentiality, privilege, and third-party disclosure. *Professional Psychology*, 1978, *9*, 458–466.

ISO official explains rate-making procedures. *MLC Commentary*, 1976, *3*(2), 2–4.

Janov, A. *The primal scream.* New York: Dell, 1970.

Johnson, A. F. Comment on Gergen. *American Psychologist*, 1974, *29*, 470.

Jones, E. *The life and work of Sigmund Freud* (Vol. 1). New York: Basic Books, 1953.

Jourard, S. M. *Self-disclosure: An experimental analysis of the transparent self.* New York: Wiley-Interscience, 1971.

Jurow, G. L. and Mariano, W. E. Law and private practice. In G. D. Goldman and G. Stricker (Eds.), *Practical problems for a private psychotherapy practice.* Springfield, Ill.: Charles C Thomas, 1972.

Kalinowsky, L. and Hippius, H. *Pharmacological, convulsive and other somatic treatments in psychiatry.* New York: Grune and Stratton, 1969.

Kanner, L. *Child psychiatry*, 3d ed. Springfield, Ill.: Charles C Thomas, 1957. (First published in 1935).

Kardener, S. H., Fuller, M., and Mensh, I. N. A survey of physicians' attitudes and practices regarding erotic and nonerotic contact with patients. *American Journal of Psychiatry*, 1973, *130*, 1077–1081.

Kilmann, P. R. and Sotile, W. M. The marathon encounter group: A review of the literature. *Psychological Bulletin*, 1976, *83*, 827–850.

King, J. H. *The law of medical malpractice.* St. Paul, Minn.: West Publishing, 1977.

Kittrie, N. N. *The right to be different.* Baltimore: Pelican Books, 1973.

Kotulak, R. Malpractice suits—Growing sickness. *Chicago Tribune*, May 11, 1975, p. 1.

Krauskopf, J. M. and Krauskopf, C. J. Torts and psychologists. *Journal of Counseling Psychology*, 1965, *12*, 227–237.

Kreitman, N., Sainsbury, P., Morrissey, J., Towers, J. and Scrivener, J. The reliability of psychiatric assessment: An analysis. *Journal of Mental Science*, 1961, *107*, 887–908.

Krouner, L. W. Shock therapy and psychiatric malpractice: The legal accommodation to a controversial treatment. *Journal of Forensic Sciences*, 1975, *20*, 404–405.

Lavin, J. H. The most discouraging countersuit verdict yet. *Medical Economics*, September 4, 1978, p. 74.

Lazarus, A. A. Multimodal behavior therapy: Treating the BASIC ID. *The Journal of Nervous and Mental Disease*, 1973, *156*, 404–411.

Lazarus, A. A. *Multimodal behavior therapy*. New York: Springer, 1976.

Ledakowich, A. Malpractice case report. *Resident and Staff Physician*, 1972, *18*(3), 84. (a)

Ledakowich, A. Malpractice case report. *Resident and Staff Physician*, 1972, *18*(4), 60. (b)

Ledakowich, A. From a malpractice lawyer's casebook. *Resident and Staff Physician*, 1974, *20*(4), 1s–2s; 4s–5s; 9s.

Ledakowich, A. Shift the blame onto the surgeon? *Resident and Staff Physician*, 1976, *22*(6), 18. (a)

Ledakowich, A. Is one specialist on a team responsible for the negligence of another? *Resident and Staff Physician*, 1976, *22*(6), 28s. (b)

Ledakowich, A. Is fear of the future compensable? *Resident and Staff Physician*, 1976, *22*(5), 18. (c)

Ledakowich, A. An erroneous prediction of death. *Resident and Staff Physician*, 1976, *22*(10), 25. (d)

Ledakowich, A. A case of unreported child abuse. *Resident and Staff Physician*, 1976, *22*(7), 37. (e)

Ledakowich, A. Child abuse decision reversed by Supreme Court of California. *Resident and Staff Physician*, 1977, *23*(1), 112.

Lennard, H. J., Epstein, L. J., Bernstein, A., and Ransom, D. C. Hazards implicit in prescribing psychoactive drugs. *Science*, 1970, *169*, 438–441.

Lentz, R. J., Paul, G. L., and Calhoun, J. F. Reliability and validity of three measures of functioning with "hard core" chronic mental patients. *Journal of Abnormal Psychology*, 1971, *78*, 69–76.

Lief, H. I. Sexual activity with patients. *Medical Aspects of Human Sexuality*, April 1978, pp. 55; 57.

Lesse, S. Editorial comment. *American Journal of Psychotherapy*, 1965, *19*, 105.

Litigation. *Law and Behavior*, 1976, *1*(3), 1–3.

Little, R. B. and Strecker, E. A. Moot questions in psychiatric ethics. *American Journal of Psychiatry*, 1956, *113*, 455–460.

London, P. Psychotherapy for religious neuroses? Comments on Cohen and Smith. *Journal of Consulting and Clinical Psychology*, 1976, *44*, 145–147.

Louisell, D. W. The psychologist in today's legal world, Part II: Confidential communication. *Minnesota Law Review*, 1957, *41*, 731–750.

Lovaas, O. I. and Bucher, B. D. (Eds.), *Perspectives in behavior modification with deviant children*. Englewood Cliffs, N.J.: Prentice-Hall, 1974.

Lowen, A. *Physical dynamics of character structure*. New York: Grune and Stratton, 1958.

Lucero, R. J. and Vail, D. J. Authors' response: Public policy and public responsibility. *Hospital and Community Psychiatry*, 1968, *19*, 232–233.

Lucero, R. J., Vail, D. J., and Scherber, J. Regulating operant-conditioning programs. *Hospital and Community Psychiatry*, 1968, *19*, 53–54.

McCartney, J. L. Overt transference. *Journal of Sex Research*, 1966, *2*, 227–237.

Macklin, R. Ethics, sex research, and sex therapy. *The Hastings Center Report*, 1976, *6*, 5–7.

McLemore, C. W. and Court, J. H. Religion and psychotherapy—ethics, civil liberties, and clinical savvy: A critique. *Journal of Consulting and Clinical Psychology*, 1977, *45*, 1172–1175.

Mann, W. E. *Orgone, Reich, and eros*. New York: Touchstone, 1973.

Marmor, J. Sexual acting-out in psychotherapy. *American Journal of Psychoanalaysis*, 1972, *32*, 3–8.

Marmor, J. Some psychodynamic aspects of the seduction of patients in psychotherapy. *The American Journal of Psychoanalysis*, 1976, *36*, 319–323.

Martin, R. *Legal challenges to behavior modification*. Champaign, Ill.: Research Press, 1975.

Masling, J. The influence of situational and interpersonal variables in projective testing. *Psychological Bulletin*, 1960, *57*, 65–85.

Masters, W. H. and Johnson, V. E. *Human sexual response*. Boston: Little, Brown, 1966.

Masters, W. H. and Johnson, V. E. *Human sexual inadequacy*. Boston: Little, Brown, 1970.

A medicolegal ruling with ominous implications. *Medical Economics*, April 17, 1978, p. 254.

Meduna, L. J. *Die konvulsions therapie der schizophrenie*. Marhold: Halle, 1936.

Meisel, A., Roth, L. H., and Lidz, C. W. Toward a model of the legal doctrine of informed consent. *American Journal of Psychiatry*, 1977, *134*, 285–289.

Messinger, S. Malpractice suits—the psychiatrist's turn. *The Journal of Legal Medicine*, April 1975, pp. 31–39.

Meyer, V. Modification of expectations in cases with obsessional rituals. *Behavior Research and Therapy*, 1966, *4*, 273–280.

Middleton, B. M. The implications of malpractice suits. *Maryland State Medical Journal*, 1970, *19*, 78–79.

Miller, D. and Burt, R. A. Children's rights on entering therapeutic institutions. *American Journal of Psychiatry*, 1977, *134*, 153–156.

Mills, D. H. Malpractice and drugs. *Resident and Staff Physician*, 1974, *20*(4), 35–39; 42; 44.

Mintz, E. E. *Marathon groups: Reality and symbol*. New York: Equinox, 1971.

Miron, N. B. The primary ethical consideration. *Hospital and Community Psychiatry*, 1968, *19*, 226–228.

Miron, N. B. A final rejoinder. In R. Ulrich, T. Stachnik, and J. Mabry (Eds.), *Control of human behavior* (Vol. 2). Glenview, Ill.: Scott, Foresman, 1970.

Mischel, W. *Personality and assessment*. New York: Wiley, 1968.

MLC news brief. *MLC Commentary*, 1975, *2*(6), 1.

Moline, R. A. Atypical tardive dyskinesia. *American Journal of Psychiatry*, 1975, *132*, 534–535.

Moore, E. Legislative control of shock treatment. *University of San Francisco Law Review*, 1975, *9*, 738–780.

Moore, M. T. and Book, M. H. Sudden death in phenothiazine therapy: A clinicopathologic study of twelve cases. *Psychiatric Quarterly*, 1970, *44*, 389–402.

Morse, H. N. The tort liability of the psychiatrist. *Syracuse Law Review*, 1967, *18*, 691–727.

Muller, C. The overmedicated society: Forces in the marketplace for medical care. *Science*, 1972, *176*, 488–492.

Myers, M. J. and Fink, J. L. Liability aspects of drug product selection. *Journal of the American Pharaceutical Association*, 1977, *NS 17*, 33–35.

Parker, D. Some legal implications for personnel officers. *Journal of the National Association of Women Deans and Counselors*, 1961, *24*, 198–202.

Paulson, G. W. Movement disorders secondary to drugs. *Ohio State Medical Journal*, 1973, *69*, 685–686.

Perr, I. N. Liability of hospital and psychiatrist in suicide. *American Journal of Psychiatry*, 1965, 122, 631–638.

Perry, J. A. Physicians' erotic and nonerotic physical involvement with patients. *American Journal of Psychiatry*, 1976, *133*, 838–840.

Pharmacists fall short of legal, professional responsibilities. *Journal of the American Pharmaceutical Association*, 1977, NS 17(1), 62.

Plachta, A. Asphyxia relatively inherent to tranquilization. *Archives of General Psychiatry*, 1965, *12*, 152–158.

Plaut, E. A. A perspective on confidentiality. *American Journal of Psychiatry*, 1974, *131*, 1021–1024.

Powledge, F. The therapist as double agent. *Psychology Today*, July 1977, pp. 44–47.

Prosser, W. L. *Law of torts* (4th ed.) St. Paul, Minn.: West Publishing, 1971.

Psychologist faces malpractice charges. *APA Monitor*, 1972, 3(9, 10), 16.

Public opinion, law limit use of ECT as data show efficacy. *Clinical Psychiatry News*, April 1978, pp. 1; 16.

Ragan, C. A., Jr. The malpractice pall over medicine. *Resident and Staff Physician*, 1974, *20*(4), 9–10.

Ravitch, M. M. Informed consent—descent to absurdity. *Resident and Staff Physician*, 1974, *20*(4), 10s–12s; 16s; 20s.

Redlich, F. C. and Freedman, D. X. *The theory and practice of psychiatry*. New York: Basic Books, 1966.

Reilly, P. J. The case against countersuits. *American Medical News*, March 28, 1977.

Rivlin, A. M. Social experiments: Promise and problems. *Science*, 1974, *183*, 35.

Robinson, G. W., Jr. Discussion. *American Journal of Psychiatry*, 1962, *118*, 779–780.

Rogers, C. R. and Skinner, B. F. Some issues concerning the control of human behavior: A symposium. *Science*, 1956, *124*, 1057–1066.

Rosenberg, C. L. The first countersuit money changes hands. *Medical Economics*, August 7, 1978, pp. 31–32; 35–36; 41; 45; 49.

Roskam, P. First-person review: CHAMPUS hit on confidentiality. *APA Monitor*, March 1979, pp. 3; 16.

Roston, R. A. Ethical uncertainties and "technical" validities. *Professional Psychology*, 1975, *6*, 50–54.

Roston, R. A. and Sherrer, C. W. Malpractice: What's new? *Professional Psychology*, 1973, *4*, 270–276.

Roth, L. H., Meisel, A., and Lidz, C. W. Tests of competency to consent to treatment. *American Journal of Psychiatry*, 1977, *134*, 279–284.

Rothblatt, H. B. and Leroy, D. H. Avoiding psychiatric malpractice. *California Western Law Review*, 1973, *9*, 260–272.

Ruebhausen, O. M. and Brim, O. G. Privacy and behavioral research. *American Psychologist*, 1965, *21*, 423–437.

Sadoff, R. L. New malpractice concerns for the psychiatrist. *Legal Aspects of Medical Practice*, 1978, *6*(3), 31–35.

Sagall, E. L. and Reed, B. C. The liability of attendings and chiefs. *Resident and Staff Physician*, 1975, *21*(3), 77; 80–81; 85–86; 89; 92.

Sales, B. D. and Grisso, T. Law and professional psychology: An introduction. *Professional Psychology*, 1978, *9*, 363–366.

Sampson, C. C. Are more controls on the way? *Journal of the National Medical Association*, 1977, *69*(1), 9.

Sandor, A. A. The history of professional liability suits in the United States. *Journal of the American Medical Association*, 1957, *163*, 459–466.

Sarbin, T. R., Taft, R., and Bailey, D. E. *Clinical inference and cognitive theory*. New York: Holt, Rinehart and Winston, 1960.

Schiele, B. C., Gallant, D., Simpson, G., Gardner, E. A. and Cole, J. O. Tardive dyskinesia: A persistant neurological syndrome associated with antipsychotic drug use. *Annals of Internal Medicine*, 1973, *79*, 99–100.

Schmidt, H. O. and Fonda, C. P. The reliability of psychiatric diagnosis: A new look. *Journal of American Sociology*, 1956, *52*, 262–267.

Schutz, W. C. *Joy*. New York: Grove Press, 1967.

Schwartz, L. L. The health care credibility gap. *Medical Tribune*, September 13, 1978, p. 22.

Schwartz, V. E. Civil liability for causing suicide: A synthesis of law and psychiatry. *Vanderbilt Law Review*, 1971, *24*, 217–256.

Schwartz, W. B. and Komesar, N. K. Doctors, damages and deterrence: An economic view of medical malpractice. *New England Journal of Medicine*, 1978, *298*, 1282–1289.

Schwitzgebel, R. K. Federal regulation of medical devices. *Harvard Law School Bulletin*, 1976, *27*, 34–36.

Schwitzgebel, R. K. Federal regulation of psychological devices: An example of medical–political drift. In B. D. Sales (Ed.), *Psychology in the legal process*. New York: Spectrum, 1977.

Schwitzgebel, R. K. Suggestions for the uses of psychological devices in accord with legal and ethical standards. *Professional Psychology*, 1978, *9*, 478–488.

Serban, G. and Gidynski, C. B. Schizophrenic patients in community: Legal misinterpretations of "right to treatment." *New York State Journal of Medicine*, 1974, *74*, 1977–1981.

Shah, S. A. Privileged communications, confidentiality, and privacy: Privileged communications. *Professional Psychology*, 1969, *1*, 56–59.

Shah, S. A. Privileged communications, confidentiality, and privacy: Confidentiality. *Professional Psychology*, 1970, *1*, 159–164. (a)

Shah, S. A. Privileged communications, confidentiality, and privacy: Privacy. *Professional Psychology*, 1970, *1*, 243–252. (b)

Shepard, M. *The love treatment: Sexual intimacy between patients and psychotherapists*. New York: Peter H. Wyden, 1971.

Siassi, I. and Thomas M. Physicians and the new sexual freedom. *American Journal of Psychiatry*, 1973, *130*, 1256–1257.

Siegal, M. Confidentiality. *The Clinical Psychologist*, 1976, *30*, 1.

Siegel, R. A. The significance for psychology of *O'Connor v. Donaldson*: A reply to Bernard. *American Psychologist*, 1978, *33*, 858–861.

Six court decisions of current interest. *Resident and Staff Physician*, 1974, *20*(4), 96; 98; 100; 102; 104–105; 119–120.

Six ways to reduce malpractice suits. *Resident and Staff Physician*, 1977, *23*(4), 25s–27s; 30s.

Slawson, P. F. Patient–litigant exception: A hazard to psychotherapy. *Archives of General Psychiatry*, 1969, *21*, 347–352.

Slawson, P. F. Psychiatric malpractice: A regional incidence study. *American Journal of Psychiatry*, 1970, *126*, 136–139.

Slawson, P. F., Flinn, D. E., and Schwartz, D. A. Legal responsibility for suicide. *Psychiatric Quarterly*, 1974, *48*, 50–64.

Slovenko, R. *Psychiatry and law*. Boston: Little, Brown, 1973.

Smith, F. M. Whose malpractice crisis? *The Journal of the Louisiana State Medical Society*, 1975, *127*, 293–297.

Spadoni, A. J. Legal rights vs. patient needs. *Illinois Medical Journal*, 1977, *151*, 86.

Spaniol, J. F. *The United States courts: Their jurisdiction and work.* Washington, D.C.: U.S. Government Printing Office, 1975.

Speaker, F. Informed consent decision offers comfort. *Pennsylvania Medicine,* 1977, *80*(1), 13.

Stampfl, T. G. and Levis, D. J. Essentials of implosive therapy: A learning theory-based psychodynamic behavioral therapy. *Journal of Abnormal Psychology,* 1967, *72,* 496–503.

Stern, H. R. The problem of privilege: Historical and juridical sidelights. *American Journal of Psychiatry,* 1959, *115,* 1071–1088.

Stokes, J. B. Comment on "Socially reinforced obsessing: Etiology of a disorder in a Christian Scientist." *Journal of Consulting and Clinical Psychology,* 1977, *45,* 1164–1165.

Stone, A. A. Recent mental health litigation: A critical perspective. *American Journal of Psychiatry,* 1977, *134,* 273–279.

Swett, C., Jr. Drug-induced dystonia. *American Journal of Psychiatry,* 1975, *132,* 532–534.

Swoboda, J. S., Elwork, A., Sales, B. D., and Levine, D. Knowledge of and compliance with privileged communication and child-abuse–reporting laws. *Professional Psychology,* 1978, *9,* 448–457.

Tarshis, C. B. Liability for psychotherapy. *Faculty of Law Review, University of Toronto,* 1972, *30,* 75–96.

Taylor, B. J. and Wagner, N. N. Sex between therapists and clients: A review and analysis. *Professional Psychology,* 1976, *7,* 593–601.

Terman, L. M. and Merrill, M. A. *Stanford–Binet intelligence scale.* Boston: Houghton Mifflin, 1960.

Testing and public policy. (Special issue) *American Psychologist,* 1965, *20,* 857–992.

Thornton, W. E. and Thornton, B. P. Tardive dyskinesia and low dosage. *American Journal of Psychiatry,* 1973, *130,* 141.

Tikare, S. K. and Tikare, S. S. Extrapyramidal motor disorders due to toxic effect of phenothiazines. *Journal of Indian Medical Association,* 1972, *58,* 39–42.

Trent, C. L. and Muhl, W. P. Professional liability insurance and the American psychiatrist. *American Journal of Psychiatry,* 1975, *132,* 1312–1314.

Turek, I., Kurland, A. A., Hanlon, T. E. and Bohm, M. Tardive dyskinesia: Its relation to neuroleptic and antiparkinson drugs. *British Journal of Psychiatry,* 1972, *121,* 605–612.

Ulrich, R., Stachnik, T., and Mabry, J. (Eds.), *Control of human behavior* (Vol. 1). Glenview, Ill.: Scott, Foresman, 1966.

U.S. News and World Report Books. *What everyone needs to know about law.* New York: Simon and Schuster, 1973.

Voth, H. M. Love affair between doctor and patient. *American Journal of Psychotherapy,* 1972, *26,* 394–400.

Waterman, A. S. The civil liberties of the participants in psychological research. *American Psychologist,* 1974, *29,* 470–471.

West, L. J. Ethical psychiatry and biosocial humanism. *American Journal of Psychiatry,* 1969, *126,* 226–230.

Wexler, D. B. Token and taboo: Behavior modification, token economies and the law. *California Law Review,* 1973, *61,* 81–109.

What to expect if your case goes to trial. *Resident and Staff Physician,* 1974, *20*(4), 65–68.

Wiskoff, M. Ethical standards and divided loyalties. *American Psychologist,* 1960, *15,* 656–660.

Zaro, J. S., Barach, R., Nedelman, D. J., and Dreiblatt, I. S. *A guide for beginning psychotherapists.* Cambridge: Cambridge University Press, 1977.

Zigler, E. and Phillips, L. Psychiatric diagnosis and symptomatology. *Journal of Abnormal and Social Psychology,* 1961, *63,* 69–75. (a)

Zigler, E. and Phillips, L. Psychiatric diagnosis: A critique. *Journal of Abnormal and Social Psychology,* 1961, *3,* 607–618. (b)

Case Index

NOTE: Included here are the cases and case numbers (in parentheses) for all of the cases cited in the text. Not included in this index are cases cited in the Appendix and cases cited in excerpted material.

CASES CITED WITH THE NAMES OF THE LITIGANTS UNAVAILABLE OR WITHHELD

Subject Index